Pediatric Resuscitation: A Practical Approach

Mark G. Roback, MD, FAAP
Associate Professor, Department of Pediatrics
University of Colorado School of Medicine
Fellowship Director, Section of Emergency Medicine
The Children's Hospital
Denver, Colorado

Stephen J. Teach, MD, MPH, FAAP
Associate Professor of Pediatrics
George Washington University School of Medicine and Health Sciences
Associate Chief, Division of Emergency Medicine
Children's National Medical Center
Washington, DC

American College of Emergency Physicians®

Disclaimer and Copyright Notice

Additional copies of this publication can be ordered from ACEP, PO Box 619911, Dallas, TX 75261-9911; toll-free 800-798-1822, touch 6, or 972-550-0911; www.acep.org/bookstore.

First printing, October 2005

Mary Anne Mitchell, Managing Editor

Mary Ostrowski, Editorial Assistant

Victor Perea, Graphic Designer

Mike C. Goodwin, Creative Services Manager

Emma Kiewice, Publications Sales and Promotions Manager

Marta Foster, Director, Educational and Professional Publications

Thomas S. Werlinich, Associate Executive Director, Educational and Professional Products

Indexing: Hughes Analytics, Chicago, Illinois

Printing: The Covington Group, Kansas City, Missouri

About the Editors

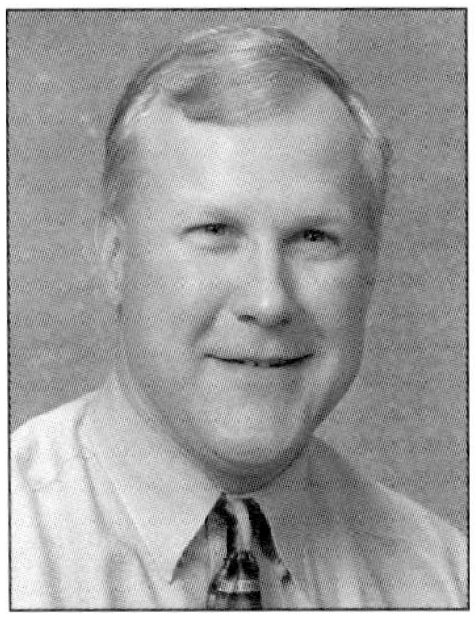

Mark G. Roback, MD, FAAP

Dr. Roback is Fellowship and Research Director for the Section of Emergency Medicine at The Children's Hospital in Denver, Colorado. He is an associate professor of pediatrics at the University of Colorado School of Medicine. He is also the director of the Mock Resuscitation Program at The Children's Hospital as well as a course director for Pediatric Advanced Life Support.

Pediatric sedation and resuscitation are topics on which Dr. Roback is a state, national, and international speaker. His interest in these and other areas has led him to author several journal articles, textbook chapters, and a prior textbook.

Dr. Roback received his undergraduate and medical degrees from the University of Minnesota. He completed residency training and chief residency in pediatrics at the University of Minnesota Hospitals and Clinics. Dr. Roback completed fellowship training in pediatric emergency medicine at Children's Hospital Boston. He is board certified in pediatrics and pediatric emergency medicine.

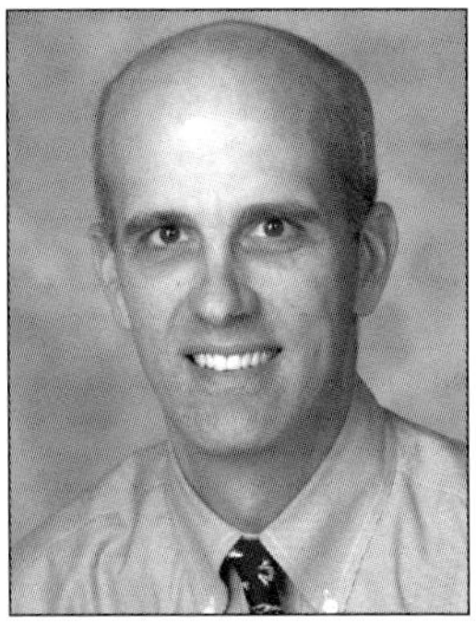

Stephen J. Teach, MD, MPH, FAAP

Dr. Teach is the Associate Chief of Emergency Medicine at Children's National Medical Center in Washington, DC. He is also an associate professor of pediatrics at the George Washington University School of Medicine and Health Sciences.

He is a national authority on the management of acute and chronic asthma and other forms of respiratory distress and has a strong interest in the evaluation and management of the child with fever and suspected invasive infections and sepsis. He has lectured and published extensively in both areas.

Dr. Teach received his undergraduate degree at Yale College and his medical degree from Harvard Medical School. He completed residency training in pediatrics and fellowship training in pediatric emergency medicine at Children's Hospital Boston. His public health degree is from the University of California at Berkeley. He is board certified in pediatrics and pediatric emergency medicine.

Contributors

Dewesh Agrawal, MD
Assistant Professor of Pediatrics and Emergency Medicine
George Washington University School of Medicine and Health Sciences
Division of Emergency Medicine
Children's National Medical Center
Washington, DC

Michael C. Bachman, MD, MBA
Assistant Medical Director
Department of Pediatric Emergency Medicine
Newark Beth Israel Medical Center
Newark, New Jersey

Richard G. Bachur, MD
Assistant Professor of Pediatrics
Harvard Medical School
Associate Chief and Fellowship Director
Division of Emergency Medicine
Children's Hospital Boston
Boston, Massachusetts

Lalit Bajaj, MD, MPH
Assistant Professor, Department of Pediatrics
University of Colorado School of Medicine
Section of Emergency Medicine
The Children's Hospital
Denver, Colorado

Katherine Bakes, MD
Assistant Professor of Emergency Medicine
University of Colorado School of Medicine
Denver Health Medical Center
Denver, Colorado

Brent J. Barber, MD
Fellow, Division of Pediatric Cardiology
Oregon Health and Science University
Portland, Oregon

Kathlene E. Bassett, MD
Associate Professor, Department of Pediatrics
University of Utah School of Medicine
Primary Children's Medical Center
Salt Lake City, Utah

F. Keith Battan, MD
Associate Professor of Pediatrics
University of Colorado School of Medicine
Associate Director, Emergency and Trauma Services
The Children's Hospital
Denver, Colorado

Jeffrey S. Blake, MD
Fellow, Division of Emergency Medicine
Children's National Medical Center
Washington, DC

David C. Brousseau, MD, MS
Assistant Professor, Pediatrics
Medical College of Wisconsin
Section of Pediatric Emergency Medicine
Children's Hospital of Wisconsin
Milwaukee, Wisconsin

Grant Burch, MD
Assistant Professor of Pediatrics
Director, Pediatric and Adult Congenital Cardiac Catheterization Laboratory
Fellowship Director, Division of Pediatric Cardiology
Oregon Health and Science University
Portland, Oregon

Ari R. Cohen, MD
Fellow, Division of Emergency Medicine
Children's Hospital Boston
Boston, Massachusetts

Frances W. Craig, MD, FAAP
Director of Resident Education
Pediatric Emergency Medicine
Children's Pediatric Group
East Tennessee Children's Hospital
Knoxville, Tennessee

Carlos A. Delgado, MD
Assistant Professor of Pediatrics
Emory University School of Medicine
Division of Pediatric Emergency Medicine
Children's Healthcare of Atlanta
Atlanta, Georgia

Amy L. Drendel, DO
Fellow, Pediatric Emergency Medicine
Medical College of Wisconsin
Children's Hospital of Wisconsin
Milwaukee, Wisconsin

Elizabeth A. Edgerton, MD, MPH
Assistant Professor of Pediatrics
George Washington University School of Medicine and Health Sciences
Washington, DC
Director of Clinical Prevention
Agency for Healthcare Research and Quality
Rockville, Maryland

Kathryn D. Emery, MD
Associate Professor, Department of Pediatrics
University of Colorado School of Medicine
Section of Emergency Medicine
The Children's Hospital
Denver, Colorado

Glenn Faries, MD
Assistant Professor, Department of Pediatrics
University of Colorado School of Medicine
Section of Emergency Medicine
The Children's Hospital
Denver, Colorado

Mario Gehri, MD
Médecin - chef
Hôpital de l'Enfance
Lausanne, Switzerland

Richard A. Greenberg, MD
Clinical Instructor, Department of Pediatrics
University of Colorado School of Medicine
Fellow, Section of Emergency Medicine
The Children's Hospital
Denver, Colorado

Karen Gruskin, MD
Instructor of Pediatrics
Harvard Medical School
Division of Emergency Medicine
Children's Hospital Boston
Boston, Massachusetts

Molly B. Hasty, MD
Fellow, Pediatric Emergency Medicine
University of Alabama School of Medicine at Birmingham
Children's Hospital
Birmingham, Alabama

Stanley H. Inkelis, MD
Professor of Pediatrics
David Geffen School of Medicine at UCLA
Director, Pediatric Emergency Medicine
Harbor-UCLA Medical Center
Torrance, California

Elizabeth S. Jacobs, MD
Assistant Professor of Pediatrics
George Washington University School of Medicine and Health Sciences
Division of Emergency Medicine
Children's National Medical Center
Washington, DC

Amir Kimia, MD
Fellow, Division of Emergency Medicine
Children's Hospital Boston
Boston, Massachusetts

Tom Langston, MD
Clinical Instructor, Department of Pediatrics
University of Colorado School of Medicine
Fellow, Section of Emergency Medicine
The Children's Hospital
Denver, Colorado

Jason A. Levy, MD
Fellow, Division of Emergency Medicine
Children's Hospital Boston
Boston, Massachusetts

Erica L. Liebelt, MD, FACMT
Associate Professor of Pediatrics and Emergency Medicine
University of Alabama School of Medicine at Birmingham
Director, Medical Toxicology Services
University of Alabama Hospital and Children's Hospital
Birmingham, Alabama

Contributors

Charles G. Macias, MD, MPH
Assistant Professor of Pediatrics
Section of Emergency Medicine, Research Director
Fellowship Director, Pediatric Emergency Medicine
Baylor College of Medicine
Attending Physician
Texas Children's Hospital Emergency Department
Houston, Texas

Shannon F. Manzi, PharmD
Department of Pharmacology
Children's Hospital Boston
Boston, Massachusetts

William M. McDonnell, MD, JD
Clinical Instructor, Department of Pediatrics
University of Colorado School of Medicine
Fellow, Section of Emergency Medicine
The Children's Hospital
Denver, Colorado

Joshua Nagler, MD
Fellow, Division of Emergency Medicine
Children's Hospital Boston
Boston, Massachusetts

Frank L. Overly, MD
Assistant Professor of Pediatrics and Emergency Medicine
Brown University School of Medicine
Hasbro Children's Hospital
Providence, Rhode Island

Holly E. Perry, MD
Assistant Professor of Pediatrics
University of Connecticut School of Medicine
Connecticut Children's Medical Center
Hartford, Connecticut

Michael Quinn, MD
Assistant Professor of Pediatrics
George Washington University School of Medicine and Health Sciences
Division of Emergency Medicine
Children's National Medical Center
Washington, DC

Arleta B. Rewers, MD, PhD, MSPH
Assistant Professor, Department of Pediatrics
University of Colorado School of Medicine
Attending Physician, Section of Emergency Medicine
The Children's Hospital
Denver, Colorado

Kristine Rittichier, MD
Associate Professor, Department of Pediatrics
University of Utah School of Medicine
Primary Children's Medical Center
Salt Lake City, Utah

Mark G. Roback, MD, FAAP
Associate Professor, Department of Pediatrics
University of Colorado School of Medicine
Fellowship Director, Section of Emergency Medicine
The Children's Hospital
Denver, Colorado

Mark G. Roddy, MD
Fellow, Division of Emergency Medicine
Children's National Medical Center
Washington, DC

Genie E. Roosevelt, MD, MPH
Assistant Professor, Department of Pediatrics
University of Colorado Health Sciences Center
Section of Emergency Medicine
The Children's Hospital
Denver, Colorado

Leticia Manning Ryan, MD
Fellow, Division of Emergency Medicine
Children's National Medical Center
Washington, DC

Richard A. Saladino, MD
Associate Professor of Pediatrics
University of Pittsburgh School of Medicine
Chief, Division of Pediatric Emergency Medicine
Children's Hospital of Pittsburgh
Pittsburgh, Pennsylvania

Carl Shaw, MD
Clinical Instructor, Department of Pediatrics
University of Colorado School of Medicine
Fellow, Section of Emergency Medicine
The Children's Hospital
Denver, Colorado

Brian H. Shear, MD
Residency in Emergency Medicine
University of Colorado School of Medicine
Denver Health Medical Center
Denver, Colorado

Anne M. Stack, MD
Assistant Professor of Pediatrics
Harvard Medical School
Division of Emergency Medicine
Children's Hospital Boston
Boston, Massachusetts

Stephen J. Teach, MD, MPH, FAAP
Associate Professor of Pediatrics
George Washington University School of Medicine and Health Sciences
Associate Chief, Division of Emergency Medicine
Children's National Medical Center
Washington, DC

William Tsai, MD
Fellow, Division of Emergency Medicine
Children's National Medical Center
Washington, DC

Guy L. Upshaw, MD
Senior Instructor, Department of Pediatrics
University of Colorado School of Medicine
Section of Emergency Medicine
The Children's Hospital
Denver, Colorado

Tien T. Vu, MD
Clinical Instructor, Department of Pediatrics
University of Colorado School of Medicine
Fellow, Section of Emergency Medicine
The Children's Hospital
Denver, Colorado

Mark L. Waltzman, MD
Assistant Professor of Pediatrics
Harvard Medical School
Division of Emergency Medicine
Children's Hospital Boston
Boston, Massachusetts

Joe E. Wathen, MD
Instructor, Department of Pediatrics
Section of Emergency Medicine
University of Colorado School of Medicine
The Children's Hospital
Denver, Colorado

Debra L. Weiner, MD, PhD
Assistant Professor of Pediatrics
Harvard Medical School
Division of Emergency Medicine
Children's Hospital Boston
Boston, Massachusetts

Ethan S. Wiener, MD
Clinical Instructor, Department of Pediatrics
University of Colorado School of Medicine
Fellow, Section of Emergency Medicine
The Children's Hospital
Denver, Colorado

Noel S. Zuckerbraun, MD
Assistant Professor of Pediatrics
University of Pittsburgh School of Medicine
Division of Pediatric Emergency Medicine
Children's Hospital of Pittsburgh
Pittsburgh, Pennsylvania

Dedications

À Emma, Casimir, Jacob, et Hélène, mes amours et ma vie.
MGR

To Eliza, Owen, and Libby, who are the centers of my world, and to Meme, who taught me to care.
SJT

Acknowledgments

We wish to acknowledge all those who care for ill and injured children, as well as the families and patients we have been privileged to help as physicians. We have learned much from them all. We would also like to thank Dr. Gary Fleisher and Dr. Lewis First, who remain important mentors and friends and who taught us that the pursuit of excellence in patient care can and should be fun. Finally, we would like to thank Dr. Joan Bothner and Dr. James Chamberlain. Their enthusiastic support of our professional lives made this book, and much more, possible.

Mark G. Roback, MD, FAAP
Stephen J. Teach, MD, MPH, FAAP

Table of Contents

Figures and Tables

PALS Algorithms

Pediatric Rhythm Strips

Chest Radiograph

Tables

Preface to *Handbook of Pediatric Mock Codes*

Society has witnessed a dramatic fall in the death rate for children during the past century. This epidemiological miracle has had a profound impact on our thinking as parents and our performance as pediatricians and emergency physicians.

It's a really big deal when a child dies, especially when it occurs suddenly or unexpectedly. Right or wrong, everyone expects to lose some adults, particularly the most senior of our citizens. Physicians accept the eventuality of death for their oldest patients, and even family members are unlikely to question nature's wisdom when ailing relatives finally succumb to long, drawn-out chronic illnesses. But it's different with infants and children. In our society, parents as well as physicians expect that every youth will survive into adulthood. Evidence of this transformation in thinking appears again and again in our daily newspapers. A single fatality in a child from meningococcemia in any small community reverberates to the four corners of a state within a day.

Excepting neonates and children with do-not-resuscitate orders, residents currently in training seldom witness the death of a child. SIDS, the number one cause of mortality in infants after they leave the newborn nursery, has declined dramatically with the discovery of the simple but elusive connection with sleeping position. Beyond the age of 1 year, when trauma takes over as the chief culprit in pediatric deaths, society has made dramatic strides as well. Passenger restraints, bicycle helmets, and safer packaging for hazardous medications have all contributed to a marked decline in fatalities. Added to these advances, the movement (perhaps ill founded) of many resuscitations into the prehospital arena has led to a generation of residents with minimal exposure to CPR in children.

Yet all these future physicians are likely to be called upon on one or more occasions in their careers to resuscitate a child. During training, one can sense the anxiety that exists around the possibility of this occurrence. Residents want, and need, competence at pediatric resuscitation.

This dichotomy, between the wants and needs of residents on the one hand and a declining opportunity to gain adequate experience on the other, confronts educators at multiple institutions. Faced with this problem 15 years ago, Dr. Lewis First combined his medical knowledge and theatrical talent to develop a program to assist residents in acquiring psychomotor and attitudinal, as well as cognitive, skills in pediatric resuscitation. With each new class of residents, the scenarios for the mock codes became more elaborate. Advancing technologies, such as arrhythmia generators, added a whole new dimension to the process.

Finally, the development of a fellowship in pediatric emergency medicine provided a seemingly endless supply of enthusiastic practitioners of the art. Eventually, Mark Roback and Stephen Teach took on the challenge of translating an oral tradition into written words. From these origins arose the present volume, *Handbook of Pediatric Mock Codes.*

While most readers are probably familiar with the concept of mock codes and some may even have had some first-hand experience, I think all users will find this text to be relatively unique. It aims to take the current practice of teaching resuscitation from an informal process of questionable value to a science with defined methods and clear-cut goals. The introduction lays down the ground rules on utilizing the material. In the core text, 37 scenarios cover the breadth of pediatric resuscitation, emphasizing the more frequent events, such as trauma and respiratory arrest, but also including less common problems, from electrocution to complications of pregnancy.

If one thinks of a mock code as a type of play, the special qualities of this book become apparent. Producers need interesting characters, creative dialogue, and detailed stage directions to put on successful shows. Similarly, educators require realistic case scenarios, interventions leading to appropriate responses, and instructions for the orchestration of various simulations to "stage" an effective mock code. In this text, each of the scenarios includes a case presentation, a description of likely suggestions for treatment and outcomes, a discussion of possible complications, and a review of the specific lessons to be learned by the participants. The depth, quality, and logical formatting of the material provide the substrate for a superb educational program in resuscitation that reflects 15 years of continuous utilization and constant refinement. We are hopeful that the *Handbook of Pediatric Mock Codes* will eventually allow for standardization of the teaching of CPR in children and, as well, provide a tool for evaluation of competency across institutions.

Gary Fleisher, MD

August 1997

Preface to *Pediatric Resuscitation: A Practical Approach*

When Drs. Roback and Teach published *Handbook of Pediatric Mock Codes,* the predecessor to the current volume, I commented that the declining experience of trainees with pediatric resuscitation and the increasing demand for medical excellence made that earlier volume an essential tool for students, residents, and fellows. As I survey the present environment, I believe that these same trends have continued unabated, creating an even more important niche for *Pediatric Resuscitation: A Practical Approach.*

Obviously, the science of resuscitation has marched forward over the past 8 years, although not as consistently or rapidly as many of us would have hoped. The accumulated data have led to updated standards, even in areas as basic as the administration of epinephrine. Thus, the authors have updated the recommended sequencing of interventions and dosages of medications, in accordance with the standard references in the field. Beyond the medicine, they have worked hard as well to provide a format that is even friendlier for the user. A particularly interesting new feature is the self-learning tool that allows the material to serve the purpose of an individual study guide while continuing as a manual for mock codes. Additionally, the authors have restructured the scenarios to encourage the readers and/or participants to think their way through the expected interventions, potential complications, and possible diagnoses.

I continue to believe that incorporation into one's armamentarium of a complex psychomotor task such as resuscitation requires constant practice, rather than lectures or reading alone. That is exactly what this text provides, in a carefully devised, clinically oriented format. I am confident that users of this material will improve their skills at resuscitation through the interactions provided by these scenarios and that the experience will prove enjoyable.

Gary R. Fleisher, MD, FAAP, FACEP
May 2005

How to Use This Book

This book is designed to provide you with a practical approach to pediatric resuscitation. Situations requiring pediatric resuscitation skills are uncommon in both inpatient and outpatient clinical settings. For this reason, most health care practitioners are only rarely required to use what they have learned in pediatric life support courses. The purpose of this text, then, is to provide you with additional exposure to real-life issues in pediatric resuscitation.

Unlike our previous text, *Handbook of Pediatric Mock Codes*, this work has two audiences. It is designed to be used by individuals to review principles of resuscitation and by teams of health care practitioners to conduct pediatric mock codes. The next section, "Guidelines for Conducting the Mock Code," is adapted from our previous text and leads you through our recommended approach. If you are using this book as a self-directed study guide, you probably will want to pass over the guidelines section. But if you are using this book to conduct mock codes, the guidelines section will help you perform them successfully in your patient care setting.

In the next section, "Principles of Pediatric Resuscitation," we review and emphasize pediatric resuscitation principles and skills learned in APLS (Advanced Pediatric Life Support) and PALS (Pediatric Advanced Life Support) courses. We stress important pediatric resuscitation concepts such as the interpretation of pediatric vital signs and the use of monitors and equipment. The evaluation and management of the "ABCs" (airway, breathing, circulation), neurologic emergencies, trauma and environmental emergencies, ingestions, and neonatal resuscitation are presented next.

These initial sections prepare you for the heart of this text, which is the 46 pediatric resuscitation scenarios. Each scenario presents a pediatric patient in distress, a clinical unknown with very little initial history. The scenarios stress the initial assessment and the ABC approach presented by APLS and PALS. Each scenario also includes an assessment based on the Pediatric Assessment Triangle. This fast, simple tool, which we have borrowed from APLS and PEPP (*Pediatric Education for Prehospital Professionals*), can be used to assess patients of all ages and works for either injury or illness. It is an "across-the-room" assessment based on only visual and auditory clues – appearance, work of breathing, and circulation to the skin. These three components reflect the patient's overall physiologic status and general state of oxygenation, ventilation, perfusion, and brain function. The Pediatric Assessment Triangle is not a diagnostic tool, but it is helpful in emergency circumstances that require rapid life support decisions.

As you read through the scenarios, the text will "ask" you questions about patient assessment and physiologic status, differential diagnosis, expected interventions, and potential complications. These questions, which appear in shaded boxes, are designed to test your knowledge and understanding of resuscitation problems that might arise. For your convenience, the answers follow directly after the questions.

You might want to read through the scenarios sequentially and tackle each one as an unknown patient whom you are required to assess and manage. Or, you might prefer to select scenarios by diagnosis, which you can do by referring to the scenarios list on page 336. Each scenario ends with a discussion of its objectives for your review, along with references for further study.

Finally, in the "Appendixes" section, we provide specific information such as normal vital sign ranges and standard equipment sizes by age, a list of commonly used abbreviations, the Glasgow Coma Scale, and a mock code review guide and checklist.

This text was written by more than 50 physicians and health care providers who frequently resuscitate infants and children and teach pediatric life support courses. Their goal was to convey their experience and expertise to you. As the editors, our goal was to standardize the assessment and treatment recommendations across the scenarios and make them evidence based, rigorously adhering to recommendations of APLS and PALS. As you read through this text, you might notice some differences between scenarios with regard to drugs administered or order of steps taken. These differences mainly represent institutional or individual preferences; they are particularly evident in instances where definitive data do not exist to support specific management recommendations. We acknowledge that, in some instances, there are treatment options we have not listed that are acceptable alternatives to our recommendations.

Whether you use this text to help you to keep the principles of pediatric resuscitation fresh in your mind or use it as the foundation for conducting mock codes, we believe this book provides a valuable approach to the assessment and management of emergently ill and injured pediatric patients.

Guidelines for Conducting the Mock Code

Objectives

The primary objective of the mock code is to give the health care provider experience in caring for seriously ill or injured pediatric patients. Participants will gain experience in situations that require immediate attention to the ABCs of pediatric resuscitation. A transition from basic to advanced life support techniques is inherent in every mock code.

Each mock code scenario stresses three or four distinct objectives. Individual mock codes stress specific aspects of resuscitation, such as airway obstruction, respiratory distress, and shock. Initial assessment and management of the ABCs is required at the onset of every mock code. This might be followed by a progression of disease or injury listed within the scenarios.

It is the responsibility of the mock code director (MCD) to interact with the code team in such a way as to focus attention on the ABCs and the objectives of the specific mock code scenario.

Participants

- Mock code director
- Reviewer(s)
- Code team
  - Team leader
  - Airway physician and other physicians
  - Nurses
  - Ancillary staff

Not all patient care facilities have the luxury of fully staffed critical care areas for a complete, formal code team. Many variations of the model described below exist, and individual institutions can easily incorporate whatever resources are available to make up their own mock code teams. For example, many of the physician positions might be filled by nurses, respiratory therapists, physician assistants, paramedics, or emergency medical technicians depending on the setting. Similarly, residents or medical students may take on roles typically filled by nursing; mock code exercises also have been successfully conducted with one nurse and one physician participating. All members of the code team are important, and their performances should be reviewed.

Mock Code Team Roles and Responsibilities

Team Leader

- Responsible for directing members of the code team
- Responsible for clearly identifying his/her role and the roles of other team members
- Responsible for asking for consulting services (general surgery, neurosurgery, orthopedics, radiology, and so on) as indicated
- Responsible for crowd and noise control
- Ensures that team members follow standard precautions for infection control

Airway Physician

- Responsible for control of the airway, with rigorous

attention to protection of the cervical spine

- Assesses mental status and pupillary response
- Assesses the head for signs of trauma

Physician on Patient's Right

- Responsible for right-side intravenous access and blood draw for laboratory tests
- Performs right-side procedures (chest tube, nasogastric [NG] tube, Foley)
- Performs cardiac compressions, when indicated

Physician on Patient's Left

- Conducts primary survey, 60-second physical examination
- Responsible for left-side intravenous access and blood draw for laboratory tests
- Performs left-side procedures (chest tube)
- Conducts secondary survey, more detailed exam including rectal, and examination of the patient's back

Float Physician

- Obtains initial history
- Communicates the history to the team leader
- Available for cardiac compression relief
- Liaison between code team and parents and family members

Medication Nurse

- Calculates patient's weight. One may use the length-based Broselow Pediatric Emergency Tape for this purpose
- Anticipates and draws up medications quickly and accurately, including first round of resuscitation medications which are hand labeled
- Communicates directly with the team leader only with regard to administration of drugs
- States aloud the name and dosage of each drug before handing it to the person administering it
- Prepares continuous infusion drugs and sets up arterial lines

Bedside Nurse

- Conducts primary survey
- Responsible for vital signs, monitors, oxygen, and suction
- Assists with procedures
- Administers intravenous medications

Documenting Nurse

- Documents dosages and times of all drugs given and informs the team leader
- Keeps track of length of the arrest and the patient's response to therapy
- Documents and labels all laboratory specimens
- Documents vital signs every 5 minutes
- Responsible for fully completing the arrest flow sheet

Circulating Nurse

- Assists with airway management and cervical spine immobilization
- Assists with intravenous access and infusions and arterial line setup
- Pages consulting services when asked by the team leader

Nursing Assistants

- Report to documenting nurse for direction, such as sending specimens to the lab or obtaining blood products from the blood bank and equipment or drugs from the pharmacy

It is helpful to give a formal lecture at various times of the year (to account for rotating staff) to orient members of the code team to their individual responsibilities and expectations regarding their performance in the mock code. Because the mock code is an educational experience, the MCD should make every effort to set a collegial tone and acknowledge the fact that participants will feel stressed.

Equipment

Equipment used for the mock code need not be elaborate and should be reused, but having the actual equipment available is essential. Actual procedures such as endotracheal intubation and intraosseous access can be performed on mannequins.

All resuscitation drugs should be available, but for the exercise the medication nurse can simply state aloud the volume of a given concentration of drug to be drawn up without actually doing it. Having the resuscitation drugs available allows participants to see the actual sizes and shapes of the vials and their volumes and concentrations; this is essential.

To keep costs down, resuscitation equipment opened and used for a mock code can be stored in a box properly labeled "Mock Code Supply Box" so that it can be reused. Institutions that conduct mock code exercises frequently might have a "Mock Code Crash Cart" so that all equipment and drugs necessary for resuscitation are readily available. In either case, precautions must be in place to ensure that the "Mock Code Supply Box" or "Mock Code Crash Cart" is never inadvertently opened and the materials used in a real resuscitation.

Recommended equipment for pediatric resuscitation is listed in "Monitors and Equipment" (see page 25). Neonatal resuscitation equipment is listed in the corresponding section of "Evaluation and Management" (see page 72).

It is the responsibility of the MCD to arrive well in advance of the scheduled start of the exercise in order to prepare the mannequin and set up the resuscitation equipment. Diligence in preparation is important to a successful program.

Scenarios

The mock code scenarios in this book are designed to be realistic and practical. If the participants believe they might actually encounter these situations someday they will be much more invested in the process. The MCD should try to keep it simple in the beginning, and then judge by the participants' responses what their level of experience is and just how complicated any scenario should become.

A mock code exercise can be designed to last either 30 or 60 minutes. The MCD should enforce a strict 15-minute time limit for the actual scenario. The rest of the time should be devoted to introduction, review and questions, and demonstration of skills (eg, intubation, vascular access) as time allows.

The recommended schedules for the codes are follows:

60-Minute Mock Code Exercise	Elapsed Time
Setup	Prior to exercise
Introduction	0-5 minutes
Scenario	5-20 minutes
Review and questions	20-40 minutes
Demonstration of skills, if time allows	40-60 minutes

30-Minute Mock Code Exercise	Elapsed Time
Setup	Prior to exercise
Scenario	0-15 minutes
Review and questions	15-30 minutes

The MCD should begin the exercise by summoning the code team to the patient (mannequin) area. A brief introduction can stress to participants the need to address the mannequin as if it were a real patient. So if a participant wants to know what the lungs sound like, he or she should have already auscultated the chest using a stethoscope. It should be stressed that all information required can be obtained through the MCD, who acts as the parents (history), gives physical findings when asked, and describes the patient's progression and response to interventions.

A useful option is to alternate between physicians and nursing staff as to who is allowed to address the "patient" first. After initial assessment, the starting group then is required to call the other for assistance. This approach emphasizes the need for a complete code team and stresses the importance to all members of the value of collaborative care.

The MCD should orchestrate the movements of the mock code, beginning with a brief initial history. As the team begins the initial assessment and management, the MCD should give additional information only when asked by the team or team leader. Requiring the team to elicit information (history, physical examination) and describe procedures (indications, landmarks, equipment) is a major objective of all mock code exercises.

When giving information, the MCD should use specific numbers and historical data. For example, "The heart rate is 190 bpm" rather than "The patient is tachycardic." The use of actual numbers gives the scenario an essence of reality and allows the MCD to readily change the vital signs as the scenario unfolds. Team members take the exercise more seriously when very specific information is offered.

The MCD must maintain a balance between giving information not elicited by the team and allowing them to stray too far afield. The MCD might nudge the team back on course by adding a timely bit of information or emphasize a point by allowing the patient's condition to progress to full cardiopulmonary arrest.

Ending the Mock Code Exercise and Patient Disposition

When the patient's condition has been stabilized, the MCD must bring the exercise to a formal end. One effective method of closure is to ask the team leader, "Now what?" At the point where the code team members recognize that patient disposition is in order, the mock code scenario has reached an acceptable end.

Alternatively, the MCD might say, "OK, let's stop," and then question the team leader regarding patient disposition. In addition to providing closure, this approach allows further insight into the team leader's assessment of the situation. For example, if the team leader believes a floor bed is adequate for a patient who obviously needs the OR, something has gone awry.

Disposition options typically include the hospital ward, ICU, CT scanner, or the OR. Mock codes should not end in death. When they do, the participants become so focused on the act of dying that the objectives of the scenario become secondary and the learning experience is compromised. If the MCD wants the code team to experience death of a patient (eg, an unsalvageable case of SIDS), the exercise should have no other objectives. The ABCs of resuscitation are lost on participants when the outcome is death. Giving participants experience dealing with the death of a patient is a worthwhile objective but is beyond the scope of this text.

Review

Whenever possible, an individual other than the MCD should be responsible for observing the mock code proceedings and reviewing the performances of the participants. This reviewer will evaluate physician and nursing staff responses in the exercise, so he or she preferably will have superior training and experience. The review itself should focus on teamwork, cover the scenario objectives, and last no more than 10 minutes. If a separate reviewer is not available, the MCD may fill this role.

Ideally, mock codes are a positive learning experience for all participants. When giving feedback, it is important to initially stress the positive aspects of each exercise and what was done correctly before addressing the areas where improvement is needed.

The "Mock Code Review Guide and Checklist" (Appendix D) can be used to facilitate an organized review. It emphasizes the ABCs as well as the primary and secondary surveys. It also includes a list of important information that the team is expected to obtain during the mock code exercise. The reviewer may wish to refer to the review guide and jot notes on it during the scenario.

When discussing a review, it is helpful for the code team to focus on no more than three main issues for future improvement. Stick to the basics! Stress the ABCs and objectives. Do not get hung up on style points or minutiae.

It is important to allow code team members the opportunity to ask questions regarding the exercise and their performance. This may take place during or after the review. The review should be conducted in an educational manner that fosters questions and discussion, but keep in mind the 10-minute time limit.

Giving feedback effectively is an art. The relative inexperience of many of the participants necessitates the review being conducted in a positive, upbeat, educational manner. Anyone conducting mock code exercises will benefit from investigating resources and ideas on effective methods of giving feedback. "Feedback in Clinical Medical Education" published in *JAMA*[1] and the "Providing Feedback" chapter in *Teaching During Rounds*[2] are two excellent and highly recommended pieces.

Closing Statements

In closing, the MCD should summarize the scenario, the team's response, and the review. He or she should again stress the objectives of the scenario, repeat the diagnosis, and briefly discuss the initial management and progression. The MCD is responsible for making sure the event ends on a positive note. If time allows, procedures encountered may be further explained and demonstrated after the closing statements.

Keeping Track

A well-organized longitudinal pediatric mock code program should have a quality assurance and improvement component. Records should be kept of the date, location, scenario used, participants, and a review of their performance in each mock code. Notes should be taken on particular strengths and weaknesses of each exercise, as well as the participants' responses. Ideally, these notes will serve as a reference and give insights on how future mock code exercises can be run better and how participants can learn and improve their resuscitation skills.

References

1. Ende J. Feedback in clinical medical education. *JAMA*. 1983;250:777-781.
2. Weinholtz D, Edwards JC. Providing feedback. In: *Teaching During Rounds*. Baltimore, Md: The Johns Hopkins University Press; 1992:85-93.

Principles of Pediatric Resuscitation

Pediatric Vital Signs

Lalit Bajaj, MD, MPH

Understanding how normal vital signs change as children grow older is extremely important in the evaluation and resuscitation of pediatric patients. Appendix A lists normal ranges for respiratory rate, heart rate, and minimal systolic blood pressure and emphasizes the wide range of age-specific norms. A heart rate of 160 can be normal in a neonate, for example, while the same heart rate in an adolescent is significantly tachycardic and signals the need for immediate attention to circulatory status.

The following sections address temperature, respiratory rate, heart rate, and blood pressure. Patient weight is a key component in pediatric resuscitation because equipment and medication doses are weight based. Pain is an emerging vital sign, and federal mandates now exist to monitor and evaluate pain in all hospitalized patients.[1]

Temperature

Normal core temperature is 37°C (98.6°F). Children can have significant individual variations in their normal core temperature (36.2°C to 38°C), as well as diurnal fluctuation with peaks between 5:00 and 7:00 PM and temperatures varying by as much as 1°C (although diurnal variation is less pronounced in infants). Rectal temperature assessment is still considered the most accurate, reproducible, and practical means of determining true core body temperature. Rectal thermometry is not always convenient for parents and triage facilities, so oral, axillary, and tympanic thermometers are often used. Oral and axillary temperature measurements have been found to be significantly lower and inconsistent compared to rectal measurement. Studies comparing infrared ear thermometers with rectal thermometers have shown conflicting results.[2,3] The routine use of ear thermometers in situations that require precise measurement, such as suspected fever in a neonate, is discouraged.

Respiratory Rate

As a child grows, normal respiratory rates change. Minute ventilation is dependent on tidal volume and respiratory rate. With growth, tidal volume increases and normal respiratory rates gradually decrease. Children primarily increase their minute ventilation by increasing their respiratory rates (tachypnea) and not their tidal volumes. Tachypnea is a common response to hypoxia, fever, and respiratory ailments such as pneumonia and asthma. Tachypnea is also seen as a compensatory response to a metabolic acidosis.

Heart Rate

Normal heart rate ranges, as shown in Appendix A, change dramatically depending on age. Cardiac output is dependent on heart rate and stroke volume. As a child grows, stroke volume increases primarily due to the growth of the left ventricle, and this results in a gradual lowering of the normal resting heart rate. Myocardial function (contractility) remains the same.[4] The most effective way for young children to increase their cardiac output is to raise their heart rates. Infants and toddlers are especially sensitive to a multitude of factors that can increase heart rate, including fever, pain, anxiety, hypovolemia, and medications. It is important to remember that a child's primary response to hypovolemia is tachycardia; blood pressure remains relatively normal until 25% to 30% of a child's blood volume is lost, at which point blood pressure falls precipitously. A child with a normal heart can tolerate much longer periods of tachycardia than an adult can.

Blood Pressure

Along with heart rate, normal blood pressure ranges change dramatically with age. As a child grows, the systemic vascular resistance (SVR) rises and, therefore, blood pressure as a measure of SVR also rises. As a child reaches adolescence, blood pressure is near adult norms. Adolescent females tend to have slightly lower normal blood pressures than their male counterparts do. Again, low blood pressure is a late finding in pediatric shock, secondary to preservation of cardiac output via increased heart rate and increased SVR. It is crucial that the evaluation of end organ perfusion be ongoing during a pediatric resuscitation.

Pain

Assessment and management of pain have become a priority in patient care in recent years, reinforced by federal mandates.[1] The assessment of a child's pain must take into account the patient's age, cognitive level, and type of pain. It has become clear that pain in both infants and young children has been underestimated and undertreated for decades.[5,6] Pain measurement tools have been developed for all ages of children. Neonatal pain scales such as the Premature Infant Pain Profile (PIPP) and the Neonatal Infant Pain Scale (NIPS) have been used in nurseries.[7] The NIPS scale uses behavioral indicators such as facial expression, cry, and breathing patterns. Pain scales for children 3 years and older have been studied in the emergency setting. In particular the seven-point Faces Pain Scale and different versions of the Visual Analog Scale have been used and shown to be effective measurement tools for pediatric pain.[8] It is essential that physicians treating pediatric patients recognize and aggressively treat pain.

Weight

A pediatric patient's weight is an especially important piece of information in a resuscitation because the medications used are all dosed by weight. The Broselow Pediatric Emergency Tape (Armstrong Medical Industries, Inc, Lincolnshire, Ill) is an effective tool for estimating weight during a resuscitation. Appendix A lists estimated 50th percentile weights by age. The growing obesity epidemic will require that these estimates be changed in the coming years.

References

1. National Pharmaceutical Council Inc, Joint Commission on Accreditation of Healthcare Organizations. *Pain: Current Understanding of Assessment, Management, and Treatments* [online publication]. December 2001. Available at: http://www.jcaho.org/news+room/health+care+issues/pain_mono_npc.pdf. Accessed on May 12, 2005.
2. Craig JV, Lancaster GA, Taylor S, et al. Infrared ear thermometry compared with rectal thermometry in children: a systematic review. *Lancet.* 2002;360:603-609.
3. Jean-Mary MB, Dicanzio J, Shaw J, et al. Limited accuracy and reliability of infrared axillary and aural thermometers in a pediatric outpatient population. *J Pediatr.* 2002;141(5):671-676.
4. Rowland TW. Children: the development of cardiac performance with exercise. Sportscience [serial online]. Available at: http://www.sportsci.org/encyc/drafts/Child_cardiac_perf.doc. Accessed on May 12, 2005.
5. Simons SH, van Dijk M, Anand KS, et al. Do we still hurt newborn babies? A prospective study of procedural pain and analgesia in neonates. *Arch Pediatr Adolesc Med.* 2003;157:1058-1064.
6. Simons J, Roberson E. Poor communication and knowledge deficits: obstacles to effective management of children's postoperative pain. *J Adv Nursing.* 2002;40(1):78-86.
7. Gallo A. The fifth vital sign: implementation of the Neonatal Infant Pain Scale. *J Obstet Gynecol Neonatal Nurs.* 2003;32:199-206.
8. Bulloch B, Tenenbein M. Validation of two pain scales for use in the pediatric emergency department. *Pediatrics.* 2002;110(3):1-6.

Monitors and Equipment

Lalit Bajaj, MD, MPH

Understanding which equipment and monitoring devices are needed for a pediatric resuscitation is very important. Children grow and change quickly, so the need for pediatric-sized resuscitation equipment is obvious. Everything from suction catheters and intravenous catheters to oxygen face masks, laryngoscope blades, and endotracheal tubes must be readily available in various pediatric sizes. Table 1 lists the minimal equipment and monitoring items recommended for the resuscitation of a pediatric patient. Standard equipment sizes by age are listed in Appendix A.

Two important monitors have become widely used in pediatric resuscitation, the pulse oximeter and the end-tidal CO_2 monitor (capnometer). These monitors, described in the following sections, have important uses and limitations.

Pulse Oximetry

Pulse oximetry was invented in Japan in the early 1970s and became widely available in the 1980s. Continuous monitoring of oxygen saturation is now considered standard of care in virtually all infants and children receiving mechanical ventilation or intensive care. Other typical uses now include monitoring of patients undergoing resuscitation, monitoring of patients undergoing procedural sedation, patients self-administering analgesia, and high-risk patients receiving supplemental oxygen. Pulse oximetry also is used as a screening tool for triage of pediatric patients in acute care settings.

A pulse oximeter estimates arterial oxygen saturation by measuring the absorption of light at two different wavelengths (approximately 660 and 940 nm) in tissue beds. The light absorption changes as the volume of blood in the tissue bed changes and the relative amounts of oxygenated and deoxygenated hemoglobin change. The pulse oximeter measures the ratio of absorption of the two wavelengths. It then averages the readings over a short period of time and correlates the ratio with a calibrated curve of arterial oxygenation. Pulse oximetry has been shown to be accurate within 4% in the range of 70% to 100%. Below 70%, there is a limited amount of calibration data.[1,2]

Several factors can alter the reliability of pulse oximeter measurements. Motion artifact is the most common cause of falsely low readings in the pediatric population. Low peripheral perfusion states such as hypovolemia, severe hypotension, hypothermia, and low cardiac output do not produce adequate signals and result in falsely low readings. Bright ambient light can alter accuracy as well; this can be corrected by wrapping the probe in an opaque

Table 1.
Equipment and Monitors Needed for a Pediatric Resuscitation

Equipment

- Backboard, cervical spine collars
- Airway equipment
  - Oxygen source/tubing with face masks
  - Suction/catheters
  - Bag-mask ventilation (BMV) apparatus with appropriately sized masks
  - Oral airway, nasal trumpet
  - Laryngoscopes, ET tubes, stylets
- Vascular access equipment
  - Intravenous catheters of various sizes
  - Intraosseous needles
  - Central venous catheter kits
  - Intravenous fluid (normal saline, lactated Ringer)
- Resuscitation medications
- Rapid sequence intubation medications
- Defibrillator with pediatric attachments
- Orthopedic splints

Monitors

- Cardiorespiratory monitor
- Pulse oximeter
- Rectal thermometer
- Sphygmomanometer
- Doppler
- End-tidal CO_2 monitor

material. Nail polish or varnish can cause falsely low readings. Dyshemoglobinemias also can affect pulse oximeter readings. Different forms of hemoglobin are indistinguishable to the machine. Carboxyhemoglobin (CO-hemoglobin) is read as 90% oxygenated hemoglobin and 10% deoxygenated hemoglobin and, therefore, overestimates true oxygen saturation. The presence of methemoglobin also produces inaccuracies in measurement; the readings tend to be close to 85% regardless of the true oxygen saturation.[1,2]

It is important to keep in mind that a pulse oximeter provides no information concerning a patient's ventilatory status (P_{CO_2}). A patient can easily maintain acceptable oxygen saturation when ventilation is impaired, especially if the patient is receiving supplemental oxygen.

End-Tidal CO_2 Monitor

Capnometry is the measurement of expired CO_2, and capnography is the graphic representation of expired CO_2 over time. End-tidal CO_2 is the measurement of CO_2 at the very end of expiration and is the maximal concentration of expired CO_2. If ventilation and perfusion are well matched, the end-tidal CO_2 will nearly equal the Pa_{CO_2} (usually 2 to 5 mm Hg less than Pa_{CO_2}).

There are two common methods of measuring end-tidal CO_2. The most common is the use of infrared spectroscopy to measure the amount of gas absorbed at the bandwidth of CO_2. This can be done either with sensors in the patient's breathing circuit (mainstream) or remote from the patient as part of a monitoring system (sidestream) that can intermittently sample a small amount of expired gas. Colorimetric devices are also available; they are pH-sensitive devices that are attached between the endotracheal (ET) tube and ventilation tubing. The device turns yellow in response to CO_2. These devices are especially useful in rapid sequence intubation (RSI) to assist in confirmation of tube placement: there will be no endotracheal CO_2 detected in a patient who has the ET tube inadvertently placed in the esophagus.[2,3] These can be falsely negative in cases of cardiorespiratory arrest where a small or no amount of CO_2 is being produced.

Endotracheal CO_2 can increase in a patient experiencing increased cardiac output, injection of bicarbonate solution, or hypoventilation. Endotracheal CO_2 decreases with hyperventilation, decreased cardiac output, pulmonary embolism, or obstruction or leakage in the ventilator circuit. A patient in full cardiac arrest might have no detectable endotracheal CO_2. Capnometry is primarily useful for confirming proper ET tube placement, early detection of respiratory complications (pneumothorax) or tube obstruction, and managing hyperventilation in patients with confirmed or suspected increased intracranial pressure.[2,3]

References

1. Salyer JW. Neonatal and pediatric pulse oximetry. *Respir Care.* 2003;48:386-398.

2. Nadkarni UB, Shah AM, Deshmukh CT. Non-invasive respiratory monitoring in a paediatric intensive care unit. *J Postgrad Med.* 2000;46:149-152.

3. Bhende MS. End-tidal carbon dioxide monitoring in paediatrics: concepts and technology. *J Postgrad Med.* 2001;47:153-156.

Evaluation and Management: Airway

Mark G. Roback, MD

The importance of proper airway evaluation and management cannot be overemphasized. It is the first and most critical of the pediatric ABCs. This section outlines the evaluation and management of typical pediatric airway problems. This outline only summarizes the information available regarding the pediatric airway; references are provided for more in-depth study.

This section begins by addressing the unique qualities of the pediatric airway compared with that of an adult. Evaluation in the emergent setting is followed by a more complete airway-directed history and physical examination. Once the airway is assessed, management and resuscitation are discussed. Basic and adjunctive airway-opening maneuvers are presented first, followed by progression to more advanced techniques such as RSI and cricothyrotomy. Indications, contraindications, and complications of each airway intervention are discussed. Airway obstruction is presented in a more in-depth manner. All descriptions of airway techniques and maneuvers take into account patients who might be victims of trauma, with a focus on appropriate airway management in the patient with potential cervical spine injury.

The material presented here is consistent with the APLS and PALS texts. However, it is important to note that there are acceptable alternatives to these recommendations, specifically with regard to the drugs used in RSI, that may be used effectively in individual resuscitation situations.

The Pediatric Airway

- The airway is proportionately smaller in children and infants, but the tongue is proportionately larger relative to the oropharynx.
- The most narrow portion of the airway in adults is the glottic inlet at the level of the vocal cords. In contrast, in infants and children younger than approximately 8 years, the most narrow part of the airway is the subglottic region, below the level of the cords.
- Pediatric vocal cords are more anteriorly positioned than in adults. Cricoid pressure (the Sellick maneuver) is helpful to visualize the cords under direct laryngoscopy.
- The pediatric epiglottis is shorter than in adults and is composed of soft, flexible cartilage. In adults, the epiglottis is longer and stiffer. Direct laryngoscopy in younger patients therefore is usually facilitated by using a straight (Miller) blade and "picking up" the epiglottis to visualize the cords rather than placing a curved (Macintosh) blade in the vallecula, as in adults.[1]
- Obstruction in the pediatric airway can occur with minimal insult such as airway swelling (croup, anaphylaxis), secretions, positioning, and decreased tone, as well as with foreign body aspiration. Because the pediatric airway is smaller than the adult airway, small changes in airway diameter cause proportionately large increases in airway resistance to air flow.
- Recognizing patients with potentially difficult airways is crucial. Patients with a history of difficult intubation, known airway anomalies, or unique airway anatomy (eg, short neck, large tongue, micrognathia, decreased tone, or redundant tissue as seen in patients with, for example, Pierre Robin sequence, Treacher Collins syndrome, or mucopolysaccharidosis) must be identified, and the proper equipment and personnel must be assembled before intubation is attempted.

Evaluation

Emergent Question

Is the patient able to speak or cry?

Look for respiratory distress (grunting, flaring, retractions), choking, and/or cyanosis, which might indicate airway obstruction.

Listen for air movement over the airway in the neck and for quality of breath sounds (stridor).

Feel for movement of air from the mouth and nose and for crepitus in the neck.

Assess whether the airway can be maintained with basic airway maneuvers, including positioning, suction, and oxygen, or if the airway requires advanced techniques, including bag-mask ventilation (BMV) or endotracheal intubation.

History

Common causes of airway obstruction to be considered include the following:

- Foreign body aspiration
- Infections including croup, which is viral, and epiglottitis and soft tissue infections of the pharynx or trachea (tracheitis), which are bacterial and much less common than croup
- Trauma, especially laryngeal fracture
- Conditions of decreased tone, especially postictal states and neuromuscular disease
- Conditions of increased secretions and/or decreased ability to clear secretions
- History of allergies or recent exposure to new drugs, foods, or insect bites, which might indicate anaphylaxis with concomitant airway swelling

Physical Examination

Look for signs of respiratory insufficiency.

- General appearance—Level of consciousness, work of breathing
- Airway—Ability to move air, audible stridor (high-pitched sound typically heard in inspiration indicative of partial obstruction). Inspiratory stridor is generally due to obstruction *outside* of the thorax; expiratory stridor is generally due to obstruction *inside* the thorax.
- Chest—Respiratory rate, inspiratory-to-expiratory phase ratio, presence of retractions or accessory muscle use
- Auscultation—Listen over the airway for air entry, stridor, or wheeze.
- Cardiac—Assess for circulatory compromise and hypoxia by evaluation of perfusion, capillary refill, skin color, or presence of mottling, as well as character of heart tones and pulses.

Management

As the airway is being addressed, assemble the following equipment:

- Oxygen, nonrebreather mask, self-inflating or standard anesthesia bag with appropriately sized masks
- Suction, with appropriately sized catheters
- Airway adjuncts—Oropharyngeal and nasopharyngeal airways
- Laryngoscope with blades and ET tubes of appropriate sizes
- Magill forceps for patients with suspected airway foreign body

Resuscitation

If the airway is deemed to be *not* maintainable, begin resuscitation immediately, as follows:

- Administer 100% oxygen initially via a nonrebreather mask.
- Position head in midline, jaw thrust, chin lift, and head tilt (except in trauma).
- Suction the airway to clear secretions, vomitus, and foreign bodies as indicated.
- Establish oropharyngeal or nasopharyngeal airways if deemed appropriate.
- Assist with BMV as needed, realizing that this might induce emesis.
- Intubate the trachea if the interventions above are not adequate.
- Consider the following alternative airway techniques (discussed later) if intubation is contraindicated or unsuccessful:
  - Laryngeal mask airway (LMA)
  - Combitube (adolescents >4 feet tall)
  - Fiberoptic scopes, lighted stylets
  - Surgical airway (percutaneous needle cricothyrotomy)

Airway Obstruction

Relieve anatomic obstruction (hypopharyngeal tissue block) by opening the airway.

- Keep the head in midline position. The occiput is prominent in infants and young children, so when they are placed supine on a flat surface, flexion of the neck and partial airway obstruction can result. A towel roll placed under the shoulders might alleviate this problem, although great care must be taken to avoid excessive extension or flexion of the neck in trauma patients.

- Head tilt and chin lift (the "sniffing position") result in slight extension of neck and opening of the airway. This maneuver is contraindicated in trauma patients with potential cervical spine injuries.[2]
- The jaw thrust maneuver opens the airway while maintaining inline cervical spine positioning and is recommended for trauma patients.

Check tongue position. Patients with decreased muscle tone (eg, postictal, neuromuscular disease) and patients with large tongues (eg, Pierre Robin sequence) are at risk for anatomic obstruction.

Clear secretions and vomitus. Suction the airway while log-rolling the patient with inline immobilization where indicated to protect the cervical spine.

Consider airway adjuncts.[3]

- **Oropharyngeal Airway:** This device circumvents soft tissue airway obstruction from the lips and teeth to the glottis. It is to be used only in unconscious patients. Patients with intact airway reflexes gag or vomit when an oropharyngeal airway is placed, possibly resulting in laryngospasm or bronchospasm. Proper sizing of the oropharyngeal airway is crucial.[1]
- **Nasopharyngeal Airway:** This is to be used when the patient has good respiratory effort but has mechanical upper nasopharyngeal obstruction despite basic airway maneuvers. It can be used successfully in conscious or semiconscious patients. Care must be taken to avoid trauma to the nasopharynx. This airway adjunct is contraindicated in patients with midface trauma, bleeding disorders, or history of previous facial surgery.

Manage foreign body obstruction.

- In the initial assessment, it must be determined whether the airway is maintainable (partially obstructed) or completely obstructed. Awake patients with partially obstructed airways should be placed in a position of comfort (usually with a parent or care provider). Oxygen should be administered in a noninvasive manner, and the patient should be transported to a facility where appropriately trained personnel can provide definitive care.
- When the airway is completely obstructed, patients younger than 12 months should receive alternating back blows and chest thrusts in an attempt to clear the obstruction. In patients older than 12 months, the Heimlich maneuver or abdominal thrusts should be performed. Blind finger sweeps are contraindicated in all age groups.[2]
- When these maneuvers are unsuccessful, attempts to provide BMV to the patient are indicated. If BMV is unsuccessful, attempts should be made to visualize and to remove the foreign body under direct laryngoscopy using a Magill forceps. In some cases, if the foreign body cannot be removed, attempts may be made to advance the foreign body into a mainstem bronchus, resulting in the ability to ventilate at least one lung.

Potential Complications in Initial Airway Management:

- Oxygen or suction tubing is not connected to wall.
- Oxygen is not set to deliver maximal percentage.
- Incorrect face mask size is used.
- Suction catheter is too small to effectively clear secretions or vomitus.
- Equipment required to remove an airway foreign body is not available or is not the correct size.
- Attempts to remove a foreign body using laryngoscopy and a Magill forceps in awake or partially awake patients can lead to complete airway obstruction.
- Blind attempts to remove a foreign body can result in trauma and bleeding or in further impaction of the foreign body.

Bag-Mask Ventilation

BMV can be performed effectively by almost any health care professional. It has been shown to be as effective as endotracheal intubation for most pediatric patients over short periods of time.[4] Because respiratory failure is the number one cause of cardiac collapse in pediatric patients, it is essential that this skill be practiced by all pediatric health care providers.

Indications: BMV is indicated whenever assisted ventilation is required—respiratory insufficiency or failure, severe head injuries, or the shock state.

Contraindications: BMV should not be performed before suctioning the airway in newborns with respiratory suppression immediately after a delivery with meconium. It should not be administered to patients with known diaphragmatic hernia.

Technique to perform BMV:

- Place the patient in good airway position (see earlier).
- Assemble proper equipment, including oxygen, suction, and appropriate monitors.
- Select the proper size of face mask and bag.
- With fingers on the angle of the mandible and the thumb around the connection of the mask and bag, place the mask over the nose and mouth, obtaining a good seal by applying gentle pressure.
- Apply cricoid pressure if the patient has lost airway protective reflexes.
- Begin ventilation with 100% oxygen while watching for chest rise and ausculating the lungs for good air exchange. Look, listen, and feel for air leak around the mask.
- Check patient response to BMV—heart rate, color, and oxygenation on pulse oximetry.

Potential Complications:

- Vomiting and aspiration pneumonitis, especially if cricoid pressure is not used
- Barotrauma from overzealous bagging, resulting in pneumothorax or tension pneumothorax
- Allergic reactions to latex-containing face mask materials
- Trauma to face and lips if excessive pressure is applied to face mask

Emergent Intubation

Indications: Emergent intubation is indicated in cardiopulmonary arrest, apnea, respiratory insufficiency, actual or potential airway obstruction, respiratory depression, severe burns, severe multiple trauma, severe head injury, increased intracranial pressure (ICP), depressed mental status, and loss of normal protective airway reflexes.

Preparation: Assemble materials required for intubation: 100% oxygen, suction, face masks, self-inflating or anesthesia bag, laryngoscope (with functioning light), and ET tube of proper size. A useful formula for determining the proper size of an ET tube is (age + 16)/4. As an alternative, one may use the length-based Broselow Pediatric Emergency Tape. Also see Appendix A, Normal Vital Sign Ranges and Standard Equipment Sizes by Age.

Medications to be administered should be drawn up, and appropriate monitors (continuous cardiorespiratory monitor and pulse oximeter) should be placed.

Rapid Sequence Intubation

RSI is performed for patients with full (or presumed full) stomachs to achieve a fully relaxed state for ease of intubation and fewer adverse effects. RSI is also used to avoid physiologic responses to laryngoscopy, such as reflex bradycardia and increased ICP.[5]

The RSI technique is as follows:

- Begin preoxygenation with 100% inspired oxygen for 2 to 5 minutes (when possible) to completely saturate hemoglobin with oxygen, providing the most reserve possible. If possible, avoid BMV, which increases the likelihood of vomiting and aspiration.
- Administer a vagal stimulation blocker (also reduces oral secretions) to prevent reflex bradycardia in children younger than 1 year, in children younger than 5 years who will receive succinylcholine, and in patients older than 5 years who receive more than one dose of succinylcholine.[6] *Note:* Atropine is frequently used empirically in patients up to 5 years old. For the purposes of this text, atropine is recommended for the indications listed above and listed as a consideration for patients aged 1 to 5 years with normal heart rates who do not receive succinylcholine.
  - **Atropine 0.02 mg/kg IV**—Minimum dose is 0.1 mg (lower doses can result in paradoxical bradycardia), and maximum dose is 0.5 mg.
- If needed, administer adjunct drugs, such as lidocaine for closed head injuries and presumed increased ICP or fentanyl for pain.
  - **Lidocaine 1 mg/kg IV**
  - **Fentanyl 2 to 5 mcg/kg IV**—A vasoactive

drug, fentanyl must be given with caution in patients of uncertain hemodynamic status. It typically is not used in patients with shock.

- Administer sedative alternatives to induce unconsciousness.
  - **Etomidate 0.3 mg/kg IV**—With a rapid onset of action and short duration of action, etomidate has minimal physiologic effects, supports blood pressure, and decreases ICP and intraocular pressure.
  - **Midazolam 0.1 mg/kg IV**—With a rapid onset of action (although longer than that of etomidate) and a longer duration of action than etomidate, midazolam has amnestic and anticonvulsant properties.
  - **Thiopental 2 to 5 mg/kg IV**—Thiopental lowers ICP but can cause hypotension; it is used in hemodynamically stable patients such as those with isolated head injuries.
  - **Ketamine 1 to 2 mg/kg IV**—The drug of choice for RSI in asthma patients due to potent bronchodilatory properties, ketamine increases heart rate, blood pressure, ICP, and secretion production. Ketamine is usually avoided in patients with head injuries and where there is concern for increased ICP.
- Administer neuromuscular blocking agents: Because of their rapid onset of action, succinylcholine and rocuronium are the two most commonly used paralytic agents for RSI.[7]
  - **Succinylcholine 1 to 1.5 mg/kg IV (2 mg/kg for infants)**—This depolarizing muscle relaxant is desirable because it has a very short duration of action (3 to 5 minutes). However, it has many undesirable effects including muscle fasciculations and increased ICP, intraocular pressure, and intragastric pressure. It also has been associated with hyperkalemia and hypertension. It should be avoided in patients with renal failure, large burns, or hyperkalemia. In children 5 years old or older, a defasciculating dose of a nondepolarizing agent should be considered.
  - **Rocuronium 0.6 to 1 mg/kg IV**—Rocuronium is a nondepolarizing agent with a rapid onset of action but a longer duration of action (30 to 60 minutes). Minimal cardiovascular effects make it a desirable choice for RSI.
- Apply cricoid pressure (the Sellick maneuver) to occlude the esophagus without compressing the airway or moving the cervical spine. Cricoid pressure should be used in patients receiving BMV who are unable to protect the airway (absent gag reflex).
- Attempt intubation when full airway muscle relaxation is achieved.
- Confirm ET tube placement as follows:

  Look—Watch the ET tube go through the cords. Look for symmetric chest rise. Condensation in the ET tube is a nonspecific finding that does not confirm proper ET tube placement.

  Listen over the chest for symmetric breath sounds and over the abdomen.

  Observe the patient's response, heart rate, and skin color.

  Monitors—Pulse oximeter and cardiorespiratory monitor. The color-change-style end-tidal CO_2 monitor is used to confirm ET tube placement in the trachea. A chest radiograph is obtained to visually confirm placement, and arterial blood gas (ABG) analysis is used to evaluate effectiveness of ventilation.
- Once ET tube placement is confirmed, secure the tube in place using tape, and place a nasogastric (NG) or orogastric (OG) tube to evacuate the stomach contents. This decreases the likelihood of aspiration and might improve ventilation if significant gastric air is present. Cricoid pressure should be maintained until placement of the ET tube is confirmed by physical findings.

Note: It should be emphasized that the drugs used in any given RSI vary depending on specific patient problem, experience of the physician administering the drugs, and individual/institutional preferences. In the mock code scenarios presented in this book, the drugs listed reflect APLS/PALS recommendations and the authors' preferences for the given situations. Other drugs may be substituted safely in most cases. Distinct contraindications are discussed.

Potential Complications:

- Laryngoscopy and intubation can result in bradycardia, pain, ICP elevation, increased risk of gastric regurgitation/aspiration, and hypoxia.
- Vomiting can occur with BMV or just before intubation, requiring proper use of suction. Patients should be log-rolled with maintenance of cervical spine immobilization in trauma. Vomiting might be seen more frequently if cricoid pressure is not properly applied, as described earlier.
- Laryngoscope light fails.
- Breath sounds are decreased or absent on the left side of the chest, indicating a right mainstem intubation.
- Patient is extubated if the ET tube is not properly handled and taped.
- Inadequate oxygenation leads to hypoxia followed by bradycardia and asystole.
- Positive-pressure ventilations can lead to barotrauma if attention is not paid to tidal volume delivered. Patients can develop pneumothorax. If barotrauma is unrecognized and positive-pressure ventilations are continued, tension pneumothorax might occur.
- Mechanical trauma of laryngoscopy and intubation can result in edema or bleeding, which might in itself cause airway obstruction.
- Aspiration pneumonitis can develop if secretions or stomach contents are aspirated. The use of cricoid pressure with BMV and intubation is recommended to prevent aspiration.

Rescue Airway Techniques

When endotracheal intubation and BMV are unsuccessful, alternative approaches must be considered using one of the methods described briefly next.

Laryngeal Mask Airway[8]**:** Available in a variety of sizes, the laryngeal mask airway is designed to be placed into the mouth and guided down so that the inflatable cuffed ventilating port covers the glottis, allowing for effective oxygenation and ventilation. Newer models are designed to serve as a conduit to intubation with a special flexible tracheal tube.

Combitube: This device is designed for patients over 4 feet tall, so it is not appropriate for preadolescents. The Combitube is a tube with two balloons. It is placed in the esophagus, and the smaller, distal balloon is inflated to occlude the esophagus. The larger, proximal balloon is then inflated to occlude the oral cavity. Oxygen 100% is then ventilated through the tube, exiting through the esophageal port located between the two balloons. This oxygen then enters the trachea to provide effective oxygenation.

Fiberoptic Scopes and Lighted Stylets: These devices assist trained airway personnel in performing endotracheal intubation by improving visualization.

Potential Complications:
These techniques are used when conventional techniques fail. The most important complication would be failure of these techniques, necessitating establishment of a surgical airway.

Surgical Airway Techniques[9]

Cricothyrotomy: Cricothyrotomy is indicated when airway obstruction results in hypoventilation and desaturation, cyanosis, bradycardia, and impending cardiorespiratory failure, but only when conventional methods of securing the airway and ventilating (BMV, endotracheal intubation, or rescue airway techniques) are unsuccessful. It should also be considered in cases of severe facial trauma or life-threatening upper airway obstruction. When trained personnel are available, this procedure is preferred to percutaneous needle or catheter cricothyrotomy because it results in much more effective ventilation.

Percutaneous Needle Cricothyrotomy Technique[10]**:**

- Place the catheter through the cricothyroid membrane for transtracheal ventilation.
- Use a 14- to 18-gauge intravenous catheter with the connector from a 3.0 ET tube.
- Attach the ventilation bag to the connector; ventilation will be very difficult due to the smaller size of the intravenous catheter compared with an ET tube.
- As an alternative, connect to a high-pressure oxygen source and provide intermittent bursts at a rate of approximately 20/min. Each burst lasts about 1 second on (inspiration) followed by 2 seconds off (exhalation). Use jet ventilator when available.

Potential Complications:

- The neck area has many vascular structures, and bleeding is a common complication.
- Puncture of the trachea can lead to subcutaneous emphysema.
- Skin organisms might be introduced, resulting in tracheal infection.

These complications should not dissuade caregivers from attempting cricothyrotomy if certain death will occur if the airway is not secured.

References

1. King BR, King C, Coates WE. Critical procedures. In: Gausche-Hill M, Fuchs S, Yamamoto L, eds. *APLS: The Pediatric Emergency Medicine Resource.* 4th ed. Sudbury, Mass: American Academy of Pediatrics, American College of Emergency Physicians, Jones and Bartlett Publishing Co; 2004:691-717.
2. Guidelines 2000 for Cardiopulmonary Resuscitation and Emergency Cardiovascular Care. Part 9: pediatric basic life support. The American Heart Association in collaboration with the International Liaison Committee on Resuscitation. *Circulation.* 2000;102(8 suppl):I-253-I-290.
3. Scarfone RJ. Airway adjuncts, oxygen delivery, and suctioning the upper airway. In: Henretig FM, King CC, eds. *Textbook of Pediatric Emergency Procedures.* Baltimore, Md: Williams & Wilkins; 1997:101-118.
4. Gausche M, Lewis RJ, Stratton SJ, et al. Effect of out-of-hospital pediatric endotracheal intubation on survival and neurological outcome. *JAMA.* 2000;283:783-790.
5. Yamamoto LG. Emergency airway management—rapid sequence intubation. In: Fleisher GR, Ludwig S, eds. *Textbook of Pediatric Emergency Medicine.* 4th ed. Philadelphia, Pa: Lippincott Williams & Wilkins; 2000:71-82.
6. Gerardi MJ, Sacchetti AD, Cantor RM, et al. Rapid-sequence intubation of the pediatric patient. Pediatric Emergency Medicine Committee of the American College of Emergency Physicians. *Ann Emerg Med.* 1996;28:55-74.
7. Zaritsky AL, Nadkarni VM, Hickey RW, et al, eds. *PALS Provider Manual.* Dallas, Tex: American Heart Association and American Academy of Pediatrics; 2002:363.
8. Pollack CV. The laryngeal mask airway: a comprehensive review for the emergency physician. *J Emerg Med.* 2001;20:53-66.
9. Walls RM, Vissers RJ. Surgical airway techniques. In: Walls RM, ed. *Manual of Emergency Airway Management.* Baltimore, Md: Lippincott Williams & Wilkins; 2000:89-104.
10. Peak DA, Roy S. Needle cricothyroidotomy revisited. *Pediatr Emerg Care.* 1999;15:224-226.

Evaluation and Management: Breathing

Stephen J. Teach, MD, MPH

Breathing is the process by which air, having passed through the large and small airways of the head, neck, and thorax, enters the alveoli, permitting gas exchange (oxygenation and ventilation). Although closely linked to the evaluation and management of the upper airway, the evaluation and management of breathing focus more on the thorax, with attention to the intrathoracic large and small airways, the alveoli themselves, the pleural spaces and surfaces, the diaphragm, and the chest wall. Its assessment always follows assessment of the airway, because oxygenation and ventilation are possible only with an intact airway.

Evaluation of Breathing

Emergent Question

Is the patient moving sufficient air in and out of the chest to maintain effective oxygenation and ventilation, or is the patient in imminent respiratory failure?

A rapid focused evaluation should help determine the child's overall respiratory status.

Look for the respiratory rate (adjusting for age-appropriate norms, see Appendix A), location of the trachea, symmetry of chest rise, use of accessory muscles, retractions, and skin color.

Listen for symmetry and quality of breath sounds, for adequacy of air movement, and for presence of extra intrathoracic sounds such as stridor, crackles, rhonchi, and/or wheezes.

Feel for subcutaneous air (crepitus), tenderness, and instability of the chest wall.

Assess by using the physical examination findings combined with the information derived from monitors and an ABG analysis (when time permits) to determine if respiratory failure is imminent. If so, positive-pressure ventilation with BMV and, ultimately, endotracheal intubation will be necessary to prevent respiratory arrest followed by circulatory collapse and death. Pulse oximetry, although a good measure of **oxygenation** (Po_2), tells us nothing about **ventilation** (Pco_2). The end-tidal CO_2 monitor is used for the noninvasive assessment of ventilation. The ABG is the gold standard by which both oxygenation and ventilation are assessed.

History

Common causes of respiratory compromise include both **obstructive** processes (those marked by small airway abnormalities that trap air in the alveoli, making ventilation especially difficult) and **restrictive** processes (those marked by stiff alveoli or interstitium that make it difficult to expand the alveoli, making oxygenation especially difficult). Important elements of the initial history include the presence of fever (suggesting an infectious process), trauma, and underlying diseases such as asthma, cystic fibrosis, sickle cell disease, neurologic disorders, metabolic disorders, and immunodeficiencies.

Key points of the history include the following:

- Obstructive disorders include asthma and cystic fibrosis, both of which are exacerbated by viral and bacterial infections. Bronchiolitis is a virally mediated obstructive process of the bronchioles that mimics asthma and can be a precursor to it. Viral illnesses frequently start as upper respiratory tract infections.
- Restrictive disorders include "alveolitis" (pneumonia or pneumonitis) that is usually infectious (with viral, bacterial, fungal, and atypical varieties), but which can be chemical (due to aspiration or drowning). Pneumonia can coexist with airway diseases such as bronchiolitis.
- Traumatic causes of respiratory compromise are numerous, and each has a unique intervention.
  - Pneumothorax—Chest tube
  - Hemothorax—Chest tube
  - Pulmonary contusion—Oxygen and possibly intubation
  - Pulmonary hemorrhage—Oxygen and possibly intubation
  - Open sucking chest wound—Occlusive dressing, usually together with a chest tube
  - Flail chest—Positive-pressure ventilation
- Remember that not all respiratory distress

originates as a pulmonary problem. Sepsis and metabolic disorders (diabetic ketoacidosis, for example) can cause metabolic acidosis, which in turn can result in hyperventilation to "blow off" CO_2 (a compensatory respiratory alkalosis). Neurologic disorders with central or peripheral nervous system etiologies can cause hypoventilation due to suppression of respiratory drive centrally (such as in a postictal state) or weakness of the muscles of respiration (such as in a muscular dystrophy).

- A myriad of ingestions can cause respiratory distress and/or respiratory failure. Salicylates, for example, induce a metabolic acidosis that can precipitate hyperventilation. Opiates, barbiturates, benzodiazepines, and certain other anticonvulsants can suppress respiratory drive and lead to respiratory arrest in overdosage.

Physical Examination

Look, listen, and feel for signs of respiratory distress and/or respiratory insufficiency. A full examination should follow the emergent assessment described earlier.

Key points of the physical examination include the following:

- General appearance reveals much about a child's respiratory status. In fact, much of the assessment of breathing is made through simple observation. Alert, talkative children are rarely in imminent danger. An anxious child with retractions, flaring, and grunting who is sitting in a tripod position with his or her nose thrust forward (the "sniffing" position) is at risk of respiratory failure. The somnolent unresponsive child who continues to labor to breathe requires emergent intervention.
- Aside from a child's general appearance, the respiratory rate might be the most important sign of respiratory status (see Appendix A for age-specific norms). Principally and initially regulated by P_{CO_2} and the acid-base status, respiratory drive becomes dependent on P_{O_2} only in situations of extreme hypoxia.
- Respiratory rates can be difficult to interpret in children. Normal rates vary tremendously by age (Appendix A), ranging from up to 60 breaths/min in infants to only 16 breaths/min in adolescents. In addition, fever, pain, and anxiety all can increase the respiratory rate. Finally, respiratory rates can paradoxically fall as respiratory distress progresses to respiratory failure, as a child fatigues from the overall work of breathing. The latter is a critically important clinical sign demanding immediate intervention, usually intubation with mechanical ventilation.
- Distinguishing tachypnea (rapid respiratory rate) from dyspnea (a sense of shortness of breath) can be crucial. The two can coexist and overlap, but the former might occur as a result of completely **extra**pulmonary factors such as fever or anxiety or as a response to a metabolic derangement such as diabetic ketoacidosis or septic shock. The latter tends to occur due to pulmonary factors such as airway inflammation, obstruction, alveolar infection, or pleural or chest wall factors.
- Auscultation of the chest in four quadrants both anteriorly and posteriorly can reveal the presence of abnormally loud or soft breath sounds, stridor, rales, crackles, or wheezes. In general, stridor suggests large airway obstruction, wheezing suggests lower airway obstruction, and crackles suggest alveolar disease. Auscultatory findings of pneumonia can be especially difficult to appreciate in young infants, making it more necessary to rely on history and other examination findings, including fever, tachypnea, and work of breathing.
- Noting symmetry of breath sounds is crucial because it can offer hints to foreign body aspiration, pneumothorax, hemothorax, or intubation of the right mainstem bronchus with an ET tube.
- Inspection and palpation of the chest wall are important in order to uncover chest wall injuries, especially after trauma.

Management of Breathing

Equipment

As described earlier in the Airway section, management of impending or actual respiratory failure begins with assembling the proper equipment for ventilation and, if necessary, for airway management as follows:

- Oxygen, face mask, nonrebreather mask, self-inflating or standard anesthesia bag with appropriately sized masks
- Suction with appropriately sized catheters
- Airway adjuncts: oropharyngeal and nasopharyngeal airways
- Laryngoscope with blades and ET tubes of appropriate sizes
- Magill forceps for patients with suspected airway foreign body

Interventions to Support Breathing

Oxygen

- Oxygen is rarely contraindicated in the child in respiratory distress or in imminent respiratory failure.
- Application of 100% oxygen by face mask or nonrebreather mask greatly increases the inspired FIO_2 and often decreases the work of breathing, especially in the hypoxic child.
- If the child is in respiratory failure, assisted ventilation with BMV or intubation will be necessary.

Bag-Mask Ventilation and Ventilating After Intubation

- Positive-pressure ventilation is delivered via a self-inflating **or** standard anesthesia bag with an appropriately sized mask using 100% oxygen. This procedure is described in more detail in the Airway section.
- Controversy exists (particularly with neonates[1,2]) regarding whether resuscitation should occur with 100% oxygen, room air, or something in between. The issue is that 100% oxygen is associated with the generation of free radicals, which can cause neurologic damage.
- BMV requires proper head positioning and a good seal with the mask on the face. Its effectiveness can be assessed by observing chest excursion, auscultating breath sounds, and following vital signs and pulse oximetry readings.
- The Sellick maneuver (cricoid pressure) is used to collapse and occlude the esophagus, preventing aspiration of stomach contents into the lungs.
- Ventilation through an ET tube with a self-inflating or standard anesthesia bag follows the same principles of careful assessment of chest excursion and breath sounds. Care must be taken to ensure a proper connection between the bag and the ET tube.
- Potential complications of BMV via an ET tube are as follows:
  - When the face mask is the wrong size for the patient, a poor seal results in ineffective oxygenation and ventilation.
  - A self-inflating or standard anesthesia bag of the wrong size can result in underventilation or overventilation.
  - Overzealous bagging or use of an oversized self-inflating or standard anesthesia bag can lead to pneumothorax.
  - Vomiting can lead to aspiration if no cricoid pressure is used.
  - Abdominal distention from air secondary to BMV can compromise ventilation; nasogastric (NG) or orogastic tube is required.
  - Air leak from a small-sized ET tube may result in ineffective ventilation.

Thoracentesis

- The indications for thoracentesis (needle thoracostomy) are suspected tension pneumothorax or suspected hemothorax that is compromising ventilation.
- Thoracentesis is a temporizing measure done before chest tube placement, but it can also be used to remove air or fluid. A chest tube is typically more effective, however, especially for fluid.
- The anterior approach is used to evacuate air. After sterile preparation, an intravenous catheter (14 to 22 gauge, depending on child's size) is passed **over** the rib in the second intercostal space in the midclavicular line. It can be connected to a large syringe via a three-way stopcock to permit continuous removal of air.[3]
  - The posterior approach is used to evacuate fluid. After sterile preparation, an intravenous

catheter is passed over the rib in the midaxillary line or, fourth or fifth intercostal space.

- Always introduce the needle superior to the rib to avoid the intercostal nerve and vessels that run deep to the thinner, inferior aspect of the rib.
- Potential complications of thoracentesis include the following.
  - Pneumothorax or hemothorax might result if the lung is punctured.
  - Pulmonary contusion can occur if the lung is traumatized.
  - Hepatic or splenic trauma can occur if the needle crosses the diaphragm.
  - Damage to neurovascular structures passing inferior to the ribs can result if positioning is incorrect.

Tube Thoracostomy

- The indications for a chest tube are to drain an abnormal collection of air (pneumothorax), blood (hemothorax), or other fluid from the pleural space. By evacuating this space, the lung is allowed to fully reexpand.[3,4]
- Some authorities recommend decompression of a suspected tension pneumothorax through thoracentesis before the placement of a chest tube.[5]
- This procedure is relatively contraindicated in the presence of severe coagulopathy, massive hemothorax, or severe pulmonary adhesions or pulmonary blebs. It should not be withheld if the perceived benefits outweigh the potential risks.
- A detailed discussion of this procedure is available elsewhere.[6] The relevant landmark is the site just anterior to the midaxillary line at nipple level, in the third, fourth, or fifth intercostal space. The tube must be placed **over** the rib to avoid the subcostal neurovascular bundle.
- Potential complications of tube thoracostomy include the following.
  - Pneumothorax or hemothorax might result if the lung is punctured.
  - Pulmonary contusion can occur if the lung is traumatized.
  - Hepatic or splenic trauma can occur if the tube crosses the diaphragm.
  - Damage to the long thoracic nerve or mammary tissue can occur when the incision is made.
  - Damage to neurovascular structures passing inferior to the ribs can result if positioning is incorrect.
  - Increased intrathoracic hemorrhage might occur after decompression of a hemothorax.

References

1. Saugstad OD, Ramji S, Vento M. Resuscitation of depressed newborn infants with ambient air or pure oxygen: a meta-analysis. *Biol Neonate.* 2004;87:27-34.
2. Tarnow-Mordi WO. Room air or oxygen for asphyxiated babies? *Lancet.* 1998;352:341.
3. King BR, King C, Coates WC. Needle thoracostomy. In: Gausche-Hill M, Fuchs S, Yamamoto L, eds. *APLS: The Pediatric Emergency Medicine Resource.* 4th ed. Sudbury, Mass: American Academy of Pediatrics, American College of Emergency Physicians, Jones and Bartlett Publishing Co; 2004:741.
4. Miller KS, Sahn SA. Chest tubes: indications, technique, management, and complications. *Chest.* 1987;91:258.
5. Hamilton AD, Archer GJ. Treatment of pneumothorax by simple aspiration. *Thorax.* 1983;38:394.
6. King BR, King C, Coates WC. Tube thoracostomy In: Gausche-Hill M, Fuchs S, Yamamoto L, eds. *APLS: The Pediatric Emergency Medicine Resource.* 4th ed. Sudbury, Mass: American Academy of Pediatrics, American College of Emergency Physicians, Jones and Bartlett Publishing Co; 2004:743-744.

Evaluation and Management: Circulation

Richard G. Bachur, MD

Circulation refers to the continuous flow of blood throughout the body. The process can be divided into the following four steps:

- Oxygenated blood is pumped by the left ventricle into the aorta to be distributed by arteries, arterioles, and the capillary circuit for exchange of gas and nutrients.
- Deoxygenated blood then returns to the right atrium through the venous system.
- Deoxygenated blood then moves from the right ventricle into the pulmonary circulation to exchange carbon dioxide for oxygen.
- Finally, newly oxygenated blood returns to the left atrium and ventricle.

Specific physiologic concepts about the circulation are important to understand. Cardiac output is the blood volume passed through the heart per time unit. Cardiac output is dependent on the **stroke volume** (volume of blood delivered by one contraction of the ventricle) and the **heart rate**. Stroke volume depends on preload (venous return, filling pressure to the ventricle), contractility of the ventricle, and afterload (left ventricular outflow resistance and systemic vascular resistance [SVR] or the tone of the arteriolar system). Oxygen delivery depends on the content of oxygen in the blood and the cardiac output. Oxygen content is a function of the concentration of hemoglobin, the hemoglobin-oxygen affinity curve, the oxygen saturation (Sao_2), and a small component of dissolved oxygen.

Ultimately, adequacy of the circulation depends on the delivery of oxygen to the end organs and tissues—hence, the essential link to adequate airway and breathing. Without adequate delivery of oxygen to tissues, the pathophysiology of shock ensues. **Compensated** shock is defined as a state in which end-organ perfusion is maintained by compensatory mechanisms and blood pressure is within normal range. **Decompensated** shock is defined as the point at which compensatory mechanisms are overwhelmed, and hypoperfusion and hypotension ensue.[1] The evaluation of circulation therefore relies on accurate assessment of the vital signs, cardiorespiratory system, pulses, perfusion, and end-organ function.

Evaluation of Circulation

Emergent Question

Does the patient have adequate circulation to support end-organ function? A focused, rapid evaluation of the circulatory status is essential for every ill patient.

Look for evidence of poor perfusion, such as cyanosis, mottling, pallor, or altered mental status; for evidence of chest trauma, such as asymmetry of chest expansion as occurs with tension pneumothorax; and for jugular venous distention (JVD), as seen with pericardial tamponade, tension pneumothorax, or congestive heart failure.

Listen for the heart rate to rapidly identify bradycardia or tachydysrhythmia; for heart tones such as a murmur, rub, or gallop to identify cardiac etiologies of poor circulation; for breath sounds such as rales or wheezing that can be heard with congestive heart failure; and for diminished breath sounds to indicate a pneumothorax or hemothorax.

Feel for central pulses, temperature of skin, and capillary refill.

Assess to determine whether circulation is adequate, inadequate, or absent (no pulses) through a combination of history and physical examination findings plus heart rhythm on the monitor and blood pressure measurement. Patients without a pulse require chest compressions and immediate assessment of the heart rhythm (Figure 1, page 46). Patients with a pulse but poor perfusion need aggressive treatment for shock to avoid cardiopulmonary arrest. Some patients who appear to be in shock with a pulse but poor perfusion have dysrhythmias and should be treated based on the rhythm as outlined in the appropriate algorithms. Additional assessment during stabilization may include continuous cardiac and respiratory monitoring, pulse oximetry, end-tidal CO_2 monitoring, ABGs, chest radiography, invasive arterial blood pressure monitoring, indwelling urinary catheter, measurement of central venous pressure, and possibly echocardiography.

History

Shock can be classified into the following categories:

- **Hypovolemic** shock: Loss of intravascular volume
- **Cardiogenic** shock: Impaired cardiac output from cardiac and extracardiac causes
- **Distributive** shock: Inappropriate vasodilation and maldistribution of blood flow with low SVR, most commonly septic in nature

Important elements to elicit in the initial history include the presence of fever (suggesting infection, heat-related illness, or toxic ingestion); illness with fluid loss through emesis, diarrhea, sweat, or urine; trauma; and/or underlying cardiac disease and/or immunodeficiency. In all causes of shock, urine production is decreased.

Hypovolemic Shock

- Gastrointestinal illness is the most common cause of hypovolemia in children with excessive losses through diarrhea, emesis, and intraluminal extravasation of fluid.
- Trauma can lead to internal hemorrhage (often into the chest, abdomen, and thigh) or external hemorrhage.[2]
- Burns can cause voluminous loss of fluid and protein.[3]
- Anaphylaxis (after exposure to a known or suspected allergen) can lead to leaky vasculature, considerable "third-spacing" (movement of fluid into an interstitial space outside the vascular system), and resultant hypovolemia.
- Toxins such as iron, heavy metals, certain envenomations, and colchicine can cause hemorrhage or third-spacing.

Cardiogenic Shock

- Cardiac causes (with key historical features)
  - Ductal-dependent congenital heart disease (neonate with sudden deterioration)
  - Myocarditis or cardiomyopathy (increasing symptoms of congestive heart failure, chest pain, and/or fever)
  - Endocarditis with acute valvular dysfunction (fever, rigors, symptoms of congestive heart failure, chest pain, prior history of cardiac problem)
  - Arrhythmia
  - Supraventricular tachycardia (SVT) (sudden change in appearance, respiratory difficulty, altered mental status, syncope, chest pain, palpitations)
  - Ventricular tachycardia (VT) (sudden change in appearance, syncope, sudden death, palpitations, chest pain, history of trauma [as in commotio cordis], ingestion, existing structural cardiac disease or prolonged QT syndrome)
  - Bradycardia (syncope, weakness, orthostasis)
- Extracardiac causes (with key historical features)
  - Pericardial tamponade (trauma, infection, postinfection, rheumatologic)
  - Tension pneumothorax or hemothorax (trauma)
  - Pulmonary embolism (abrupt onset of chest pain, syncope, respiratory distress, leg swelling, history of hypercoagulability)
  - Dissection of the aorta (sudden, searing back pain, chest pain, sudden collapse)
  - Intrathoracic/mediastinal tumor (increasing shortness of breath, positional dyspnea, chronic cough, chest pain)

Distributive Shock

- The patient with sepsis syndrome[4] usually presents with a history of fever. Immunocompromised patients are especially vulnerable to sepsis. Septic shock can also have elements of hypovolemic and cardiogenic shock.
- Anaphylaxis, which might overlap with hypovolemic shock, can present with urticaria, vomiting, swelling, and respiratory difficulty. There is not always a clear allergen exposure.
- Spinal cord injury can be accompanied by neuronally mediated disruption in vascular tone.[5]

Physical Examination

The focus of the physical examination is to identify signs of cardiovascular compromise. Key elements are described as follows:

- General appearance can indicate whether a patient is in shock. Patients who are alert and interacting appropriately with the environment and who have normal color cannot have significant circulatory compromise. At the other extreme, patients with lethargy, altered consciousness, and evidence of poor perfusion based on color (cyanosis, pallor, mottling) might be in shock and in need of emergent intervention. Especially in pediatric patients, early shock can present with subtle signs of anxiety, mild respiratory distress, quietness, or lethargy. In the child who is not ill or toxic, further examination is necessary to determine if the patient is in the early stages of shock.
- After rapid assessment of the airway and breathing, **central pulses** (brachial or femoral in infant; carotid or femoral in child) must be palpated. The presence, quality, and rate of the central pulses provide valuable information before information is available from monitors. Perfusion can be further assessed by comparing central and peripheral pulses and assessing the skin for temperature, color, and capillary refill time. Fast, weak pulses with cool, acrocyanotic extremities imply a shock state. Fast, strong pulses with warm extremities can be seen in compensated forms of early distributive shock in the presence of low SVR.
- **Vital signs** must be interpreted with other clinical information. Patients with compromised but compensated circulation initially have tachycardia as the only clue to an early shock state. Patients with low blood pressure in addition to tachycardia have decompensated shock. Interpretation of heart rate is very age dependent and must be considered in the context of anxiety, pain, and temperature. Patients with tachycardia and evidence of poor perfusion must be treated aggressively for shock. Blood pressure is maintained in early shock and therefore is not a good indicator of circulatory status in children. Compensatory peripheral vasoconstriction (high SVR) can lead to narrow pulse pressures (especially with hypovolemic and cardiogenic shock), whereas pulse pressure is increased in early distributive shock. A low diastolic pressure in a seemingly well-perfused patient with tachycardia must be recognized as distributive shock. Pulsus paradoxus can be seen with pericardial tamponade. Patients in shock usually are tachypneic (effortless tachypnea) due to acidosis and compensatory hyperventilation. Such patients should not have increased work of breathing unless they have a primary pulmonary problem (such as pneumonia with sepsis) or a cardiogenic etiology for shock. Accurate SaO_2 might be difficult to obtain in states of poor perfusion; end-tidal CO_2 might reveal compensatory hyperventilation **or** the hypercarbia associated with decompensated shock.
- Physical examination of key systems in shock states might provide evidence of the etiology.

Pulmonary System

Auscultation of the chest is performed to assess for any adventitial noises. The lungs are usually clear despite the tachypnea, although diffuse rales or decreased breath sounds symmetrically can be seen with cardiogenic shock. Wheezing might suggest anaphylaxis. Absence of breath sounds in one hemithorax should raise concern for a pneumothorax or hemothorax. Examination of the chest wall should identify any signs of trauma.

Cardiac System

Auscultation of the heart might identify murmurs (outflow tract obstruction, such as coarctation of the aorta in a neonate), rubs (pericarditis), decreased heart sounds (pericardial effusion), or gallop (myocardial dysfunction, such as in myocarditis). JVD can be noted with congestive heart failure, pericardial tamponade, or tension pneumothorax. Diminished or absent femoral pulses in the presence of upper extremity pulses can be a sign of coarctation of the aorta in an ill neonate.

Neurologic System

Altered mental status can be secondary to poor cerebral perfusion and should be part of the early assessment. Primary neurologic conditions also associated with shock include meningitis with concomitant sepsis, certain intoxications/ingestions, metabolic disturbances with severe dehydration, and multiple trauma. Patients with hypotension, relative bradycardia, and absent deep tendon reflexes should be evaluated for spinal cord injury. This syndrome is more common with high spinal cord injuries.[6] A bulging fontanel can be seen with meningitis or intracranial hemorrhage.

Skin

Decreased perfusion as manifested by cool, pale, or cyanotic extremities is present in most shock states (except for early distributive shock). Decreased skin turgor can be seen with hypovolemia due to dehydration. Petechiae and purpura can be found with sepsis. Unexplained bruises might be seen with inflicted trauma, especially in the afebrile infant presenting in shock. Urticaria or angioedema might be noted in anaphylaxis.

Other Findings

Dry mucous membranes and sunken eyes can be seen with severe dehydration. Abdominal tenderness or distention can be seen with peritonitis or hemorrhage associated with trauma. An enlarged liver might be seen with congestive heart failure, and a massively enlarged spleen might be seen with splenic sequestration in patients with sickle cell anemia. In the trauma victim, a careful secondary survey should identify any penetrating injuries.

Management

Familiarity with the PALS algorithms is essential for managing patients with compensated or decompensated shock and cardiac arrest. Early recognition of shock and aggressive treatment result in improved prognosis. Patients with shock must receive careful attention first to airway and breathing. Even if there is not immediate evidence of respiratory failure requiring emergent positive-pressure ventilation, these patients should be frequently reassessed. Interventions to improve circulation are futile in the absence of proper oxygenation and ventilation. Positive-pressure ventilation can actually complicate shock by decreasing venous return to the heart (preload). This should be anticipated when a patient in early compromised shock is intubated.

Interventions to Support and Evaluate Circulation

Oxygen

- All patients with circulatory compromise should receive supplemental oxygen regardless of the etiology. A normal assessment of airway and breathing along with a normal Sa_{O_2} does not obviate the need for supplemental oxygen.
- For patients who have severe, refractory hemodynamic instability, endotracheal intubation should be considered to protect the airway, maximize oxygen delivery, and decrease metabolic demands.

Fluid Resuscitation

- Patients with compromised circulation need appropriate intravenous access and aggressive fluid resuscitation.[7] Cardiogenic shock due to myocardial dysfunction is the only relative contraindication to fluid administration. Given the rarity of this etiology, rapid fluid administration should not be withheld.
- Initial fluid administration should be with isotonic normal saline or lactated Ringer solution; initial boluses should be 20 mL/kg with reassessment between boluses. Improvement, even if transient, is helpful in determining the course of therapy. For patients with tachycardia and adequate blood pressure but poor perfusion, normalization of heart rate and improved perfusion are indicators of success. Patients with hypotension can be more refractory to early interventions.
- Initial fluid resuscitation might require up to 80 mL/kg of crystalloid. In cases where there is no improvement of perfusion or vital signs after 40 mL/kg, additional therapy should be considered. Infusions of vasoconstrictor and inotropic medications should be prepared to treat distributive shock.[8] Inotropes are needed for some forms of cardiogenic shock.
- Prostaglandin E_1 should be considered for cardiogenic shock in neonates to maintain the patent ductus arteriosus.
- Blood products should be considered for patients with hemorrhagic shock unresponsive to 40 to

60 mL/kg of crystalloid boluses. Vasopressor agents have no role in early hemorrhagic shock.

- Measurement of urine output via an indwelling urinary catheter and central venous pressure monitoring can also be useful to judge effectiveness of volume resuscitation.

Chest Radiography

A chest radiograph can be helpful in managing shock. Small heart size might indicate relative hypovolemia. Large heart size can suggest congenital heart disease in the young infant or acquired heart disease (eg, myocarditis) in the older child. A large cardiac silhouette can also be seen with pericarditis or pericardial tamponade. Absence of pulmonary vasculature or prominent vasculature with fluid might help identify a cardiogenic etiology.

Specific Pediatric Resuscitation Algorithms[9]

Bradycardia (Figure 2, page 47)

If bradycardia is causing hemodynamic compromise, oxygen should be provided with assessment of the airway and breathing. For infants and young children with persistent bradycardia despite management of the airway, chest compressions should be considered if the heart rate is less than 60 beats per minute and the patient has poor perfusion. Epinephrine and atropine should be considered. Cardiac pacing (transcutaneous or transvenous) can be considered. Specific etiologies should be considered: hypoxemia, hypothermia, head injury, heart block, toxins, or drugs.

Tachycardia With Adequate Perfusion (Figure 3, page 48)

Patients with tachycardia and normal perfusion should be assessed carefully because unexplained tachycardia can progress to shock. SVT and VT must be distinguished from sinus tachycardia. SVT might respond to vagal maneuvers or adenosine or require cardioversion at an initial dose of 0.5 to 1 J/kg (in the awake patient, administer sedation and analgesia unless contraindicated by hemodynamic status). VT with pulses might respond to amiodarone, procainamide, or lidocaine. Attempts at cardioversion might be necessary if there is no response to medications.

Tachycardia With Poor Perfusion (Figure 4, page 49)

Evaluation of the rhythm dictates treatment. Underlying causes—the **four Hs and four Ts** —should be considered: hypoxia, hypothermia, hypovolemia, and hyperkalemia/hypokalemia and tamponade, tension pneumothorax, toxins, and thromboembolism. For SVT or VT, immediate cardioversion should be performed.

Pulseless Arrest (Figure 1, page 46)

- Treatment again is guided by the rhythm. Patients with VF/VT require immediate defibrillation up to three times (2 J/kg, 2 to 4 J/kg, 4 J/kg) followed by epinephrine, repeat attempt at defibrillation, and subsequent attempts after successive medications (amiodarone, lidocaine, and magnesium). Careful reassessment should follow each intervention.
- Pulseless electrical activity and asystole should be treated with rapid volume resuscitation, epinephrine, and the identification and treatment of underlying causes (the four Hs and four Ts, as given earlier). Both require epinephrine every 3 to 5 minutes.

Medications

Adenosine

Adenosine is indicated for SVT with adequate perfusion and is administered in a dose of 0.1 mg/kg (maximum of 6 mg for initial dose) via rapid infusion, ideally in a proximal, large vein such as in the antecubital fossa. The repeat dose is 0.2 mg/kg (maximum, 12 mg).

Amiodarone

Amiodarone is indicated for VT with adequate perfusion and VT/VF with poor perfusion/absent pulses that is unresponsive to cardioversion/defibrillation. It is given as 5 mg/kg IV over 20 to 60 minutes (adequate/poor perfusion) or bolus IV/IO (pulseless).

Atropine

Atropine is indicated for bradycardia due to suspected increased vagal tone or primary atrioventricular block. It is dosed as 0.02 mg/kg IV (minimum, 0.1 mg).

Dopamine

Dopamine is indicated for hypotension; it is a weak inotrope. Infusion starts at 5 to 10 mcg/kg/min, and it is titrated up to 20 mcg/kg/min.

Dobutamine

Dobutamine is indicated for hypotension; it is a moderately strong inotrope. Infusion starts at 5 to 10 mcg/kg/min, and it is titrated up to 20 mcg/kg/min.

Epinephrine

Epinephrine is indicated for bradycardia, asystole, pulseless electrical activity, and pulseless VT/VF that is unresponsive to defibrillation. As a bolus, it is dosed at 0.01 mg/kg IV/IO (0.1 mL/kg of 1:10,000); 0.1 mg/kg ET (0.1 mL/kg of 1:1,000). For refractory hypotension, infusion of epinephrine starts at 0.1 to 1.0 mcg/kg/min. High-dose epinephrine (0.1 mL/kg of 1:1,000 IV/IO) is no longer recommended as a first-line agent in pediatric resuscitation. Its value remains in doubt.[10] The PALS protocol allows for consideration of high-dose epinephrine under special circumstances.[9]

Lidocaine

Lidocaine is indicated for ventricular arrhythmia. As a bolus, it is dosed at 1 mg/kg IV/IO/ET.

Magnesium

Magnesium is indicated for torsade de pointes or hypomagnesemia. As a bolus, it is dosed at 50 mg/kg IV/IO.

Procainamide

Procainamide is recommended for VT with a normal perfusion or refractory VT with poor perfusion. As a bolus, it is dosed at 15 mg/kg IV over 30 to 60 minutes.

Prostaglandin E_1

Prostaglandin E_1 can be used in ductal-dependent congenital heart disease to reopen a closing ductus. It can be infused at 0.05 mcg/kg/min with an increase to 0.2 mcg/kg/min over several minutes. Side effects include apnea, pulmonary congestion, and hypotension.

Central Venous Catheter Placement[11]

The indications for placement of a percutaneous central venous line are as follows:

- Lack of peripheral venous access during a resuscitation
- Tenuous peripheral access and administration of medications with serious consequences of extravasation (vasopressors, calcium)
- Need to measure central venous pressure
- Need for transcutaneous pacing

Common sites include femoral, subclavian, and internal jugular veins. The umbilical vein may be used in the immediate postnatal period.

The femoral site is the most commonly used in pediatric patients because of the readily identifiable landmarks and low complication rate. The femoral vein is easiest to access in the proximal medial thigh just distal to the inguinal ligament. The vein lies just medial and slightly posterior to the femoral artery. After a sterile preparation of the skin and stabilization of the leg in the frog-leg position (consider placing a towel roll under the ipsilateral buttock), a needle with an attached syringe should be used to enter the vessel (45 degrees to skin, aspirating while advancing). A guidewire can then be placed before removal of the needle (Seldinger technique) to facilitate passing the catheter into the vessel. Central lines require radiographic confirmation of position.

Potential complications of central line placement are numerous and include the following:

- Local hemorrhage and hematoma might occur. In the femoral area, compression controls bleeding, but this is more difficult in the subclavian or jugular area.
- Infection might occur, but the risk can be reduced by using sterile technique.
- False tracking of catheter into surrounding soft tissues can occur, with the risk of extravasation of infused fluid and medications.
- Line might be placed into an artery instead of a vein.
- The vessel can thrombose.
- Injury to adjacent nerve might occur during placement.
- There can be inadvertent penetration into the bladder, peritoneum, or rectum when using the femoral approach.

- Pneumothorax can occur with subclavian and internal jugular attempts.

Intraosseous Needle Placement[12]

The indications for intraosseous placement are either

- When immediate fluid administration and medications are critical in the moribund child while identifying other means of access or
- When vascular access is needed urgently and attempts at peripheral access have failed.

Intraosseous access should be replaced by more secure access after immediate stabilization.

The most common site for intraosseous placement is in the proximal medial tibia. After sterile preparation, the intraosseous needle is placed approximately 1 cm below and medial to the tibial tuberosity. A sudden decrease in resistance is usually felt after penetration of the cortex. After removal of the stylette, blood should be aspirated to confirm placement in the marrow. If no blood can be aspirated, infusion of fluid without evidence of extravasation can also confirm placement. The needle should be stabilized to avoid being dislodged. Secondary sites include the distal tibia and distal femur.

Potential complications of intraosseous placement include the following:

- Failure to place the needle into the marrow space with extravasation of fluids or medications, which can potentially lead to compartment syndrome
- Causing a fracture during placement, especially in young infants
- Injury to a nearby growth plate
- Infection

Pericardiocentesis[13]

The indication for pericardiocentesis is emergent drainage of pericardial fluid that is causing life-threatening cardiac tamponade.

Under sterile conditions, a needle (1 inch for an infant, 2 inches for a child, 3 inches for an adolescent) attached to a syringe is directed just to the left and inferior to the xiphoid process. The needle should enter the skin at approximately 45 degrees to the skin surface and aiming for the left acromion while aspirating for fluid. Echocardiography can be used to guide the needle.

Potential complications of pericardiocentesis include the following:

- Pneumothorax or hemothorax
- Injury to the coronary arteries
- Hemorrhage into the pericardium leading to worsened tamponade

References

1. Fitzmaurice L, Gerardi MJ. Cardiovascular system. In: Gausche-Hill M, Fuchs S, Yamamoto L, eds. *APLS: The Pediatric Emergency Medicine Resource.* 4th ed. Sudbury, Mass: American Academy of Pediatrics, American College of Emergency Physicians, Jones and Bartlett Publishing Co; 2004:137-140.
2. Gutierrez G, Reines HD, Wulf-Gutierrez ME. Clinical review: hemorrhagic shock. *Crit Care.* 2004;8:373-381.
3. Sheridan RL. Comprehensive treatment of burns. *Curr Probl Surg.* 2001;38:657-756.
4. Butt W. Pediatric critical care, septic shock. *Pediatr Clin North Am.* 2001;48:601-625.
5. Atkinson PP, Atkinson JL. Spinal shock. *Mayo Clin Proc.* 1996;71:384-389.
6. Bilello JF, Davis JW, Cunningham MA, et al. Cervical spinal cord injury and the need for cardiovascular intervention. *Arch Surg.* 2003;138:1127-1129.
7. Dellinger RP, Carlet JM, Masur H, et al. Surviving Sepsis Campaign guidelines for management of severe sepsis and septic shock. *Crit Care Med.* 2004;32:858-873.
8. Sessler CN, Perry JC, Varney KL. Management of severe sepsis and septic shock. *Curr Opin Crit Care.* 2004;10:354-363.
9. Rhythm disturbances. In: Hazinski MF, Zaritsky AL, Nadkarni VN, et al, eds. *PALS Provider Manual.* Dallas, Tex: American Heart Association, 2002:185-228.
10. Perondi MB, Reis AG, Paiva EF, et al. A comparison of high-dose and standard-dose epinephrine in children with cardiac arrest. *N Engl J Med.* 2004;350:1722-1730.
11. King BR, King C, Coates WC. Central venous catheter placement. In: Gausche-Hill M, Fuchs S, Yamamoto L, eds. *APLS: The Pediatric Emergency Medicine Resource.* 4th ed. Sudbury, Mass: American Academy of Pediatrics, American College of Emergency Physicians, Jones and Bartlett Publishing Co; 2004:730-735.
12. King BR, King C, Coates WC. Intraosseous needle placement. In: Gausche-Hill M, Fuchs S, Yamamoto L, eds. *APLS: The Pediatric Emergency Medicine Resource.* 4th ed. Sudbury, Mass: American Academy of Pediatrics, American College of Emergency Physicians, Jones and Bartlett Publishing Co; 2004:736-738.
13. King BR, King C, Coates WC. Pericardiocentesis. In: Gausche-Hill M, Fuchs S, Yamamoto L, eds. *APLS: The Pediatric Emergency Medicine Resource.* 4th ed. Sudbury, Mass: American Academy of Pediatrics, American College of Emergency Physicians, Jones and Bartlett Publishing Co; 2004:745-746.

Figure 1.
Pediatric Pulseless Arrest Algorithm. Reproduced with permission from: Hazinski MF, Zaritsky AL, Nadkarni VN, et al, eds. *PALS Provider Manual.* Dallas, Tex: American Heart Association; 2002:216. Copyright 2002, American Heart Association.

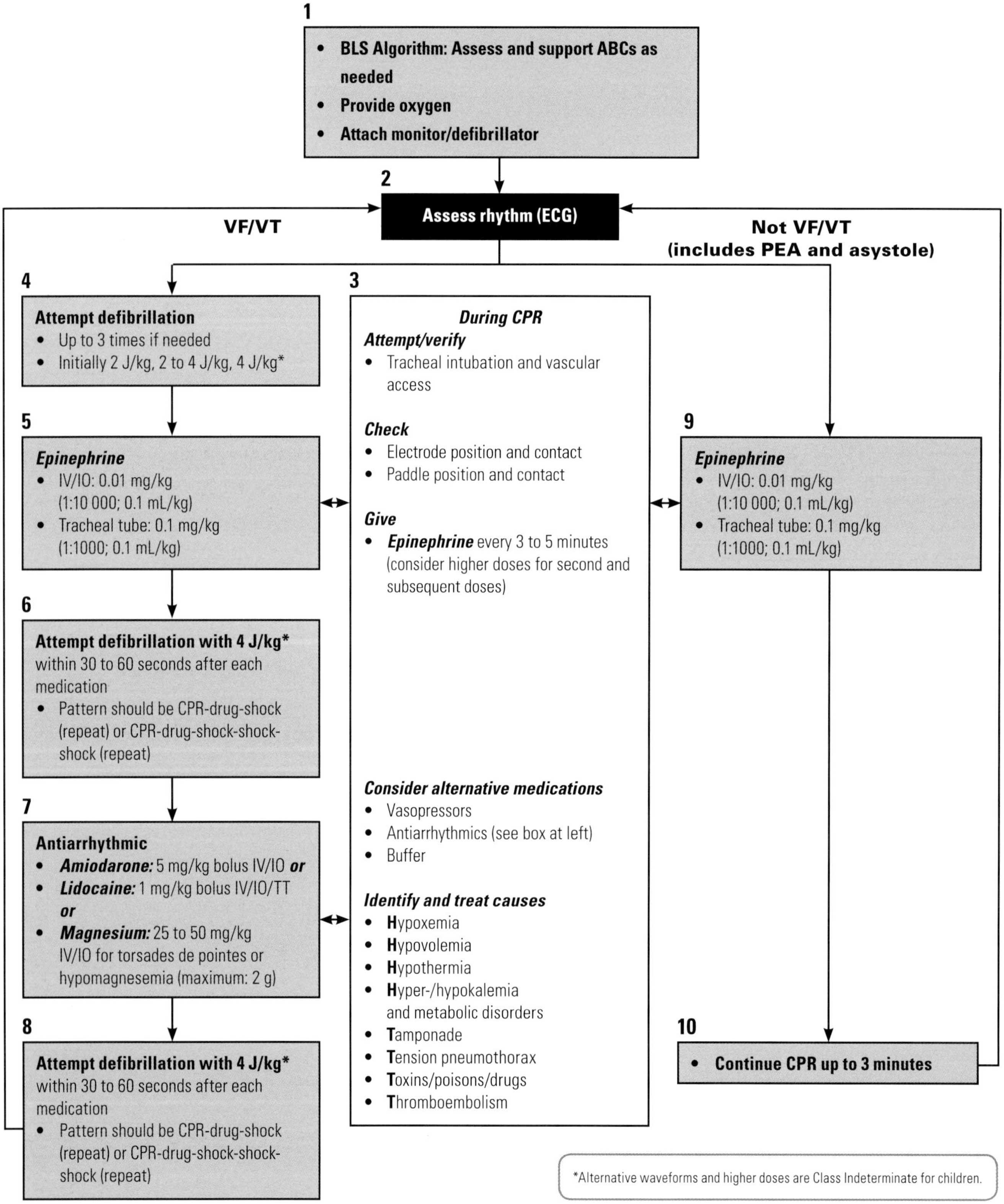

Figure 2.
Pediatric Bradycardia Algorithm. Reproduced with permission from: Hazinski MF, Zaritsky AL, Nadkarni VN, et al, eds. *PALS Provider Manual*. Dallas, Tex: American Heart Association; 2002:199. Copyright 2002, American Heart Association.

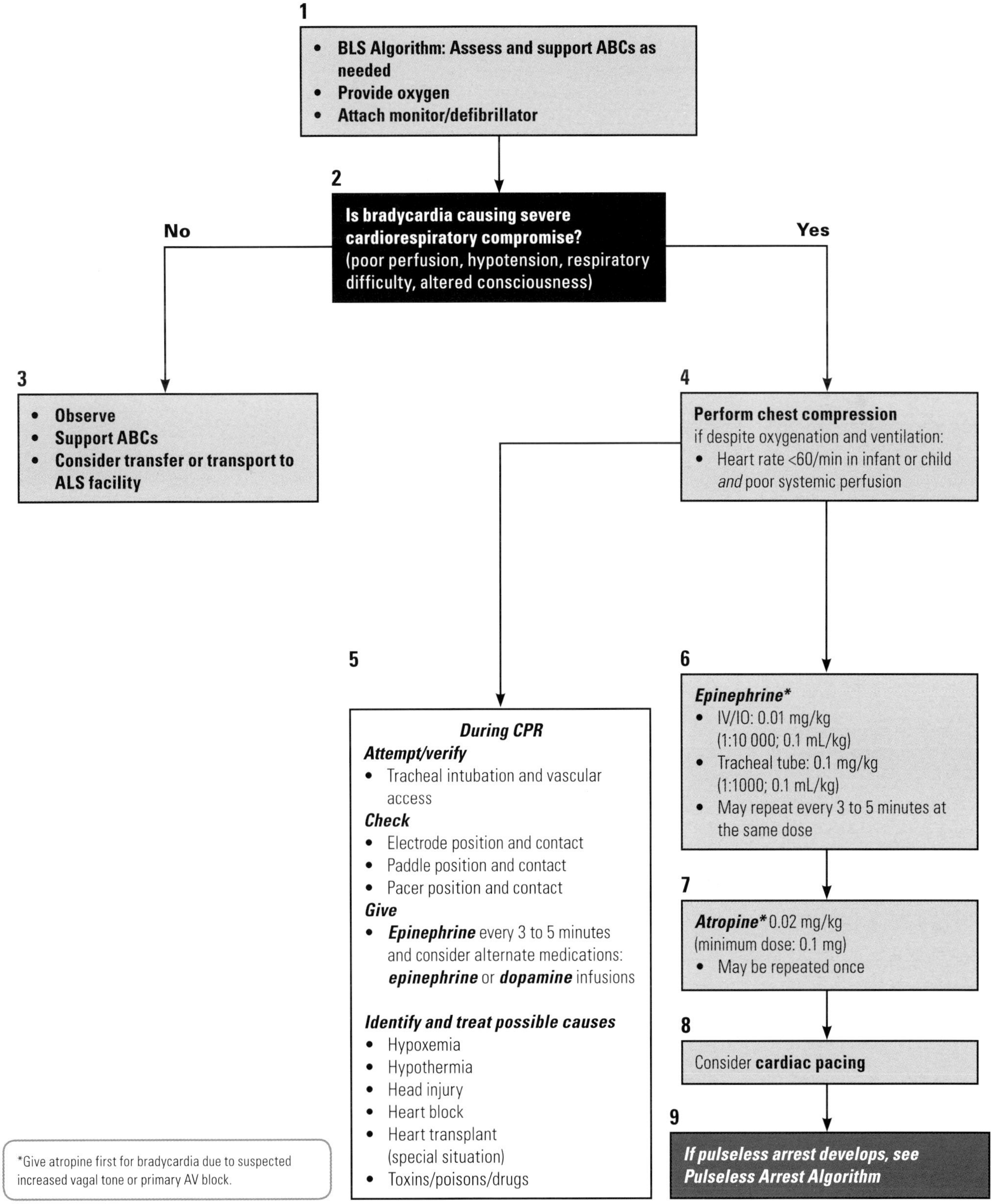

Figure 3.
Tachycardia With Adequate Perfusion. Reproduced with permission from: Hazinski MF, Zaritsky AL, Nadkarni VN, et al, eds. *PALS Provider Manual.* Dallas, Tex: American Heart Association; 2002:209. Copyright 2002, American Heart Association.

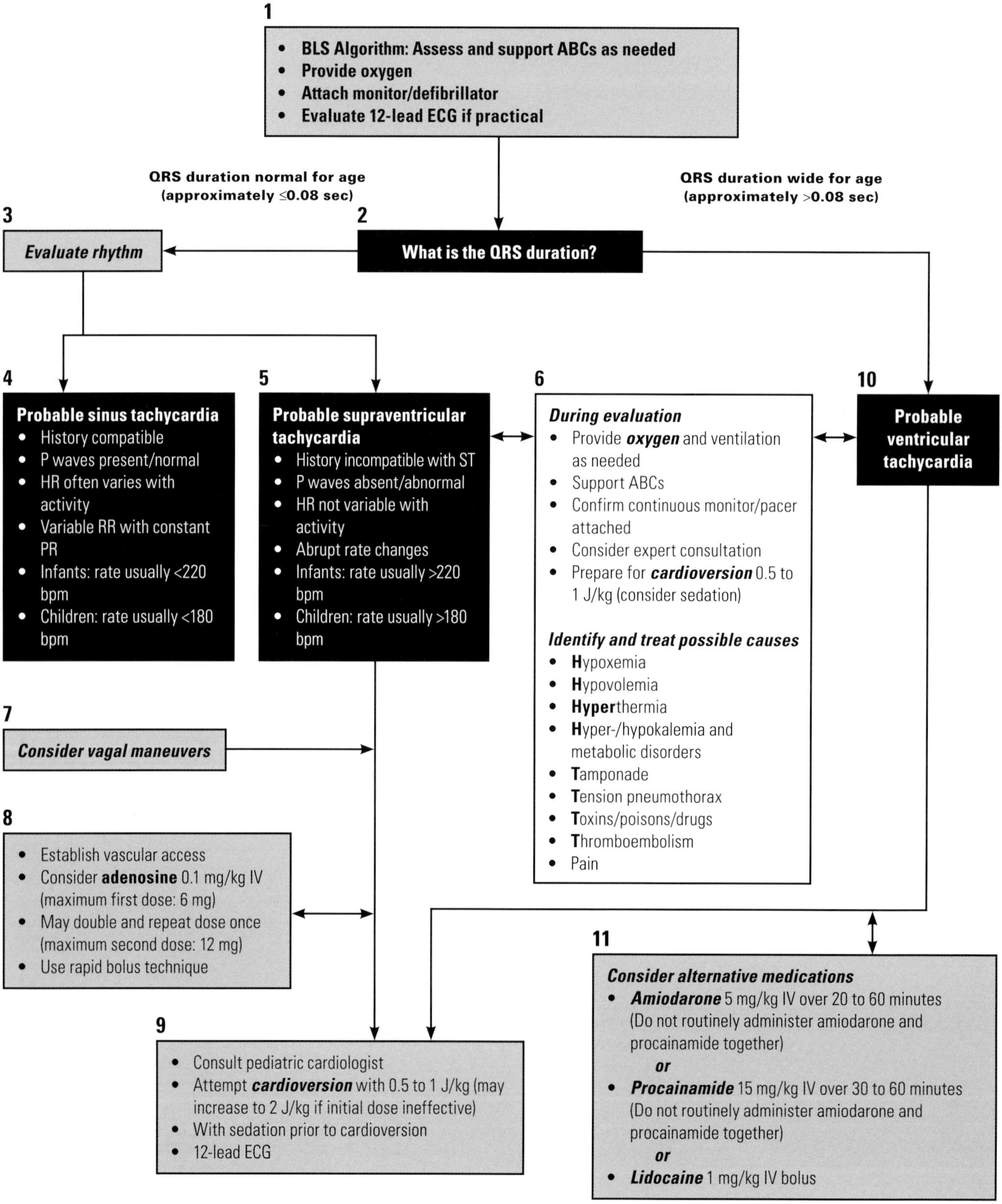

Figure 4.
Tachycardia With Poor Perfusion. Reproduced with permission from: Hazinski MF, Zaritsky AL, Nadkarni VN, et al, eds. *PALS Provider Manual.* Dallas, Tex: American Heart Association; 2002:207. Copyright 2002, American Heart Association.

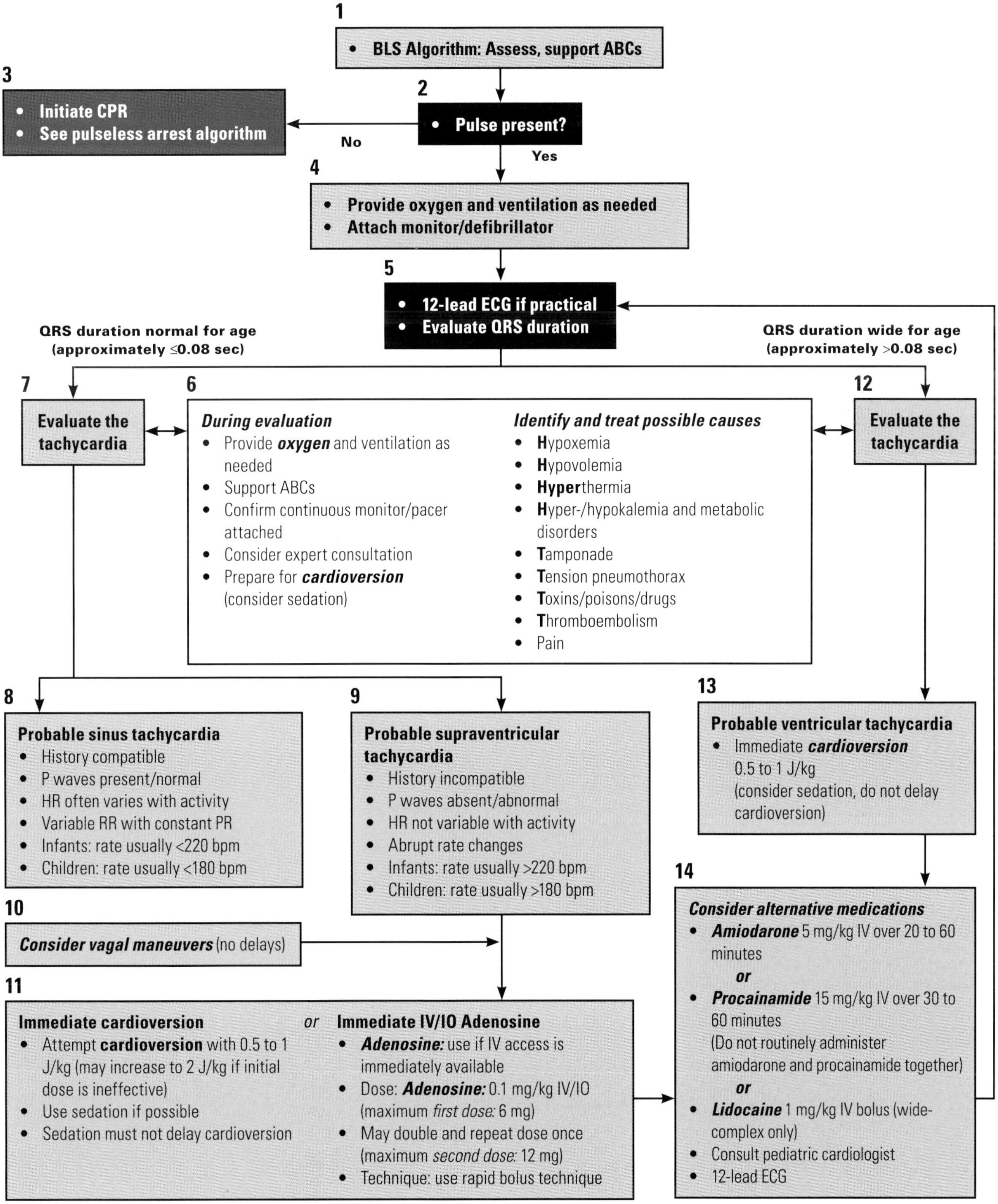

Evaluation and Management: Neurologic Emergencies

Genie E. Roosevelt, MD, MPH

Altered Mental Status

Altered mental status presents a difficult diagnostic and management challenge in pediatric emergency medicine. The differential diagnosis for a child with altered mental status includes a wide spectrum of disease processes with potential for significant morbidity and mortality. The health care provider must react quickly and systematically to the situation. As always, initial management of the ABCs of resuscitation is paramount.

Evaluation

The **history** should be directed to consider the common causes of altered mental status. The AEIOU TIPS mnemonic can be helpful[1]:

Alcohol, abuse; **E**lectrolytes (hypoglycemia, diabetic ketoacidosis, electrolyte abnormality), encephalopathy; **I**nfection (meningitis, encephalitis, abscess); **O**verdose, ingestion; **U**remia; **T**rauma (head injury, intracranial hemorrhage, nonaccidental trauma); **I**nsulin (hypoglycemia), intussusception, inborn errors of metabolism; **P**sychogenic (behavioral); **S**hock, stroke, seizure (postictal state), shunt.

The **physical examination** should proceed as follows:

- Attention to the ABCs
- Complete vital signs, including blood pressure
- General appearance—An objective assessment of the child's level of consciousness using the AVPU system[2] (Alert, responds to Voice, responds to Pain, Unresponsive) or the Glasgow Coma Scale score (see Appendix C).
- Respiratory pattern
  - Hyperventilation (anxiety, metabolic acidosis, midbrain or pons lesion)
  - Kussmaul respiration (deep breathing associated with metabolic acidosis; rate can be fast, normal, or slow)
  - Bradypnea (diabetic coma, drug-induced respiratory depression, increased intracranial pressure)
  - Cheyne-Stokes respiration (periods of deep breathing alternating with period of apnea; drug-induced respiratory depression, diffuse brain injury, metabolic encephalopathy)
- Head—Evidence of trauma, quality of anterior fontanel if age appropriate
- Eyes
  - Pupil size and responsiveness
  - Spontaneous eye movements
  - Ophthalmoscopic examination for papilledema or retinal hemorrhages
- Neck—Nuchal rigidity
- Skin—Evidence of trauma

Management and Interventions

- Secure airway (consider jaw thrust, airway adjuncts, suction secretions).
- Maintain in-line cervical spine control if trauma is a concern.
- Administer 100% oxygen via face mask.
- Assess ventilation and supplement as needed with BMV and intubation. Most anticonvulsants are respiratory suppressive, so the team must be prepared to manage the airway and breathing.
- Establish vascular access.
- Perform rapid bedside glucose determination.
- Monitor, including pulse oximetry.
- Consider empiric medications as follows:
  - **Dextrose 0.5 to 1 g/kg IV** delivered as **2 to 4 mL/kg $D_{25}W$**
  - **Thiamine 50 to 100 mg IV** in alcoholic and/or malnourished adolescents to prevent Wernicke encephalopathy; not required in infants and young children
  - **Naloxone 0.1 mg/kg** ≤20 kg, **2 mg** >20 kg **IV/IM/ET tube**, repeat every 2 to 3 minutes as needed or based on response for reversal of central nervous system (CNS) and respiratory depression associated with narcotic ingestion.
  - **Flumazenil 0.01 mg/kg** ≤20 kg, **0.2 mg** >20 kg **IV/IM**, repeat doses **0.01 mg/kg** up

to a maximum of **0.05 mg/kg** or consider **continuous infusion 0.005 to 0.01 mg/kg/hr** for reversal of CNS and respiratory depression associated with benzodiazepine ingestion: **contraindicated** in cyclic antidepressants and in patients with seizures treated with benzodiazepines

- Order laboratory workup for altered mental status of unclear etiology, as follows:
  - Complete blood cell count (CBC)
  - Electrolytes, including serum glucose, blood urea nitrogen (BUN), creatinine
  - Venous or arterial blood gas analysis
  - Toxicology screen, including acetaminophen, aspirin, and ethanol levels
- Order laboratory workup for suspected metabolic etiology, as follows:
  - Liver function testing, including ammonia
  - Measured and calculated serum osmolality
- Order computed tomography (CT) scan for focal neurologic abnormalities or signs of increased intracranial pressure once the patient is stabilized.
- Administer air contrast enema in a patient with signs of intussusception (vomiting, abdominal pain, blood in the stool).

Seizures

Seizures are a common presenting complaint in children coming to the emergency department. The approach varies depending on age, prior history of seizures or neurologic symptoms, and presence of an acute intercurrent illness. Febrile seizures, afebrile seizures, and status epilepticus are discussed separately because the approach to each is different.

Febrile Seizures

History

A simple febrile seizure is a nonfocal, generalized seizure lasting less than 15 minutes in a child between the ages of 6 months and 5 years who has a temperature greater than 38°C.[3] In addition, the seizure does not recur within 24 hours, and a subsequent neurologic examination shows no abnormalities. The prognosis after a simple febrile seizure is excellent. Febrile seizures in children that last longer than 15 minutes, have any focal component, or recur within 24 hours are termed **complex febrile seizures** and are associated with a higher risk of recurrent febrile seizures and epilepsy.[4] The history in a patient with a febrile seizure should be focused on the duration and nature of the seizure (focal versus generalized) and the child's behavior after the seizure.

Physical Examination

A careful physical examination looking for signs of infection is essential. The elements are as follows:

- Attention to the ABCs
- Complete vital signs, including blood pressure
- Head—Quality of anterior fontanel if age appropriate
- Neurologic examination—Level of consciousness, focal findings, pupillary response
- Neck—Nuchal rigidity

Management and Interventions

- Most children return to a normal level of consciousness within 1 hour after a febrile seizure. If the patient is nontoxic and hemodynamically stable, a period of observation without intervention is appropriate.
- Routine diagnostic evaluation of children presenting with simple febrile seizures is not indicated; the presence of a simple febrile seizure does not increase the likelihood of a serious bacterial infection such as bacteremia compared with children presenting with fevers without febrile seizures.[5]
- In patients who continue to have altered mental status or who have stiff neck or persistent lethargy, a lumbar puncture should be performed to rule out meningitis.
- An emergent or outpatient electroencephalogram is not indicated for a patient with a simple febrile seizure.
- Antibiotics are not indicated unless there is a specific bacterial infection to treat.
- Anticonvulsants do not have a role in the treatment of simple febrile seizures.[6]
- Around-the-clock antipyretics such as ibuprofen or acetaminophen have never been shown to

prevent the recurrence of febrile seizures.

- The recurrence rate of febrile seizures is approximately 33%. The four factors that predict recurrence are a positive family history of febrile seizures in a first-degree relative, young age (<18 months), shorter duration of fever before presentation (<1 hour), and lower temperature on presentation (<40°C).[7]

Afebrile Seizures

The patient must have two or more afebrile seizures before the diagnosis of epilepsy (seizure disorder) is made.[8]

History

Seizures can be confused with other conditions such as breath-holding spells, gastroesophageal reflux with apnea, vasovagal episodes, arrhythmias, and pseudo-seizures. Thirteen behavioral descriptors that have been found to discriminate between seizures and nonseizure events are not remembering what happened, moving mouth in a "funny" way, fidgeting in seat, drooling, jerking/twitching, becoming stiff, changes in breathing, staring off, biting or chewing tongue, eyes that look glassy, not responding, mumbling or slurring words, and turning eyes or head to one side.[9]

History-taking should be directed to elicit the following common causes of seizures:

- History of epilepsy
- Changes in medications—both anticonvulsants and other medications that can affect anticonvulsant levels
- Recent history of trauma
- Mental status change in the days preceding the seizure
- History of fever or symptoms of infectious disease
- History of ingestion
- Pertinent past medical history: hemoglobinopathies (eg, sickle cell disease, hemophilia), inflammatory conditions (eg, hemolytic uremic syndrome, systemic lupus erythematosus, other vasculitis), hypertension, renal disease, metabolic disease
- History of carbon monoxide exposure

Physical Examination

- Attention to the ABCs
- Complete vital signs, including blood pressure
- Head—Evidence of trauma, quality of anterior fontanel if age appropriate
- Neurologic examination—Level of consciousness, focal findings, pupillary response, ophthalmoscopic examination
- Neck—Nuchal rigidity

Management and Interventions

- Diagnostic evaluation is not routinely indicated in children older than 6 months unless dictated by a history of significant volume loss (vomiting and diarrhea) or ingestion; these studies have not been shown to be helpful.[8] Infants younger than 6 months are at increased risk for hypoglycemia, hyponatremia, and hypocalcemia, so laboratory evaluation is appropriate in this younger age group.
- A rapid bedside glucose determination might be helpful, especially in the context of ingestion of alcohol, ingestion of hypoglycemic agents, and insulin administration.
- Measuring anticonvulsant levels in patients with known epilepsy is helpful only to document toxicity or noncompliance; these levels will not be trough levels and will not be helpful in guiding the decision to change dosing regimens.
- A toxicology screen can be helpful if ingestion is in the differential. The mnemonic for toxin-induced seizures is OTIS CAMPBELL[10]: **O**rganophosphates; **T**ricyclic antidepressants; **I**soniazid, insulin; **S**ympathomimetics; **C**amphor, cocaine; **A**mphetamines; **M**ethylxanthines, such as theophylline and caffeine; **P**hencyclidine (PCP, propoxyphene, phenol, propranolol); **B**enzodiazepine withdrawal, botanicals; **E**thanol withdrawal; and **LL** (lithium, lidocaine, lindane, lead).
- Lumbar punctures are not helpful in patients with afebrile seizures without persistence of an abnormal neurologic examination.
- Electroencephalography is indicated on an outpatient basis. The electroencephalogram (EEG) should be performed at least 48 hours

after the event because initially the EEG will just show changes consistent with a postictal state. A normal EEG does not exclude the diagnosis of epilepsy.

- Routine neuroimaging is not indicated in a child presenting with a first-time afebrile seizure provided there is no suspicion of head trauma and the patient returns to baseline within several hours of the event.[8] Emergent neuroimaging (computed tomography [CT]) should be considered for children with a predisposing condition (hemoglobinopathies, malignancy, hydrocephalus, travel to an area endemic for cysticercosis) and in patients younger than 33 months with a focal seizure.[11] Nonurgent magnetic resonance imaging (MRI) should be considered in patients younger than 1 year, those with focal seizures, and those in whom an EEG is not consistent with a benign partial epilepsy or primary generalized epilepsy.[8]
- A first-time afebrile seizure does not warrant the initiation of anticonvulsant therapy.
- If the current afebrile seizure is a recurrence of a seizure disorder and the patient is not on anticonvulsant therapy, consultation with a pediatric neurologist should occur regarding the initiation of anticonvulsant therapy.
- If the child is on anticonvulsant therapy, consultation with the child's neurologist should occur to discuss changing the dosing regimen. Rectal **diazepam** (**5 mg PR** for children <3 years, **7.5 mg PR** for children ≥3 years every 12 hours for 4 doses) might be prescribed during an acute febrile illness to prevent breakthrough seizures.[12]
- See the next section on status epilepticus regarding the management of seizures persisting after arrival to the emergency department.

Status Epilepticus

Status epilepticus is defined by continuous or repetitive seizure activity of at least 30 minutes' duration. Because most self-limited seizures stop within 5 minutes and the attempts to control the seizure are more likely to be successful early in the seizure, any patient with seizure duration of longer than 10 minutes should have anticonvulsant therapy initiated.[13]

History

Approximately half of all patients presenting to the emergency department in status epilepticus are children. One third of these episodes of status epilepticus occur in children with established epilepsy; one third are the initial presentation of a seizure disorder, and one third occur as a result of an acute event.[14]

History-taking should be directed to elicit the following common causes of status epilepticus:

- History of epilepsy
- Changes in medications—Anticonvulsants, as well as the addition of other medications that can affect anticonvulsant levels
- Recent history of trauma
- Mental status change in the days preceding the seizure
- History of fever or symptoms of infectious diseases
- History of ingestion
- Pertinent past medical history: hemoglobinopathies (eg, sickle cell disease, hemophilia), inflammatory conditions (eg, hemolytic uremic syndrome, systemic lupus erythematosus, other vasculitis), hypertension, renal disease, metabolic disease
- History of carbon monoxide exposure

Physical Examination

- Attention to the ABCs
- Complete vital signs, including blood pressure
- Head—Evidence of trauma, quality of anterior fontanel if age appropriate
- Neurologic examination—Level of consciousness, focal findings, pupillary response, ophthalmoscopic examination
- Neck—Nuchal rigidity

Management and Interventions

- Evaluate the airway; consider jaw thrust and airway adjuncts, and suction secretions as needed.
- Maintain in-line cervical spine control if trauma is a concern.
- Administer 100% oxygen via face mask.

- Assess ventilation and supplement as needed with BMV and intubation. Most anticonvulsants are respiratory suppressive, so the team must be prepared to manage the airway and breathing.
- Establish vascular access.
- Perform rapid bedside glucose testing.
- Place patient on monitors, including pulse oximetry.
- Administer medications.[13]
  - **Dextrose 0.5 to 1 mg/kg (2 to 4 mL/kg of** D_{25}) for hypoglycemia
  - Benzodiazepines as first-line therapy

    Lorazepam 0.1 mg/kg IV, maximum dose **4 mg/dose**, may repeat once in 5 to 10 minutes

    Diazepam 0.1 to 0.3 mg/kg IV, maximum **10 mg/dose**, may repeat once in 5 minutes

    Diazepam 0.5 mg/kg PR, maximum **20 mg/dose** if vascular access is unavailable
  - Fosphenytoin as second-line therapy for children

    Fosphenytoin 20 mg PE/kg IV/IM, maximum rate of **3 mg PE/kg/min**, maximum **1,000 mg/dose**

    Fosphenytoin is preferred to phenytoin because fosphenytoin is less likely to cause cardiovascular side effects such as hypotension and arrhythmias that can occur with rapid infusion of phenytoin. Fosphenytoin may also be given intramuscularly and is compatible with all types of intravenous fluids.

    If fosphenytoin is not available, **phenytoin 20 mg/kg IV**, maximum rate of **1 mg/kg/min**, maximum **1,000 mg/dose** can be used.
  - Phenobarbital as second-line therapy for neonates

    Phenobarbital 20 mg/kg IV, rate of **1 mg/kg/min**; respiratory suppressive; be prepared to ventilate, especially when given in addition to benzodiazepines

    Repeat **phenobarbital 10 mg/kg IV** 10 minutes after first infusion if seizures persist.

Refractory seizures

- Consider **pyridoxine 100 mg IV** empirically for neonates with first-time seizure.
- Consider pyridoxine for isoniazid ingestion: **1 mg pyridoxine/1 mg of isoniazid ingested.**
- Perform RSI.
- Admit to ICU.
- Consider continuous electroencephalographic monitoring.
- Medication options (there is no consensus, and data are lacking):
  - **Midazolam continuous infusion 0.2 mg/kg IV load**, followed by **1 mcg/kg/min drip**, increase by **1 mcg/kg/min** every 15 minutes until burst suppression is achieved
  - **Pentobarbital continuous infusion 5 to 15 mg/kg IV load**, followed by **0.5 to 5 mg/kg/hr continuous infusion**

Increased Intracranial Pressure

Evaluation

History-taking should be directed to elicit the following common causes of ICP.

- Trauma (intracranial hemorrhage, diffuse injury)
- Infection (meningitis, encephalitis, cerebral abscess)
- Nontraumatic cerebral edema (diabetic ketoacidosis)
- Nontraumatic hemorrhage (ruptured aneurysm, arteriovenous malformation [AVM])
- Intracranial mass or tumor

Symptoms of increased ICP include the following:

- Vomiting
- Headache
- Irritability
- Altered level of consciousness
- Failure to thrive

Physical Examination

- Attention to the ABCs
- Complete vital signs, including blood pressure. Cushing triad (bradycardia, hypertension, and abnormal respiratory pattern) is a late finding

indicative of impending brainstem herniation or chronic increased ICP.

- Head—Evidence of trauma, bulging anterior fontanel in an infant, large head circumference
- Neurologic examination:
  - Level of consciousness
  - Pupillary response (dilation of pupils with sluggish or no response to light)
  - Ophthalmoscopic examination (papilledema)
  - Upward gaze paralysis ("setting sun" sign)
  - Cranial nerve deficits
  - Alterations in gait
  - Seizure
  - Abnormal posturing

Management and Interventions

The goal is to maintain cerebral perfusion pressure (CPP) while lowering ICP; CPP = MAP + ICP where MAP = mean arterial pressure and normal ICP <15 mm Hg.

- Secure airway via RSI.
- Maintain in-line cervical spine control if trauma is a concern.
- Administer 100% oxygen via ET tube.
- Support blood pressure with volume through isotonic crystalloid and blood products as needed.
- Specific interventions (recommendations based on consensus panel for pediatric head trauma; there are no data regarding other etiologies of pediatric increased ICP)[15]:
  - Hyperventilation to maintain P_{CO_2} at approximately 30 to 35 (do not aggressively hyperventilate except in cases of impending herniation; the literature from adult studies suggests that hyperventilation reduces CPP).
  - Sedation and analgesia are appropriate because pain and stress increase ICP. There are no specific recommendations on the drug choice and dosing; however, continuous **propofol** infusion should be avoided because it has been associated with increased mortality and morbidity (acidosis, rhabdomyolysis).[16,17]
  - Hyperosmolar therapy

    Mannitol 0.25 to 1 g/kg in intermittent boluses

    a. Place Foley catheter to monitor urine output.

    b. Maintain serum osmolarity below 320 mOsm/L.

    Consider **hypertonic saline (3% NaCl) 0.1 to 1 mL/kg/hr.**

    a. Minimal dose needed to keep ICP <20 mm Hg.

    b. Effective for control of increased ICP acutely, but long-term benefit on neurologic function is unclear[18]
  - No data exist to support the use of prophylactic barbiturates.
- No pediatric data exist to support therapeutic hypothermia for traumatic brain injury, and adult studies have yielded conflicting results.[15,19]
- No data exist to support the routine use of steroids.
- Prophylactic anticonvulsant therapy is not recommended to prevent late posttraumatic seizures in children. Anticonvulsant therapy to prevent the occurrence of early posttraumatic seizures in high-risk children during the first week following severe total brain injury is recommended as a treatment option.

References

1. Issacman DJ, Trainor JL, Rothrock SG. Central nervous system. In: Gausche-Hill M, Fuchs S, Yamamoto L, eds. *APLS: The Pediatric Emergency Medicine Resource.* 4th ed. Sudbury, Mass: American Academy of Pediatrics, American College of Emergency Physicians, Jones and Bartlett Publishing Co; 2004:146-185.
2. Zaritsky AL, Nadkarni VM, Hickey RW, et al, eds. *PALS Provider Manual.* Dallas, Tex: American Heart Association and American Academy of Pediatrics; 2002:261.
3. Provisional Committee on Quality Improvement, Subcommittee on Febrile Seizures. Practice parameter: the neurodiagnostic evaluation of the child with a first simple febrile seizure. *Pediatrics.* 1996;97:769-772.
4. Technical report summary: the neurodiagnostic evaluation of the child with a first simple febrile seizure. American Academy of Pediatrics. Provisional Committee on Quality Improvement, Subcommittee on Febrile Seizures. *Pediatrics.* 1996;97:773-775.
5. Trainor JL, Hampers LC, Krug SE, et al. Children presenting with first-time febrile seizures are at low risk of serious bacterial illness. *Acad Emerg Med.* 2001;8:781-787.
6. Practice parameter: long-term treatment of the child with simple febrile seizures. American Academy of Pediatrics. Committee on Quality Improvement, Subcommittee on Febrile Seizures. *Pediatrics.* 1999;103:1307-1309.
7. Berg AT, Shinnar S, Darefsky AS, et al. Predictors of recurrent febrile seizures. A prospective cohort study. *Arch Pediatr Adolesc Med.* 1997;151:371-378.
8. Hirtz D, Ashwal S, Berg A, et al. Practice parameter: evaluating a first nonfebrile seizure in children. *Neurology.* 2000;55:616-623.

9. Williams J, Grant M, Jackson M, et al. Behavioral descriptors that differentiate between seizure and nonseizure events in a pediatric population. *Clin Pediatr.* 1996;35:243-249.

10. Erickson TB, Aks SE, Gussow L, et al. Toxicology update: a rational approach to managing a poisoned patient. *Emerg Med Pract.* 2001;3(8):1-28.

11. Sharma S, Riviello JJ, Harper MB, et al. The role of emergent neuroimaging in children with new-onset afebrile seizures. *Pediatrics.* 2003;111:1-5.

12. Knudsen FU. Recurrence risk after first febrile seizure and effect of short-term diazepam prophylaxis. *Arch Dis Child.* 1985;60:1045-1049.

13. Hanhan UA, Fiallos MR, Orlowski JP. Status epilepticus. *Pediatr Clin North Am.* 2001;48:683-694.

14. Pellock JM. Status epilepticus in children: update and review. *J Child Neurol.* 1994;9(suppl):2S27-2S35.

15. Society of Critical Care Medicine. Guidelines for the acute medical management of severe traumatic brain injury in infants, children, and adolescents. *Crit Care Med.* 2003;31(6 suppl):S407-S491.

16. Hanna JP, Ramundo ML. Rhabdomyolysis and hypoxia associated with prolonged propofol infusion in children. *Neurology.* 1998;50:301-303.

17. Cray SH, Robinson BH, Cox PN. Lactic acidemia and bradyarrhythmia in a child sedated with propofol. *Crit Care Med.* 1998;26:2087-2092.

18. Cooper DJ, Myles DS, McDermott FT, et al. Prehospital hypertonic saline resuscitation of patients with hypotension and severe traumatic brain injury. *JAMA.* 2004;291:1350-1357.

19. Clifton GL, Miller ER, Sung CC, et al. Lack of effect of induction of hypothermia after acute brain injury. *N Engl J Med.* 2001;344:556-563.

Evaluation and Management: Trauma and Environmental Emergencies

Carl Shaw, MD, and F. Keith Battan, MD

Trauma Emergencies

The previous evaluation and management sections address the primary considerations of airway, breathing, circulation, and disability (neurologic emergencies). The goal of this section is to revisit these fundamental steps in pediatric resuscitation with an emphasis on priorities specific to the care of the trauma patient.

Evaluation of the Pediatric Trauma Patient

Emergent

Identify and treat life-threatening conditions while further information is obtained. Address the following sequentially.

- **Airway**—Look, listen, feel, and assess. Assess the patient's ability to speak or cry. Open the airway (jaw thrust as needed); position, suction, and protect the cervical spine with in-line immobilization.
- **Breathing**—Determine if the patient is moving sufficient air for adequate oxygenation and ventilation. Use the pulse oximeter. Look for evidence of pneumothorax or hemothorax (unilateral diminished breath sounds, deviation of trachea, hyperresonance to percussion) requiring an immediate intervention.
- **Circulation**—Identify active bleeding that requires direct pressure. Establish intravenous access and draw blood for initial laboratory tests. Evaluate for signs of shock and, if present, begin fluid resuscitation with 20 mL/kg isotonic crystalloid.
- **Disability**—Determine level of consciousness and evaluate pupillary response to see if there is evidence of increased ICP or herniation (Cushing triad) that may require immediate intervention.

History

In trauma patients, the mechanism of injury can be predictive of patterns of injury. This information can be helpful in directing evaluation, particularly in patients who are too young or too injured to communicate with care providers. Although mechanism is a poor predictor of severity of injury,[1] certain events can coincide with more severe injuries. Vehicle rollovers, ejection from a vehicle, fatalities in the same vehicle, and falls from heights of two stories or higher often correlate with more severe injuries. Other information that can be particularly helpful in directing further care is the child's appearance at the scene, how much time has passed since the event, and what interventions have been performed up to this point. A helpful mnemonic for taking a focused history is SAMPLE: **S**igns and symptoms, **A**llergies, **M**edications, **P**ast illnesses, **L**ast meal, **E**vents preceding the injury.[2,3]

Physical Examination

Complete the full primary survey.

- **Airway**—Evaluate the patient for ability to speak and evidence of tracheal air exchange or tracheal deviation. Examine for evidence of damage to the upper airway, midface, jaw, or soft tissues of the neck.
- **Breathing**—Note the patient's respiratory rate and work of breathing. Evaluate chest excursion and breath sounds for symmetry. Asymmetric findings in a trauma patient raise concerns for pulmonary contusion, pneumothorax, hemothorax, or tension pneumothorax. Evaluate further for evidence of a flail segment.
- **Circulation**—Perfusion may be evaluated by assessing pulses, capillary refill, and skin temperature. Note the skin color and mental status. (Mental status as an indicator of cerebral perfusion, and thus of circulation, will be difficult to interpret in a patient with a closed head injury as a primary cause of altered mental status.)
- **Disability**—Initial neurologic examination should include pupillary reflexes and mental status. The AVPU scale (**A**lert, responsive to

Verbal or Painful stimulus, or Unresponsive) or Glasgow Coma Scale (see Appendix C) is helpful in the initial rapid assessment.[4,5]

- **Exposure**—Remove the patient's clothing, cutting it as necessary, for a thorough examination.
- **Environment**—Check the patient's temperature, and warm or cool the patient as appropriate.

Follow with a complete head-to-toe secondary survey, and place monitors, lines, and tubes as appropriate. Frequent reassessment of vital signs and the primary survey is essential until the patient is stable.

Management

Resuscitation

- Administer 100% oxygen, applied initially via nonrebreather mask. Provide BMV as needed; apply cricoid pressure with positive-pressure ventilation.
- Monitoring—Cardiorespiratory monitor, pulse oximeter, blood pressure, and temperature probe
- Suction—Clear airway of secretions, vomitus, loose teeth, and foreign bodies.
- Control external hemorrhage with direct pressure.
- Establish intravenous access (intraosseous, cutdown, or central venous access if peripheral intravenous access is not available). Initial laboratory tests to be considered include hematocrit, blood gases, urinalysis, amylase, liver function tests, blood type and cross-match, and coagulation studies, especially if head injury is suspected.
- Fluid resuscitation: isotonic crystalloid **20 mL/kg IV/IO** if the circulation is compromised.
- Check pupils and mental status—If there is evidence of increased ICP or herniation, perform RSI.
- Initial portable radiographs as indicated—Lateral cervical spine, chest, and anteroposterior pelvis.[5]
- Remove patient's clothing and assess for other injuries.
- Obtain further history, repeat primary survey, and reassess.
- Institute passive rewarming measures to prevent hypothermia.
- Determine need for further imaging of head, abdomen, or other sites of potential injuries.

Airway Management in the Trauma Patient

Although the details of airway management have been discussed previously (see "Evaluation & Management: Airway"), there are several concerns that are specific to an injured child.

- Until a cervical spine injury has been ruled out, maintain immobilization of the entire spine during all airway maneuvers.[3,5,6] Cervical spine immobilization is immediately secured by manual in-line stabilization. It is particularly important that a provider be continually dedicated to this task during airway manipulation. **A cervical collar alone does not provide adequate immobilization during resuscitation.**
- Relieve anatomic obstruction (hypopharyngeal tissue block) by opening the airway:
  - Keep the head in midline position.
  - A **jaw thrust is the method of choice** for opening the airway in a trauma patient while maintaining in-line cervical spine positioning.
  - **Head tilt and chin lift are contraindicated in trauma patients with potential cervical spine injuries.**
- Vomiting can jeopardize the airway of a patient in cervical spine immobilization. Vomiting should be managed by log-rolling the patient on the spine board to protect the cervical spine while suctioning to clear the airway.
- Airway adjuncts—Oropharyngeal and nasopharyngeal airways have limited use in the trauma patient, because those with significant airway compromise will typically require a more definitive airway in the form of an ET tube. Airway compromise is rarely due to blockage of the upper nasopharynx in an injured child, except in newborns, and thus the patient will not usually benefit from a nasopharyngeal airway. Nasopharyngeal airways are contraindicated in cases of midface trauma.
- Intubation

Indications for intubation[3]:

- Inadequate ventilation with BMV
- Airway protection required as a result of injury to the head or neck, or waning mental status typically with a Glasgow Coma Scale score of 8 or less.
- Control of ventilation required due to increased ICP.
- Flail chest resulting in inability of chest to generate negative inspiratory pressure and proper air exchange
- Shock unresponsive to volume resuscitation

Assembly of necessary equipment and preparation of the patient are essential. Preoxygenation and adequate suction are important as well. Patients requiring BMV for preoxygenation should receive cricoid pressure. Consider **lidocaine 1 mg/kg IV** in patients who might have increased ICP.[7] Sedative selection in the trauma patient is guided by the patient's injuries. **Etomidate 0.3 mg/kg IV** is a good choice because it has a rapid onset of action, decreases ICP, and has relatively few effects on blood pressure. **Succinylcholine 1 mg/kg IV** is commonly used for muscle relaxation in trauma. **Rocuronium 0.6 to 1 mg/kg IV** is a rapid-acting, nondepolarizing paralytic that has several advantages over succinylcholine. It does not increase intracranial, intraocular, or intragastric pressure and does not contribute to hyperkalemia in patients with large burns or significant crush injuries.

- Airway obstruction—In the event of airway obstruction that cannot be resolved, whether due to trauma or immovable foreign body, available rescue techniques are needle cricothyrotomy in the patient younger than 12 years and surgical cricothyroidotomy in the older patient (see "Evaluation and Management: Airway").

Breathing Management in the Trauma Patient

The trauma patient's ability to breathe can be diminished by alterations of mental status or direct injury to the chest. Consider pneumothorax, hemothorax, and pulmonary contusions.

- **High-flow 100% oxygen via nonrebreather face mask.** High-flow oxygen via face mask rapidly increases PaO_2 and is mandatory in seriously injured children.
- **Positive-pressure ventilation.** BMV is a temporizing measure in trauma patients. Trauma patients who require more than transient positive-pressure ventilation require intubation.[3]
- **Thoracentesis/tube thoracostomy.** Immediate needle thoracentesis is indicated before a chest radiograph is obtained in patients with clinical evidence of tension pneumothorax. This should then be followed by tube thoracostomy, also indicated in patients with hemothorax or pneumothorax leading to respiratory compromise. See "Evaluation and Management: Breathing" for a description of how to perform these two procedures.

Circulation Management in the Trauma Patient

- **Control external hemorrhage.** A complete physical examination is essential to detect all sites of significant bleeding. Apply direct pressure and elevate the site of bleeding when possible. Clamping of hemorrhaging vessels should not be done in any areas other than the scalp because of the risk of damaging adjacent nerves. Although cessation of external hemorrhage is essential, it should not distract providers from ongoing resuscitation.
- **Achieve vascular access.** Ensure that adequate intravenous access is present. Two peripheral intravenous lines, large bore relative to the size of the patient, should be obtained whenever possible. If peripheral access cannot be obtained quickly, proceed immediately to intraosseous, cutdown, or central access. An intraosseous line is useful for the delivery of crystalloid, colloid, and drugs. Intraosseous lines are contraindicated in a fractured extremity, because intravenous fluid will extravasate from the fracture site.
- **Supply appropriate volume resuscitation.** Begin volume resuscitation with 20 mL/kg of isotonic crystalloid such as normal saline or lactated Ringer solution. Treat decompensated hypovolemic shock with rapid intravenous infusions. If shock persists after the administration of 40 mL/kg of isotonic crystalloid, consider giving colloid. O-negative blood may be given in emergent conditions

before the availability of type-specific, cross-matched blood.

- **Identify sites of internal hemorrhage.** Identification of significant internal hemorrhage requires ongoing observation of changes in the patient's clinical status and physical examination findings. Five areas of the body that can contain life-threatening internal hemorrhage are the chest, abdomen, retroperitoneum, pelvis, and thigh. Usually, it is only in infants with nonfused sutures that intracranial bleeding can lead to compromised perfusion.

Disability (Neurologic) Management in the Trauma Patient

- **Head injury.** Children with evidence of head injury should have a CT scan of the head to look for evidence of intracranial pathology. Neurologic status is the most important indicator of a multiply injured child's return to function. The goal in management of the head-injured patient is to preserve cerebral perfusion and oxygen delivery. Support mean arterial pressure with volume to maintain cerebral perfusion. Prevent excessive elevation of ICP. Those with evidence of impending herniation should be treated with hyperventilation (target P_{CO_2} <30), elevation of the head of the bed 30°, and mannitol.[7] See "Evaluation and Management: Neurologic Emergencies." Patients with traumatic brain injury but no signs of herniation can be mildly hyperventilated (target P_{CO_2} ≥35) to decrease ICP while preventing extreme vasoconstriction.[7] Other potential treatment modalities for increased ICP due to traumatic brain injury include hyperosmolar therapy with 3% saline and hypothermia. Evidence for these interventions remains mixed, and further studies are required—particularly in children.[8,9]
- **Spinal Cord Injury.** Evidence of spinal cord injury is demonstrated by numbness, weakness, or paresthesias and requires that the utmost care be taken to maintain spinal cord immobilization. Initial imaging of the spine is by plain radiographs. When a fracture is seen or suspected, CT will provide more detailed information. MRI also allows visualization of hematomas or soft tissue impingement on the spinal cord. In patients with evidence of spinal cord injury, consider **methylprednisolone**, which is best administered within 8 hours after the injury.[10] For a more in-depth discussion of spinal cord injuries, see "Scenario #39, Trauma."

Exposure in the Trauma Patient

As has been mentioned, it is essential that clothing be removed to allow a complete primary and secondary survey. Also, wet garments should be removed to facilitate preservation of core temperature. Passive rewarming (warm blankets, radiant warmers, air convection units) is helpful as soon as the patient's clinical condition and the priorities of resuscitation permit. Hypothermic patients will not respond normally to resuscitative efforts. Avoidance of hypothermia in trauma patients is recommended.[11] Efforts to maintain core body temperature are particularly important in smaller children, who have a high surface area–to–body weight ratio and therefore can become hypothermic very quickly.

Environmental Emergencies

Environmental emergencies range from extremes of temperature, to exposures such as smoke inhalation, submersion, and electrical injuries, to envenomations.

The fundamental principles in the approach to the critically ill patient with an environmental emergency remain constant. Once it is safe to do so, the aim of prehospital providers is to rapidly transport the patient to definitive medical care, while providing accurate assessment and management of the ABCs.[12] Failure to reverse hypoxia, hypercarbia, and hypoperfusion from the outset can allow the patient to progress to a level of irreparable injury. Although the principles of resuscitation remain constant across this wide range of exposures, the details of management can vary considerably. This section briefly summarizes some early management priorities of common environmental emergencies.

Management

Submersion

- **Airway, Breathing**—Apply oxygen, monitor for respiratory distress, and obtain blood gases and chest radiographs, especially if evidence of aspiration or pulmonary compromise exists, which can take hours to develop.

- **Circulation**—Volume resuscitation as indicated
- **Disability**—Perform serial examinations, rule out cervical spine injuries, and consider toxic ingestion or alcohol intoxication.
- **Exposure**—Remove wet clothes and rewarm. Look for evidence of associated trauma. See "Scenario #42, Environmental Emergencies."

Hypothermia

- **Airway, Breathing**—Provide support as needed.
- **Circulation**—Fluid resuscitation will likely be required to prevent cardiovascular collapse as patient rewarms. Low core temperatures (<30°C) result in a myocardium that is resistant to defibrillation. For patients who present with ventricular fibrillation or ventricular tachycardia without a pulse, if initial defibrillation is unsuccessful, continue CPR until core temperature is above 30°C.
- **Disability, Exposure**—Remove all clothing and institute rewarming measures. Passive measures are adequate for core temperatures from 32° to 35°C. At temperatures less than 32°C, more aggressive core rewarming (eg, extracorporeal) is required. See "Scenario #42, Environmental Emergencies."

Smoke Inhalation and Burns

- **Airway**—Intubate to secure airway before the development of airway edema if there is evidence of heat injury to the airway (singed facial or nose hair, carbonaceous sputum, airway edema on direct laryngoscopy).
- **Breathing**—Administer 100% oxygen and check carbon monoxide level.
- **Circulation**—Provide volume resuscitation for significant burns and resultant poor perfusion due to capillary leak.
- **Disability, Exposure**—Expose completely to look for other burns. See "Scenario #41, Environmental Emergencies."

Heat Stroke

- **Airway, Breathing**—Provide support as indicated in severe cases.
- **Circulation**—Shock may result from dehydration or vasodilation. Treat shock with isotonic crystalloid and vasopressors as needed.
- **Disability**—Check for hypoglycemia and if present treat with dextrose; treat seizures with benzodiazepines.
- **Exposure**—Remove clothing to facilitate prompt cooling, most effectively with sprayed water and fans. Check electrolytes and renal function. Check urinalysis for evidence of rhabdomyolysis. See "Scenario #43, Environmental Emergencies."

Electrocution/Lightning Strike

Separate victim from the source of current in a safe manner.

- **Airway**—Examine airway for evidence of burn injury; intubate if there is evidence of burn injury or airway is believed to be not maintainable. Immobilize cervical spine if patient was thrown by the current.
- **Breathing**—Administer oxygen and assist breathing with BMV if respiratory effort is depressed or oxygenation/ventilation is compromised.
- **Circulation**—Confirm presence of a perfusing rhythm.
- **Disability**—Evaluate mental status.
- **Exposure**—Examine extremities for fractures and burns. See "Scenario #44, Environmental Emergencies."

References

1. Dowd MD, McAneney C, Lacher M, et al. Maximizing the sensitivity and specificity of pediatric trauma team activation criteria. *Acad Emerg Med.* 2000;7:1119-1125.
2. Extremes of age. In: *American College of Surgeons Committee on Trauma. Advanced Trauma Life Support for Doctors. Student Course Manual.* 7th ed. Chicago, Ill: American College of Surgeons; 2004:243-246.
3. Tepas JT, Fallat ME, Moriarty TM. Trauma. In: Gausche-Hill M, Fuchs S, Yamamoto L, eds. *APLS: The Pediatric Emergency Medicine Resource.* 4th ed. Sudbury, Mass: American Academy of Pediatrics, American College of Emergency Physicians, Jones and Bartlett Publishing Co; 2004:269-323.
4. Recognition of respiratory failure and shock. In: Zaritsky AL, Nadkarni VM, Hickey RW, et al, eds. *PALS Provider Manual.* Dallas, Tex: American Heart Association and American Academy of Pediatrics; 2002:36.
5. Ziegler MM, Gonzalez Del Rey JA. Major trauma. In: Fleisher GR, Ludwig S, eds. *Textbook of Pediatric Emergency Medicine.* 4th ed. Philadelphia, Pa: Lippincott Williams & Wilkins; 2000:1259-1269.
6. Trauma resuscitation and spinal immobilization. In: Zaritsky AL, Nadkarni VM, Hickey RW, et al, eds. *PALS Provider Manual.* Dallas, Tex: American Heart Association and American Academy of Pediatrics; 2002:266-268.
7. Adelson PD, Bratton SL, Carney NA, et al. Guidelines for the acute medical management of severe traumatic brain injury in infants, children, and adolescents. *Pediatr Crit Care Med.* 2003;4(3 suppl):S1-S75.

8. Cooper DJ, Myles DS, McDermott FT, et al. Prehospital hypertonic saline resuscitation of patients with hypotension and severe traumatic brain injury. *JAMA*. 2004;291:1350-1357.

9. Clifton GL, Miller ER, Sung CC, et al. Lack of effect of induction of hypothermia after acute brain injury. *N Engl J Med*. 2001;344:556-563.

10. Bracken MB. Steroids for acute spinal cord injury. *Cochrane Database Syst Rev*. 2002;(3):CD001046. Review.

11. Shock. In: *American College of Surgeons Committee on Trauma. Advanced Trauma Life Support for Doctors. Student Course Manual*. 7th ed. Chicago, Ill: American College of Surgeons; 2004:81-82.

12. Pediatric assessment. In: Dieckmann R, Brownstein D, Gausche-Hill M, eds. *Pediatric Education for Prehospital Professionals*. Sudbury, Mass: American Academy of Pediatrics, Jones and Bartlett Publishing Co; 2000:30-56.

Evaluation and Management: Ingestions

Erica L. Leibelt, MD

The evaluation and management of a child or adolescent with a known or suspected toxic exposure involves four phases: initial stabilization (life support), evaluation (history and physical examination), management, and supportive care.

Phase One: Initial Stabilization

The initial management of a known or suspected ingestion begins with the same approach used for any critically ill child, attention to the ABCs using the principles outlined in those sections of this book. Level of consciousness is an additional early concern. If a patient presents early after an ingestion, the level of consciousness could change rapidly, necessitating rapid escalations in care and culminating in intubation, ventilation, and cardiac support. In addition, specific drugs may be needed to treat emergent side effects of many poisonings (Table 1). Early use of these agents can be lifesaving or prevent severe neurologic sequelae.

Emergent decontamination is the other crucial element in initial stabilization. The goal is to decrease or eliminate ongoing exposure to toxic elements. For ocular toxic exposures, saline lavage with repeated aliquots of normal saline is required. At least **1 liter** should be used for each affected eye. Check the pH of the eye to make sure it is normal before and after irrigation, particularly in cases of alkali or acidic exposures. For dermal exposures, decontamination begins with removal of clothing followed by rinsing with copious amounts of water and then washing with soap and water. For enteral ingestions, decontamination has evolved to focus on the early administration of activated charcoal, which is covered in more depth later in this chapter.

Table 1.
Drugs Used in Initial Stabilization of Certain Toxic Ingestions

Toxic Exposure	Drug
Carbon monoxide	Oxygen
Oral hypoglycemic agents, ethanol	Glucose
Opioids, clonidine, imidazoline	Naloxone
Calcium channel antagonists, β-blockers, organophosphates	Atropine
Benzodiazepines	Flumazenil

Phase Two: Evaluation (History and Physical Examination)

The history should be brief and focused on recent events that involved the toxic exposure. Early identification of the drug, toxin, or substance involved is obviously ideal, and the local poison control center can be a useful resource if the family presents with an unknown pill or other commercial product. Route and time of exposure and an estimate of the amount ingested are all critical and may guide laboratory testing, decontamination efforts, and antidotes. Early symptoms are important, especially if they form part of a recognizable toxidrome. Efforts at home treatment, especially use of "antidotes" or syrup of ipecac, should be noted.

Often, patients present in distress without a clear history of ingestion. One should suspect an ingestion if one or more of the following are present:

- Acute onset of symptoms
- Age younger than 5 years
- History of pica or previous ingestions
- Household or environmental stress
- History of mental health disorders
- "Story does not make sense."

Especially with an unknown ingestion, the physical examination can be crucial in establishing the specific class of agents. Certain clinical signs are associated with specific drugs and chemicals (Table 2).

A toxidrome[1] is a constellation of signs and symptoms that is typical of a certain poisoning or class of poisoning. Identifying a toxidrome can suggest the diagnosis and direct the therapeutic approach when the specific agent is unknown. Table 3 lists several of the most common toxidromes.

Laboratory evaluation should be focused and individualized. Several drugs can be identified on quantitative serum drug levels to confirm and guide therapy; these drugs include acetaminophen, salicylates, ethanol, several anticonvulsants, digoxin, carboxyhemoglobin, methemoglobin, and theophylline. Comprehensive toxicology screens are rarely helpful in the initial management of patients. They are qualitative, and the absence of an agent does not rule out an ingestion. In addition, several important drugs are not detected by most "drug screens"— clonidine, cyanide, organophosphates, β-blockers, calcium channel antagonists, and oral hypoglycemic agents.

Determining the **anion gap**[2] (difference between serum cations [Na^+] and anions [$Cl^- + HCO_3^-$]) can be helpful in cases involving metabolic acidosis by revealing if an unmeasured anion is involved. A normal gap is approximately 8 to 12 mEq/L. Examples of ingestions causing metabolic acidosis with a high anion gap include salicylate, methanol, ethylene glycol, isoniazid, iron, lactic acid, and metformin.

Table 2.
Selected Clinical Signs of Toxic Exposures

Clinical Sign	Toxic Exposure
Coma	Anticonvulsants, barbiturates, carbon monoxide, clonidine, cyanide, ethanol, γ-hydroxybutyrate (GHB), opioids
Seizures	Amphetamines, antihistamines, bupropion, cocaine, camphor, isoniazid, tricyclic antidepressants, theophylline
Delirium/ psychosis	Anticholinergics, drugs of abuse (LSD, peyote, cocaine, PCP, ecstasy), sympathomimetics, over-the-counter cold remedies containing pseudoephedrine and dextromethorphan
Miosis	Opioids, organophosphates, phenothiazines, clonidine, valproic acid
Mydriasis	Amphetamines, anticholinergics, antihistamines, cocaine, sympathomimetics
Hyperpyrexia	Amphetamines, cocaine, dinitrophenol, salicylates, anticholinergics, phenothiazines, serotonergic agents, monoamine oxidase inhibitors
Hypothermia	Barbiturates, carbamazepine, clonidine, ethanol, sedative-hypnotics
Garlic odor	Arsenic, organophosphates, thallium
Wintergreen odor	Methylsalicylate

An elevated **osmolar gap** can help determine the presence of methanol, ethylene glycol, ethanol, and isopropyl alcohol **early** in the course of an ingestion. It is the difference between measured osmolality and calculated osmolality [calculated osmolality = (2Na)+(BUN/2.8) + (glucose/18)]. The normal osmolar gap is -2 ± 6.[3]

Finally, abdominal radiographs can reveal radiopacities seen with lead, iron, and other foreign bodies. An ECG can assess the QRS and QT durations and evaluate for heart block and other dysrhythmias.

Phase Three: Management

Gastrointestinal decontamination is a crucial early part of management of many ingestions. The use of syrup of ipecac has been abandoned.[4,5] In addition, there has been a gradual movement away from gastric lavage and whole-bowel irrigation and toward the use of activated charcoal alone.[6] In fact, **gastric lavage** should no longer be used routinely for most ingestions. It should be considered if ingestion occurred within 60 minutes and if ingestion involved a potentially lethal amount of toxic substances (for example, β-blockers, calcium channel antagonists, tricyclic antidepressants, digoxin, chloroquine). In patients who are somnolent or who may have ingested agents that can cause a rapid decline in the level of consciousness, endotracheal intubation to protect the airway may be necessary before lavage. Several substances with the propensity to form bezoars (large amounts of salicylate tablets, calcium channel antagonists) will not be removed with lavage. Lavage is generally less effective in removing liquids because they are more rapidly absorbed than solids. In general, the practitioner should consider all of the risks involved and the time elapsed since the ingestion before undertaking this procedure for unintentional ingestions in young children.

With its enormous surface area, **activated charcoal** acts to bind many ingestants, allowing them to be passed in the feces. It is indicated for most serious ingestions, particularly if it can be administered within 1 hour. It is not effective for iron, lithium, alcohols, common electrolytes, hydrocarbons, and most solvents.[7] It is relatively contraindicated in the presence of severe ileus or obstruction and after caustic alkali or acid ingestions because it makes endoscopy more difficult. Activated charcoal should be given with extreme caution to patients with altered mental status and a tenuous ability to protect the airway. In these cases, strong consideration must be given to elective intubation before the administration of activated charcoal to prevent pulmonary aspiration.[8] Activated charcoal also decreases the absorption of certain enteral antidotes such as acetylcysteine. The initial dose of activated charcoal is **1 g/kg**; adolescents should receive **50 g**. Repeated oral doses of activated charcoal are indicated for drugs with an enterohepatic circulation and for drugs that diffuse into the gastrointestinal lumen from the intestinal circulation (phenobarbital and theophylline are examples).

Whole-bowel irrigation involves intestinal irrigation with iso-osmotic solutions (GoLYTELY or Colyte) for significant iron, lead, or lithium ingestions (all of which are poorly bound by activated charcoal); for ingestions of sustained-release products; and for ingestions of cocaine, heroin, or amphetamine vials or packets. It is contraindicated in ileus, obstruction, and perforation. The dosage is **500 mL/hr** for toddlers via nasogastric tube and **1 to 2 L/hr** for adolescents.

Other methods of **enhanced elimination** are beyond the scope of this chapter but include forced diuresis with or without alkalinization of the urine, hemodialysis, hemoperfusion, and peritoneal dialysis.

Urgent antidotal therapy is indicated for a growing number of known or suspected ingestions. Regional poison control centers can be especially valuable resources in guiding their use. Table 4 lists the common antidotes available for several specific exposures.

Phase Four: Supportive Care

This phase is not highly individualized for specific ingestants. It involves continued monitoring of the ABCs with additional attention to fluid and electrolyte status. Admission to pediatric ICUs is often indicated for ingestions with the potential for neurologic or cardiac toxicity. A cardiorespiratory monitor, pulse oximeter, and frequent neurologic checks including assessment of level of consciousness are often essential. Some toxic effects can be quite delayed (for example, the hepatic damage following acetaminophen overdose). Discharge after an unintentional ingestion should include counseling on home safety. Psychiatric evaluation is typically indicated after intentional ingestions.

References

1. Abbruzzi G, Stork CM. Pediatric toxicologic concerns. *Emerg Med Clin North Am.* 2002;20:223-247.
2. Emmet M, Narins RG. Clinical use of the anion gap. *Medicine.* 1977;56:38-54.
3. Hoffman RS, Smilkstein MJ, Howland MA, et al. Osmol gaps revisited. *J Toxicol Clin Toxicol.* 1993;31:81-93.
4. American Academy of Pediatrics Committee on Injury, Violence, and Poison Prevention. Poison treatment in the home. *Pediatrics.* 2003;112:1182-1185.
5. Bond GR. Home syrup of ipecac use does not reduce emergency department use or improve outcome. *Pediatrics.* 2003;112:1061-1064.
6. Krenzolek EP. New developments in the therapy of intoxications. *Toxicol Lett.* 2002;127:299-305.
7. Erickson TB. Toxicology: ingestions and smoke inhalation. In: Gausche-Hill M, Fuchs S, Yamamoto L, eds. *APLS: The Pediatric Emergency Medicine Resource.* 4th ed. Sudbury, Mass: American Academy of Pediatrics, American College of Emergency Physicians, Jones and Bartlett Publishing Co; 2004:235-240.

Table 3.
Common Toxidromes

Toxidrome	Signs and Symptoms	Examples
Sympathomimetic	Increased temperature; tachycardia; hypertension; mydriasis; diaphoresis; delirium/agitation; seizures	Amphetamines, ecstasy, cocaine, ephedrine, pseudoephedrine
Anticholinergic	Increased temperature; tachycardia; hypertension; mydriasis; delirium/psychosis; seizures; coma; flushed, dry skin; urinary retention; paralytic ileus	Antihistamines, phenothiazines, tricyclic antidepressants, muscle relaxants, antiparkinsonism drugs, jimson weed, antispasmodics
Opioid/clonidine	Decreased temperature; bradycardia; bradypnea/apnea; hypotension; miosis; lethargy/coma	Opioids, clonidine, imidazolines, valproic acid
Cholinergic	Bradycardia; miosis; lacrimation; salivation; vomiting/diarrhea; diaphoresis; confusion; coma	Organophosphates, carbamates, nerve gases

8. Osterhoudt KC, Alpern ER, Durbin D, et al. Activated charcoal administration in a pediatric emergency department. *Pediatr Emerg Care.* 2004;20:493-498.

Table 4.
Antidotes for Specific Toxic Exposures

Toxin	Antidote
Acetaminophen	*N*-Acetylcysteine
β-Blockers	Glucagon
Calcium channel antagonist	Calcium, glucagons, insulin/glucose
Carbon monoxide	Oxygen
Cyanide	Sodium nitrite, sodium thiosulfate
Crotalid snake bite	CroFab (Crotalidae polyvalent immune Fab [ovine])
Digoxin	Digibind (digoxin immune Fab [ovine] fragments)
Iron	Deferoxamine [also desferrioxamine]
Isoniazid	Pyridoxine
Methanol; ethylene glycol	Fomepizole or ethanol
Methemoglobinemia-producing agents	Methylene blue
Opioids/clonidine	Naloxone
Organophosphates/nerve agents	Atropine/pralidoxime
Phenothiazines	Diphenhydramine, benztropine
Sulfonylureas	Glucose, octreotide

Evaluation and Management: Neonatal Resuscitation

Debra Weiner, MD, PhD

Delivery and resuscitation of a newborn should take place in an emergency department or clinic setting **only** when time does not permit transport to a delivery room or neonatal ICU. The pregnant woman and the neonate each requires a separate care provider team. Ideally, each team should have a minimum of two health care professionals with at least one physician per team. The focus in this section is on the neonate. It is important to recognize the equipment requirements for delivery and newborn resuscitation.[1]

Evaluation of the Neonate

Emergent Questions

- Is there an adequate airway?
- Is the newborn infant exercising enough respiratory effort to move sufficient air in and out of the chest, or is respiratory failure imminent?
- Does this patient have adequate perfusion of the vital organs and the peripheral circulation?
- Is the patient warm enough?
- Is the patient manifesting evidence of neurologic compromise?

A focused but detailed evaluation of the maternal history and the maternal and fetal physical examinations should help to determine the neonate's overall status and to guide resuscitative efforts.

Maternal History

Maternal history begins with maternal age, determination of parity, and history of prenatal care. The predicted due date (estimated date of confinement [EDC]) can be rapidly estimated based on last menstrual period (LMP) or early ultrasound examination. Important elements of maternal medical history that can affect the neonate include a history of HIV, hepatitis B, or syphilis infection or colonization with group B streptococci. History of previous pregnancy problems, including prior gestational diabetes, preeclampsia, and previous cesarean section, is important as well. Finally, a review of the current pregnancy including complications such as anemia, diabetes, pregnancy-induced hypertension, bleeding, infections, chronic maternal illness, medications, and tobacco, alcohol, and drug use is important to elicit conditions that can affect the neonate.

The labor history includes time of onset and frequency of contractions. It is crucial to determine if and when rupture of membranes occurred, because it can be predictive of the risk of ascending infection. Presence of fetal movement, any history of vaginal bleeding, and any antecedent trauma are also important.

Maternal Physical Examination

Several elements are crucial:

- Assessment of ABCs
- Vital signs, including temperature
- Physical examination, including palpation of abdomen to establish fetal position
- Fetal monitoring to assess fetal heart rate and nature and frequency of maternal contractions
- Assessment of vaginal discharge for amniotic fluid, blood, and meconium
- Avoidance of speculum or digital examination of vagina or rectum if vaginal bleeding is present. It may represent a placenta previa, and mechanical manipulation can worsen hemorrhage.

Delivery

Numerous potential complications and concerns accompany precipitous or unanticipated deliveries, particularly when they occur outside of a delivery room or other structured setting. These can include the presence of distress as documented on fetal monitoring, maternal hemorrhage, passage of meconium, presence of a nuchal cord or shoulder dystocia, failure to progress, an unanticipated multiple gestation, and breech or transverse presentation.

Neonatal Resuscitation

Normal vital signs for a newborn vary widely depending on gestational age and state of depression or stimulation (see Appendix A). In general, a neonate's heart rate varies from 90 to 160 beats per minute, the respiratory rate varies from 35 to 60 breaths per minute, and the temperature (axillary) varies from 36.5° to 37.4°C. Most term infants are vigorous and pink on delivery and require minimal intervention. If possible, when the child is being delivered, one should use a bulb to suction the mouth and nose immediately after delivery of the head and before delivery of the shoulders. Once delivered, newborns who are vigorous, with a heart rate of 100 or more beats per minute, spontaneous and unlabored respirations, and pink mucous membranes can be dried, wrapped in a warm towel, and given directly to the mother if possible. Continue to clear the airway by wiping secretions from the mouth and nose using a gauze or towel, and if necessary, use bulb suction or 8- to 10-French nasal catheter with 100 cm H_2O or less suction pressure. Wet towels are to be avoided.

Approximately 10% of newborns require additional resuscitative interventions. The need for resuscitation is determined by an integrated simultaneous evaluation for meconium, the presence and quality of cry or respirations, heart rate, muscle tone, color, and whether gestation is term or preterm. The presence of meconium, poor or absent responses, impaired respirations or low heart rate, cyanosis, and preterm delivery are indications for further evaluation and possible further intervention.

Steps in Neonatal Resuscitation[2]

Basic steps in neonatal resuscitation are the same as for older patients, with an emphasis on the ABCs.

- Place newborn on radiant heater/warming table, dry, and stimulate. Acceptable methods of tactile stimulation include gentle rubbing of the back or flicking or slapping the heels once or twice.
- Throughout resuscitative efforts, remember the importance of drying the neonate and maintaining the neonate's body temperature. Hypothermia and hyperthermia should be avoided.
- Position and clear the airway. Place the infant in supine position, head neutral or slightly extended, using a rolled blanket or towel under the shoulders if necessary. In the absence of meconium, and if secretions are minimal, wipe the mouth and nose with gauze or a towel. If secretions are more than minimal, suction the mouth and then the nose using bulb suction or 8- to 10-French catheter at 100 cm H_2O or less suction pressure. Deep or prolonged suctioning may result in laryngospasm and/or bradycardia and should be avoided.
- Meconium is present in the amniotic fluid in 13% of deliveries.[3] If meconium is present, clearing the airway is the first priority. Every effort should be made to suction the mouth, including the posterior pharynx, and nose with a bulb or 12- to 14-French suction catheter immediately after delivery of the head and before delivery of the shoulders whether the meconium is thick or thin. Once the infant is delivered, the airway should be cleared as soon as the child is placed on the warming table. If respirations are absent or depressed, heart rate is less than 100, or muscle tone is decreased,[4] laryngoscopy should be performed by direct visualization to suction the hypopharynx, the newborn should be intubated orally, and the trachea should be suctioned. If necessary, the baby should be reintubated and further suctioned with a new ET tube until the meconium is cleared. An orogastric tube should then be placed to suction any meconium from the stomach so that gastric meconium is not aspirated.
- After initial warming, stimulation, and suctioning of the airway, the next step is to evaluate respirations, heart rate, and color. Respiratory distress, especially apnea, slow respirations, or gasping respirations, is an indication for intervention (assisted ventilation). Heart rate is assessed by counting the pulse at the base of the umbilicus or through auscultation of the precordium; the heart rate should be 100 beats per minute or greater. A persistent heart rate of less than 100 beats per minute is an indication for intervention. A newborn's color can vary widely. Acrocyanosis involving only the hands and feet is usually normal; although it may be a sign of cold stress, it is not usually a sign of hypoxia. Central cyanosis involves the trunk, extremities, and mucous membranes, sometimes including the tongue. Pallor can indicate anemia, hypovolemia, hypothermia, acidosis, and/or depressed cardiac output. Both central cyanosis and pallor are indications for further intervention.

- Interventions for neonatal distress are based on the initial assessment.[1]
  - If the heart rate is more than 100, respirations are spontaneous, and the skin is pink, then provide routine neonatal care.
  - If the heart rate is more than 100, respiration spontaneous, but there is cyanosis, then provide blow-by oxygen.
  - If the heart rate is more than 100, but there are no spontaneous respirations, then provide positive-pressure ventilation (PPV) by BMV at a rate of 30 to 40 breaths per minute.
  - If the heart rate is 60 to 100, then provide PPV by BMV at a rate of 40 to 60 breaths per minute.
  - If the heart rate is less than 60, then provide PPV by BMV at a rate of 30 breaths per minute and chest compressions at a rate of 90/min.
  - If the heart rate is less than 60 after 30 seconds of BMV and chest compressions, then perform endotracheal intubation, establish intravascular access, and administer medications and/or fluid resuscitation as indicated.
- Reassess 30 seconds after each intervention, withdrawing support if clinical improvement makes support unneccesary, or advancing to next phase of resuscitation if there is no improvement or there is deterioration.

Interventions in Neonatal Resuscitation

Free-Flow (or Blow-by) Oxygen

- Free-flow oxygen is indicated in the presence of central cyanosis with a heart rate of greater than 100. It is provided as 100% O_2 at 5 to 10 L/min and can be delivered via face mask, nasal cannula, or tubing held close to the newborn's nose and mouth. An anesthesia bag will passively deliver oxygen but many self-inflating bags will not.
- If oxygen is to be delivered for a prolonged period of time, it should be humidified and heated. When oxygen is no longer needed, it should be withdrawn gradually.
- If the child remains cyanotic despite blow-by oxygen, consider the presence of congenital heart disease. Perform preductal and postductal determinations of oxygen saturation.

Positive-Pressure Ventilation

- PPV (alternatively known as BMV) is indicated in the presence of apnea or a sustained heart rate of less than 100.[5]
- PPV should be delivered using an anesthesia or self-inflating bag with a capacity of at least 450 to 500 mL but not greater than 750 mL.[1] The bag should have a pressure release valve with an override and an in-line manometer to prevent inadvertent delivery of breaths at excessive inspiratory pressures. Rate should be 40 to 60 breaths per minute, or 30 breaths per minute if chest compressions are being delivered.
- Initial breaths may require pressures of 30 to 60 cm H_2O and longer inflation times because of the stiffness of uninflated lungs. Subsequent breaths should require lower pressures (25 to 40 cm H_2O).[6] Reassessment of respiratory effort and heart rate should occur every 30 seconds.
- Effectiveness of PPV can be assessed by chest wall movement, breath sounds, and improvement in heart rate and color. If a child requires prolonged PPV, an 8-French orogastric tube should be placed to decompress the stomach.
- An unresolved clinical issue is the use of 100% oxygen versus room air in neonatal resuscitation. The concern is that high concentrations of oxygen might precipitate brain injury.[7,8]

Endotracheal Intubation[9]

- Endotracheal intubation is indicated if meconium is present (under circumstances discussed earlier); if there are depressed respirations, heart rate, or muscle tone (see earlier); if PPV is ineffective or required for a prolonged period; or if chest compressions are required.
- It might also be necessary in the presence of extreme prematurity, congenital heart disease, diaphragmatic hernia, pneumothorax, omphalocele, gastroschisis, or other fetal

anomalies that affect respiratory effort or effectiveness.

- Endotracheal intubation also facilitates delivery of resuscitation medications and/or surfactant as necessary.
- Initially, almost all infants are intubated orally because it can be done more quickly. Tubes are then electively changed to the nasal orifice once the neonate is stabilized.
- Table 1[10] is helpful in determining proper equipment and ET tube depth. An appropriate ET tube size (internal diameter) can be estimated by the following: ET tube size (in mm) = gestational age (in weeks)/10. Depth (in cm) can be estimated as follows: depth = 3 × ET tube size, or depth = weight (in kg) + 6 cm.

Chest Compressions

- Chest compressions are indicated if the heart rate remains less than 60 despite PPV by BMV for 30 seconds.
- The preferred technique is the two-thumb technique in which the hands encircle the neonate's chest supporting the back. Thumbs are then placed adjacent or superimposed on the lower third of the sternum. The two-finger technique is an alternative in which the fingertips of the second and third or third and fourth fingers are placed on the lower third of the sternum at a right angle to the chest, and the other hand supports the back. The two-thumb technique may generate better coronary perfusion and peak systolic pressure than the two-finger technique.[11]
- Compression depth should be approximately one third of the anteroposterior diameter of the chest. Compressions should be delivered at 90/min and compression phase should be slightly shorter than the relaxation phase.
- Breaths delivered at a rate of 30 per minute should occur after every third compression. Compressions should be delivered during the exhalation phase of each breath. Reevaluation should take place after 30 seconds of chest compressions, and compressions should be discontinued when the spontaneous heart rate is 60 or greater.
- When compressions are discontinued, PPV rate should be increased to 40 to 60 breaths/min. PPV support should be withdrawn gradually when no longer needed.

Vascular Access

- Vascular access is indicated if delivery of medications or fluids is required or if repeated blood sampling is required.
- The preferred site for access in the neonate is the umbilical vein.[12] It is readily accessible, and line placement is usually successful. The normal neonate has 1 umbilical vein and 2 umbilical arteries. The vein is the larger, more thinly walled structure located superiorly.
- Using sterile technique, the procedure is accomplished as follows:
  - Loosely tie umbilical tape at the base of the cord.
  - Clean the cord with povidone-iodine and cut below the cord clamp, approximately 1 to 2 cm from skin surface; cannulate the vein with a 3.5 or 5 French umbilical catheter filled with normal saline and attached to a stop-cock and syringe.
  - Insert the catheter until there is a free flow of blood, usually at a depth of 2 to 4 cm.

Table 1.
Resuscitative Equipment by Gestational Age and Weight

Gestational age (wk)	Weight (g)	Laryngoscope	ET tube size (mm)	ET tube insertion depth (cm at upper lip)
<28	<1,000	Miller 0	2.5	6.5-7
28-34	1,000-2,000	Miller 0	3	7-8
34-38	2,000-3,000	Miller 0, 1	3.5	8-9
>38	>3,000	Miller 1	3.5-4.0	>9

  - Deep insertion of the umbilical venous line should be avoided so that medications are not infused directly into the liver.
- If both umbilical and peripheral vascular access attempts are unsuccessful, an intraosseous line may be placed using a 20- to 22-gauge spinal needle.[13]

Medications and Fluids (Table 2)

- Medications are indicated for asystole or bradycardia (unresponsive to PPV), CNS or respiratory depression, hypoglycemia, and severe metabolic acidosis.
- Fluids are indicated for hypovolemia, shock, and large volume of blood loss.
- High-dose epinephrine is not recommended because of possible brain and cardiac injury.[14] Epinephrine delivered via ET tube should be followed with 0.5 to 1 mL normal saline and several PPV breaths. Delivery may be improved by inserting a catheter through the ET tube.
- Volume expansion using 5% albumin is not recommended because of higher mortality rates associated with its use and because of the risk of transmission of infectious diseases.[15]
- Sodium bicarbonate use is controversial because it might be harmful to cerebral and cardiac function, and it has not been shown to improve survival.[16] It should not be given unless adequate ventilation and circulation have been established. It is very caustic and therefore should be given only through a vein with good blood return. It is not to be given via ET tube.
- Naloxone is contraindicated if maternal narcotic abuse is suspected, because it could precipitate acute withdrawal in the neonate.
- Atropine is not indicated because vagal stimulation usually does not cause bradycardia in newborns, and bradycardia is an important assessment parameter in resuscitation.

Assessment With the Apgar Score

- The Apgar score is an ordinal scale from 0 to 10 (see page 124). It is conventionally assigned to newborns at 1 and 5 minutes after delivery. Its greatest value is as a means to assign a global physiologic score to the child at that particular moment.[17]
- The 1-minute Apgar score aids in the clinical assessment of a newborn's response to the extrauterine environment and guides resuscitative efforts. It has no long-term prognostic value as a measure of neurologic outcome. Scores may be interpreted as follows:
  - 7 to 10: Excellent; neonate requires only drying, warming, stimulation, and suction.
  - 4 to 7: Moderately depressed; neonate may require resuscitation.
  - 0 to 3: Severely depressed; neonate requires immediate resuscitation.
- The 5-minute Apgar score also aids in assessment of resuscitation efforts. It is also

Table 2.
Medications and Fluids in Neonatal Resuscitation

Medication/Fluid	Dose/Route	Indications
Epinephrine 1:10,000	0.1-0.3 mL/kg (0.01-0.03 mg/kg) IV/ET tube/IO q3-5 min PRN	Asystole, heart rate <60 after 30 seconds of PPV and chest compressions
Sodium bicarbonate	1-2 mEq/kg (2-4 mL/kg of 4.2% solution) IV/IO over >2 minutes	Severe metabolic acidosis, failure of resuscitative measures
Naloxone	0.1 mg/kg (0.4 mg/mL or 1 mg/mL solution) IV/ET tube/IO given rapidly (or if perfusion poor, IM/SQ)	CNS or respiratory depression due to maternal narcotics within past 4 hours
Dextrose	0.2-0.5 g/kg IV/IO, 2-5 mL/kg 10% dextrose solution	Hypoglycemia
Normal saline or lactated Ringer	10 mL/kg IV/IO over 5-10 minutes	Hypovolemia, shock
O-negative packed red blood cells	10 mL/kg IV/IO over 5-10 minutes	Large-volume blood loss

correlated with survival, and it may be correlated with long-term neurologic outcome.[18]

- The Apgar score should be assigned every 5 minutes up to 20 minutes if it remains at less than 7.

References

1. Niermeyer S, Kattwinkel J, VanReempts P, et al. International guidelines for neonatal resuscitation: an excerpt from the Guidelines 2000 for Cardiopulmonary Resuscitation and Emergency Cardiovascular Care: International Consensus on Science. *Pediatrics.* 2000;106:e29.

2. Niermeyer S, Van Reempts P, Kattwinkel J, et al; American Heart Association; International Liaison Committee on Resuscitation. Resuscitation of newborns. *Ann Emerg Med.* 2001;37(suppl):S110-S125.

3. Gelfand SL, Fanaroff JM, Walsh MC. Meconium-stained fluid: approach to the mother and the baby. *Pediatr Clin North Am.* 2004;51:655-667.

4. Wiswell TE, Gannon CM, Jacob J, et al. Delivery room management of the apparently vigorous meconium-stained neonate: results of the multi-center, international, collaborative trail. *Pediatrics.* 2000;105:1-7.

5. Saugstad OD. New guidelines for the resuscitation of the newly born infant. *J Matern Fetal Neonatal Med.* 2002;11:2-3.

6. Burchfield DJ, Boychuck RB. Neonatal emergencies. In: Gausche-Hill M, Fuchs S, Yamamoto L, eds. *APLS: The Pediatric Emergency Medicine Resource.* 4th ed. Sudbury, Mass: American Academy of Pediatrics, American College of Emergency Physicians, Jones and Bartlett Publishing Co; 2004:480.

7. Tarnow-Mordi WO. Room air or oxygen for asphyxiated babies? *Lancet.* 1998;352:341.

8. Saugstad OD, Ramji S, Vento M. Resuscitation of depressed newborn infants with ambient air or pure oxygen: a meta-analysis. *Biol Neonate.* 2004;87:27-34.

9. King BR, King C, Coates WC. Emergent intubation. In: Gausche-Hill M, Fuchs S, Yamamoto L, eds. *APLS: The Pediatric Emergency Medicine Resource.* 4th ed. Sudbury, Mass: American Academy of Pediatrics, American College of Emergency Physicians, Jones and Bartlett Publishing Co; 2004:700-710.

10. Alessandrini EA. Neonatal resuscitation. In: Fleisher GR, Ludwig S, eds. *Textbook of Pediatric Emergency Medicine.* 4th ed. Philadelphia, Pa: Williams & Wilkins; 2000:39.

11. Menegazzi JJ, Auble TE, Nicklas KA, et al. Two-thumb versus two-finger chest compression during CRP in a swine infant model of cardiac arrest. *Ann Emerg Med.* 1993;22:240-243.

12. King BR, King C, Coates WC. Umbilical vein catheterization. In: Gausche-Hill M, Fuchs S, Yamamoto L, eds. *APLS: The Pediatric Emergency Medicine Resource.* 4th ed. Sudbury, Mass: American Academy of Pediatrics, American College of Emergency Physicians, Jones and Bartlett Publishing Co; 2004:734-736.

13. King BR, King C, Coates WC. Intraosseous needle placement. In: Gausche-Hill M, Fuchs S, Yamamoto L, eds. *APLS: The Pediatric Emergency Medicine Resource.* 4th ed. Sudbury, Mass: American Academy of Pediatrics, American College of Emergency Physicians, Jones and Bartlett Publishing Co; 2004:736-738.

14. Ziino AJ, Davies MW, Davis PG. Epinephrine for the resuscitation of apparently stillborn or extremely bradycardic newborn infants. *Cochrane Database Syst Rev.* 2003(2):CD003849.

15. Roberton NR. Use of albumin in neonatal resuscitation. *Eur J Pediatr.* 1997;156:428-431.

16. Lokesh L, Kumar P, Murki S, et al. A randomized controlled trial of sodium bicarbonate in neonatal resuscitation—effect on immediate outcome. *Resuscitation.* 2004;60:219-223.

17. Apgar V. The newborn (Apgar) scoring system. Reflections and advice. *Pediatr Clin North Am.* 1966;13:645-650.

18. Sato M, Aotani H, Hattori R, et al. Behavioral outcome including attention deficit hyperactivity disorder/hyperactivity disorder and minor neurological signs in perinatal high-risk newborns at 4-6 years of age with relation to risk factors. *Pediatr Int.* 2004;46:346-352.

SCENARIO #1

Airway Obstruction

Mario Gehri, MD

Brief Presenting History

A 14-month-old boy is brought to the emergency department from home at 10 PM with the complaint of an abrupt onset of noisy, labored breathing and barky cough.

Pediatric Assessment Triangle

Appearance: Awake and alert, but anxious and inconsolable

Work of Breathing: Labored with moderate intercostal and suprasternal retractions, long inspiratory phase, and inspiratory stridor

Circulation to the Skin: Extremities warm, no evidence of cyanosis

Initial Vital Signs

Pulse: 148

Respiratory Rate: 32

Blood Pressure: Not obtainable because of agitation

Temperature: 37.5°C (99.5°F) axillary

Oxygen Saturation: 93% in room air

ASK YOURSELF

- **How much should this 14-month-old child weigh?**

  An estimated weight for a 14-month-old child is 10 kg. One can use the length-based Broselow Pediatric Emergency Tape or a pediatric table to determine weight based on age. See Appendix A. (All medication dosages are derived using weight [or body surface area], and in this age group, a 1- or 2-kg difference in estimated weight could cause a 10% to 20% error in the dose administered.)

Physical Examination on Arrival to the Emergency Department

Airway: Mouth open, nasal congestion and clear rhinorrhea, inspiratory stridor with each breath

Breathing: Moderate retractions, symmetric breath sounds, no wheezes

Circulation: Capillary refill measured in a warm finger is less than 2 seconds

Disability: Eyes open, agitated, vigorously moving all extremities, refuses oxygen mask

ASK YOURSELF

- **What is the initial assessment? What is the patient's physiologic status?**

  The child exhibits marked increased work of breathing with retractions and audible stridor consistent with respiratory distress and with a potential for respiratory failure.[1] There is no evidence of shock at this time.

■ What is the differential diagnosis?

Although this child presents with a history and clinical presentation typical of croup, the differential diagnosis that must be considered includes other infectious conditions (epiglottitis, tracheitis, retropharyngeal abscess), allergic conditions, foreign body aspiration, and glottic injury (thermal burns or blunt trauma).[2]

■ What additional history and physical findings would help you?

Stridor, barky cough, low-grade fever, and a nontoxic appearance in this age group suggest croup. The exclusion of other conditions is imperative. A history of high fever, drooling, absence of cough, and toxic appearance points toward epiglottitis. A history of trauma, ingestion of corrosive products, or foreign body aspiration is relevant. Recent medication ingestion or exposure to known allergens that results in rash or edema suggests anaphylaxis.[3]

A history of prematurity or previous endotracheal intubation suggests an underlying airway abnormality such as tracheomalacia or subglottic stenosis. The presence of these conditions in a patient with croup increases the likelihood of more severe presentations. Croup is frequently recurrent; a previous history of severe croup is also important to obtain.

The physical examination must be carefully completed: a muffled voice ("hot potato voice") is compatible with a higher obstruction like retropharyngeal abscess. Hemangiomas of the skin must be noted and may be indicative of airway vascular anomalies.

Additional History

For the past 2 days, the patient has experienced upper respiratory infection symptoms without documented fever. He developed a barky cough on the previous evening but seemed well today, eating and drinking normally. This evening, he awoke suddenly with respiratory distress. There is no history of trauma.

Past Medical History: Uncomplicated pregnancy and delivery; ICU hospitalization at 3 months of age for croup

Medications: None

Allergies: None known

ASK YOURSELF

■ What is the most likely diagnosis?

The history and clinical presentation are compatible with moderate to severe croup with a potential for respiratory failure. The patient's airway is currently maintainable.

■ What interventions are needed at this time? What complications might be expected?

Interventions:

- Given a maintainable airway, the child may be placed in the arms of the parents, allowing him to assume a position of comfort.
- Place humidified oxygen or mist but avoid excessive stimulation, which could agitate the child and lead to worsening of his respiratory distress. Mist is traditionally used as it is thought to moisten thick secretions and decrease airway inflammation, although there are little data to support the efficacy of this practice.[4,5]
- While the patient is being held in the parent's arms, place the patient on a cardiorespiratory monitor with pulse oximetry if this can be accomplished without agitating the patient.
- Administer **dexamethasone 0.6 mg/kg PO** and then nothing further by mouth until respiratory distress diminishes.[6-9]
- Nebulized **epinephrine 0.05 mL/kg 1:1,000** dilution with oxygen, maximum dose 0.5 mL

Potential Complications:

- Agitation brought on by interventions results in worsening of respiratory distress.
- Intravenous access attempts result in severe distress.
- Patient refuses to take or vomits the dexamethasone.

■ Which patients with croup should be treated with steroids?

For patients with moderate or severe croup, treatment with corticosteroids has been shown to be effective in reducing the frequency and duration of intubation and hospitalization, as well as in decreasing the use of nebulized epinephrine.[7,8] Steroids have been shown to be effective in these patients when administered intramuscularly, orally, or as a nebulized suspension. A recent multicenter, randomized trial of oral dexamethasone for mild croup demonstrated that such treatment results in quicker resolution of croup symptoms, less lost sleep, less parental stress, and fewer patient returns for medical care.[9]

■ **Which patients with croup should be treated with nebulized epinephrine?**

Nebulized epinephrine is typically reserved for those patients with signs of moderate to severe respiratory distress.[6,10-13] Patients need not be hypoxic; rather, significantly increased work of breathing is sufficient to implement nebulized epinephrine treatment.

Progression

The patient initially improved with administration of epinephrine, but now the retractions have become more pronounced and the child appears to be exhausted.

Repeat Vital Signs

Pulse: 180

Respiratory Rate: 16

Blood Pressure: Not obtainable

Oxygen Saturation: 90% despite blow-by oxygen

ASK YOURSELF

■ **What has happened?**

Partial airway obstruction is still present and the patient is tiring. Initial interventions have not significantly improved his condition. The child is displaying signs of impending respiratory failure: diminished mental status and decreased respiratory effort and rate. The tachycardia could be due to treatment with epinephrine or to the development of shock.

Progression

Patient now responds to pain only, with a respiratory rate of 8.

ASK YOURSELF

■ **What interventions are needed at this time? What complications might be expected?**

Interventions:

- At this point the child should be removed from the arms of his parent and placed on a bed. The parents should be encouraged to remain close to him.
- Establish intravenous access: Begin fluid bolus with **normal saline 20 mL/kg IV.**
- Administer **dexamethasone 0.6 mg/kg IM** if oral dose is unsuccessful.
- Repeat nebulized **epinephrine 0.05 mL/kg 1:1,000 dilution with oxygen,** to a maximum dose of 0.5 mL.
- Prepare to assist breathing with BMV or establish an airway with RSI.
- Consider obtaining ABGs to assess respiratory insufficiency. However, an arterial blood draw could increase the patient's agitation and make his condition worse. If the child is too tired to struggle, it is probably time for RSI, and the ABG results would only support what is already known: the patient has impending respiratory failure.

Potential Complications:

- Intravenous access attempts are unsuccessful. If respiratory failure appears imminent (as evidenced by decreasing respiratory rate, agitation giving way to somnolence, and/or progressive hypoxia), an intraosseous line should be placed.
- Vomiting is quite often seen with patients in great distress. Be prepared to assist vomiting patients, especially ones with altered mental status, in protecting their airway by proper positioning and suctioning of the mouth and nose. Keep a suctioning system (large system device) readily available.
- Respiratory failure is imminent, and RSI should be instituted.

■ How would you classify the airway of this patient with croup? What considerations must be made before intubation?

When evaluating a child for emergency airway management, it is important to determine if the patient has any features that would make BMV, endotracheal intubation, or cricothyrotomy difficult to achieve.[6] The croup patient can be considered to be a "difficult airway" or to have the potential to become one because of airway edema and resultant obstruction that could impede BMV or endotracheal intubation. Prior to RSI, several smaller-than-expected-sized endotracheal tubes should be made readily available, and the ability to effectively perform BMV must be established.

■ What interventions are needed at this time? What complications might be expected?

Interventions:

- RSI
  1. #1 Miller blade, 4.5 ET tube (4.0 and 5.0 ready)
  2. Preoxygenate
  3. Cricoid pressure (with BMV or when muscle relaxation has occurred)
  4. Consider atropine **0.02 mg/kg IV**, minimum dose 0.1 mg
  5. **Etomidate 0.3 mg/kg IV** or **midazolam 0.1 mg/kg IV**
  6. **Rocuronium 0.6 to 1 mg/kg IV** or **succinylcholine 1 to 1.5 mg/kg IV**
- End-tidal CO_2 monitor
- Call for chest radiograph to confirm ET tube placement.
- Secure ET tube and place an NG tube.
- Obtain ABGs to follow pH. A VBG would be acceptable in this patient if hypoxia is not a concern and pulse oximeter readings have been verified.

Potential Complications:

- Vomiting: Requires suctioning, especially if cricoid pressure is not used
- Inability to visualize cords if not properly suctioned
- Lack of NG tube results in abdominal distention and impaired ventilation.
- Endotracheal intubation is unsuccessful and BMV is ineffective, resulting in the need for percutaneous cricothyrotomy.

Progression

With RSI and volume resuscitation, the boy's condition improves. Transfer in stable condition to the ICU is now possible.

Objectives of This Scenario

1. Distinguish upper from lower airway obstruction, and recognize that these entities are treated differently.

The patient described in this scenario has a presentation consistent with that of severe croup: sudden onset of difficult breathing, suprasternal retractions, low-grade fever, stridor at rest, and a barky cough with a previous history of severe croup. The initial response to treatment is poor, and the child progresses to impending respiratory failure. This scenario is quite common in emergency departments, even though less than 5% of croup patients can be expected to be hospitalized and only 1% to 2% of hospitalized patients are intubated.[14] This patient's symptoms are most notable during inspiration, signifying an extrathoracic or upper airway obstruction. It is important to distinguish the upper airway obstruction of croup from lower airway obstruction of asthma, because the emergent treatment for each differs. Croup is treated emergently with nebulized epinephrine rather than with albuterol, which is used in asthma. Other causes of upper airway obstruction and distinction from croup were discussed previously.

2. Initiate management of severe croup.

The priorities of managing patients with severe croup are the same as those for other critically ill patients: assess and support the ABCs with a special emphasis on the airway.

Airway: Initially, assess whether the airway is maintainable without further interventions. If the airway is maintainable, attempt supportive measures such as clearing secretions from the mouth and nose, positioning the head in the midline, and providing humidified oxygen (only if tolerated by the patient). These interventions are best attempted while the child is in the arms of the parent or guardian. If the child becomes more agitated, respiratory distress can worsen.

Breathing: Support breathing. In this scenario, no active support of ventilation is necessary until the patient tires, as evidenced by decreased respiratory rate and effort with desaturations despite oxygen treatment. It is important to be prepared to assist breathing with BMV.

Circulation: This patient presents with a normal circulatory examination. Intravenous access should not be attempted until the patient shows signs of worsening distress and potential respiratory failure, as such attempts can increase patient agitation and worsen respiratory distress.

For patients with moderate to severe upper airway obstruction, the initial intervention is to give nebulized **epinephrine** *with* oxygen.[6] Corticosteroids have been shown to be effective in the management of mild to severe croup, and their use was discussed previously.[7-9]

3. Anticipate possible complications of severe croup.

Most importantly, some patients with severe croup progress to impending respiratory failure despite therapy with nebulized epinephrine and steroids, necessitating the use of BMV followed by RSI. Preparations must be made to address the potentially difficult airway, especially in patients with underlying conditions or syndromes that predispose them to airway abnormalities. Patients with croup and concomitant conditions such as bacterial tracheitis or pneumonia may have more severe presentations. Even uncomplicated viral croup can occasionally result in death, particularly in infants.[15]

References

1. Recognition of respiratory failure and shock. In: Zaritsky AL, Nadkarni VM, Hickey RW, et al, eds. *PALS Provider Manual.* Dallas, Tex: American Academy of Pediatrics and American Heart Association; 2002:23-42.
2. Dieckmann RA. Pediatric assessment. In: Gausche-Hill M, Fuchs S, Yamamoto L, eds. *APLS: The Pediatric Emergency Medicine Resource.* 4th ed. Sudbury, Mass: American Academy of Pediatrics, American College of Emergency Physicians, Jones and Bartlett Publishing Co; 2004:27-32.
3. Fleisher GR. Infectious disease emergencies. In: Fleisher GR, Ludwig S, eds. *Textbook of Pediatric Emergency Medicine.* 4th ed. Philadelphia, Pa: Lippincott Williams & Wilkins; 2000:745-746.
4. Bourchier D, Dawson KP, Fergusson DM. Humidification in viral croup: a controlled trial. *Aust Paediatr J.* 1984;20:289-291.
5. Neto GM, Kentab O, Klassen TP, et al. A randomized controlled trial of mist in the acute treatment of moderate croup. *Acad Emerg Med.* 2002;9:873-879.
6. Stenklyft PH, Cataletto ME, Lee BS. The pediatric airway in health and disease. In: Gausche-Hill M, Fuchs S, Yamamoto L, eds. *APLS: The Pediatric Emergency Medicine Resource.* 4th ed. Sudbury, Mass: American Academy of Pediatrics, American College of Emergency Physicians, Jones and Bartlett Publishing Co; 2004:58-64.
7. Johnson DW, Jacobson S, Edney PC, et al. A comparison of nebulized budesonide, intramuscular dexamethasone, and placebo for moderately severe croup. *N Engl J Med.* 1998;339:498-503.
8. Ausejo M, Saenz A, Pham B, et al. The effectiveness of glucocorticoids in treating croup: meta-analysis. *BMJ.* 1999;319:595-600.
9. Bjornson CL, Klassen TP, Williamson J, et al. A randomized trial of a single dose of oral dexamethasone for mild croup. *N Engl J Med.* 2004;351:1306-1313.
10. Kelley PB, Simon JE. Racemic epinephrine use in croup and disposition. *Am J Emerg Med.* 1992;10:181-183.
11. Pendergast M, Jones JS, Hartman D. Racemic epinephrine in the treatment of laryngotracheitis: can we identify children for outpatient therapy? *Am J Emerg Med.* 1994;12:613-616.
12. Waisman Y, Klein BL, Boenning DA, et al. Prospective randomized double-blind study comparing L-epinephrine and racemic epinephrine aerosols in the treatment of laryngotracheitis (croup). *Pediatrics.* 1992;89:302-306.
13. Ledwith CA, Shea LM, Mauro RD. Safety and efficacy of nebulized racemic epinephrine in conjunction with oral dexamethasone and mist in the outpatient treatment of croup. *Ann Emerg Med.* 1995;25:331-337.
14. Osmond M. Croup. *Clin Evid.* 2002;8:319-328.
15. Fisher JD. Out-of-hospital cardiopulmonary arrest in children with croup. *Pediatr Emerg Care.* 2004;20:35-36.

SCENARIO #2

Airway Obstruction

Stephen J. Teach, MD, MPH

Brief Presenting History

An 18-month-old boy presents to the emergency department by ambulance. His babysitter had called 911 because the boy suddenly developed noisy breathing and "turned kinda blue."

Pediatric Assessment Triangle

Appearance: Awake, alert, extremely anxious, diaphoretic, agitated, inconsolable

Work of Breathing: Labored with a long inspiratory phase, loud inspiratory stridor with severe retractions (intercostal and suprasternal)

Circulation to the Skin: Cyanosis of the extremities and perioral area

Initial Vital Signs

Pulse: 140

Respiratory Rate: 44

Blood Pressure: Not obtainable due to agitation

Temperature: 37°C (98.6°F) axillary

Physical Examination on Arrival to the Emergency Department

Airway: Loud, stridulous inspiratory sounds with each breath

Breathing: Severe retractions; symmetric but greatly diminished breath sounds without crackles, rhonchi, or wheezes

Circulation: Capillary refill time less than 2 seconds with strong peripheral pulses

Disability: Eyes open, attempts to cry without success, highly agitated, moves all extremities

ASK YOURSELF

- **What is the initial assessment? What is the patient's physiologic status?**

  This child presents with abrupt onset of impending airway obstruction. He is in severe respiratory distress with severe inspiratory stridor and cyanosis.

- **What could be causing his distress?**

  The inspiratory stridor suggests airway obstruction that is extrathoracic, at the level of the immediate subglottic area and above. The differential diagnosis of such obstruction includes croup, epiglottitis, foreign body, and glottic injury such as a thermal burn or a laryngeal fracture.

- **What additional history would help you establish the diagnosis?**

  The presence or absence of fever and other signs of viral upper respiratory infection at home or in the emergency department would help distinguish an infectious cause. The presence of trauma (house fire, ingestion of hot liquid or corrosive, direct blow to the larynx) would help establish a diagnosis of airway injury. The abrupt onset suggests a foreign body or a traumatic etiology.

Additional History and Physical Examination Findings

The child was home with the babysitter while his parents were at the movies. He wandered into a room where his mother keeps her craft projects. The babysitter heard strange choking and gasping noises and found the child highly agitated and breathing heavily.

Past Medical History: Healthy child with no history of respiratory problems

Medications: None

Allergies: None known

Physical Examination: No rhinorrhea or evidence of upper respiratory tract infection, no bruising of the neck or evidence of oropharyngeal trauma

ASK YOURSELF

- **What is the most likely diagnosis?**

  History of abrupt onset of symptoms while unsupervised strongly suggests a foreign body.[1-5]

- **What interventions are needed at this time? What complications might be expected?**

  Interventions:

  - At this point, one should determine whether this is a maintainable or an unmaintainable airway. If the airway is maintainable, then positioning, oxygen, and gentle suction might be sufficient. Avoid excessive stimulation under all circumstances. Notify the surgical and anesthesia services so that they can prepare the OR for laryngoscopy/bronchoscopy. If the airway is unmaintainable, then plans for an emergent alternative surgical airway are paramount.
  - Administer 100% O_2 by face mask.
  - Place the patient on a cardiorespiratory monitor with pulse oximetry if it does not agitate the child too much.
  - Attempt to establish intravenous access.

  Potential Complications:

  - Agitation due to monitors and venipuncture might worsen the degree of airway obstruction and could cause complete airway obstruction. Stimulation should be kept to a minimum, as should interventions (oxygen only, for example).

Repeat Vital Signs

Pulse: 170

Respiratory Rate: 20

Blood Pressure: Not obtainable

Oxygen saturation: 88% with 100% blow-by oxygen

Progression

The child's breathing becomes increasingly slower, more labored, and noiseless, with progressive loss of muscle tone and loss of consciousness.

ASK YOURSELF

- **What has happened?**

  Impending respiratory failure due to complete airway obstruction caused by a foreign body at the level of the larynx or below. Remember, the narrowest part of the upper airway in children younger than about 8 years lies at the level of the upper extrathoracic trachea just below the glottis. In contrast, the narrowest part of the airway in older children and adults lies at the level of the glottis.

- **What interventions are needed at this time? What complications might be expected?**

  Interventions:

  - Direct visualization of the oropharynx and removal of any visible foreign body. Performing blind airway sweeps with fingers is contraindicated.
  - Abdominal thrusts to dislodge the foreign body
  - Attempt BMV with repositioning of the airway if necessary.

  Potential Complications:

  - Attempting to remove an airway foreign body with your fingers always risks further impaction in the upper airway and/or trauma and bleeding.
  - Abdominal thrusts can rupture abdominal viscera.

- Under these circumstances, BMV can precipitate emesis by forcing air through the esophagus into the stomach.

Progression

High-volume emesis of gastric contents followed by full respiratory arrest.

Repeat Vital Signs

Pulse: 80 (sinus bradycardia) and dropping

Respiratory Rate: 0

Blood Pressure: Unobtainable and pulses not felt

Oxygen Saturation: Unobtainable

ASK YOURSELF

■ What interventions are needed at this time? What complications might be expected?

Interventions:

- Attempt visualization of the airway and foreign body removal using direct laryngoscopy with a #1 Miller (straight) blade after clearing the oropharynx of emesis with suction. Magill forceps can be used for attempts at foreign body removal.[6]
- Attempt BMV.
- Continue attempts to obtain intravenous access.

Potential Complications:

- Inability to visualize or to remove the foreign body. Under these circumstances, one option is to attempt passage of an ET tube to force the foreign body into a mainstem bronchus, permitting ventilation of one lung.
- If subsequent attempts to ventilate the patient are unsuccessful, emergent percutaneous cricothyrotomy or consultation with a surgeon for emergent tracheostomy would be necessary.

Progression

Laryngoscopy permits removal of the foreign body with Magill forceps. It was a round glass bead with a hole in the middle, and it was lying on top of the vocal cords and completely occluding the boy's airway.

Repeat Vital Signs

Pulse: 0

Respiratory Rate: 0

Blood Pressure: Unobtainable and pulses not felt

Oxygen Saturation: Unobtainable

ECG Monitor: The ECG reveals asystole.

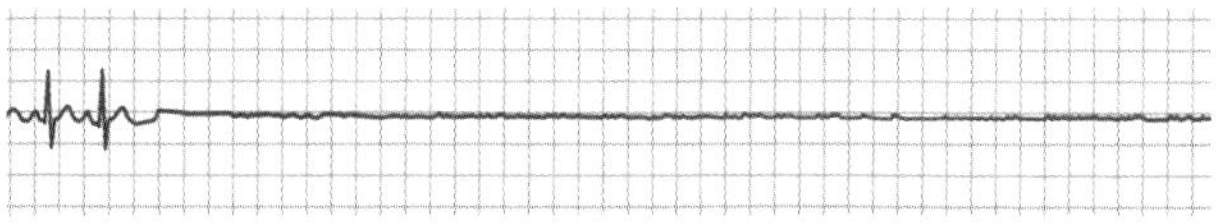

ASK YOURSELF

■ What interventions are needed at this time? What complications might be expected?

Interventions:

- Initiate algorithm for asystolic pulseless arrest ("Evaluation and Management: Circulation," Figure 1).
- Position airway and initiate BMV with cricoid pressure at a rate of 20 with 100% oxygen. Additional suctioning might be required if emesis material is still present in the patient's mouth.
- Begin chest compressions at rate of 100, pausing for each ventilation in a ratio of 5:1.
- Perform endotracheal intubation with a #1 Miller (straight) blade and 4.0 or 4.5 ET tube after further clearing the oropharynx of emesis with suction and using cricoid pressure.
- If intravenous access has not been obtained yet, insert an intraosseous needle.
- **Administer epinephrine 1:10,000 (0.1 mL/kg IV or IO)** with saline flush.

Potential Complications:

- Inability to visualize the airway if it is not properly suctioned or positioned
- Failure to verify tube position with either intubation of esophagus with auscultation of breath sounds over stomach or intubation of right mainstem bronchus
- Barotrauma induced by excessive tidal volume could precipitate a pneumothorax requiring percutaneous anterior needle aspiration or chest tube placement.

Progression

Pulses return after airway and breathing are controlled and a single dose of intravenous epinephrine is administered. Monitor now reveals sinus tachycardia.

Repeat Vital Signs

Pulse: 160

Respiratory Rate: Ventilated at 30

Blood Pressure: 60/33 with weak peripheral pulses

Oxygen Saturation: 100%

ASK YOURSELF

- **What additional complications might be expected for this patient?**

  Depending on the duration and severity of the hypoxia, transient cardiogenic shock could be expected, necessitating volume and possible inotropic support. Neurologic recovery could occur swiftly or slowly, again depending on the magnitude of the hypoxic insults received by the brain. Spontaneous respirations might resume immediately or after a period of up to several hours.

Objectives of This Scenario

1. Recognize this unique presentation of airway obstruction.

This patient presented with the hallmarks of an airway foreign body: the very abrupt onset of severe respiratory distress with loud inspiratory stridor, retractions, very poor air movement, and severe agitation.[1-5,7,8] The differential diagnosis is limited but includes acute airway trauma such as thermal or caustic injury to the epiglottis or aryepiglottic folds or laryngeal fracture. An older child might have presented with the universal choking sign (hands to neck), but this sign is likely to be absent in younger children. Foreign body aspiration is a common cause of accidental death among children in the United States, accounting for up to 300 fatalities per year.[9]

2. Recognize evolving hypoxia and hypercarbia with progression to respiratory arrest.

The agitation, duskiness, cyanosis, and severe distress are all characteristic of hypoxia and hypercarbia. Failure to intervene rapidly and to gain control of the airway in such situations allows the condition to worsen with subsequent respiratory and cardiac arrest and death.

3. Manage acute airway obstruction.

Management of foreign body aspiration depends on the patient's age, history, signs, and symptoms. The airway must be secured, and this necessitates either removal of the foreign body or creation of an artificial airway around it. Initially, the oropharynx should be visualized and the foreign body removed if possible. Performing blind finger sweeps is contraindicated in infants and young children because of the risk of further impacting the foreign body and causing complete obstruction. If visualization is unsuccessful, then back blows followed by chest thrusts (for patients younger than 12 months) are indicated; for patients older than 12 months, abdominal thrusts (no back blows) are indicated. If these are not successful, then the next step is direct visualization of the airway using laryngoscopy with removal of the foreign body if possible with forceps. BMV may be attempted if removal of the foreign body is not possible and the airway is not maintainable.

At each step in the management algorithm, one must be ready to circumvent the obstruction with a surgical airway.[10] This is controversial in the pediatric population. The most narrow part of the airway in children younger than 8 years is just below the glottis in the cricoid ring inferior to the cricothyroid membranes. As such, percutaneous cricothyrotomy might not be effective, leaving open tracheostomy as the only alternative. However, attempts at percutaneous cricothyrotomy should not be withheld when other methods fail to provide a suitable airway and when open tracheostomy is not an immediate option.

References

1. Halvorson DJ, Merritt RM, Mann C, et al. Management of subglottic foreign bodies. *Ann Otol Rhinol Laryngol.* 1996;105:541-544.
2. Silva AB, Muntz HR, Clary R, et al. Utility of conventional radiography in the diagnosis and management of pediatric airway foreign bodies. *Ann Otol Rhinol Laryngol.* 1998;107:834-838.
3. Reilly J, Thompson J, MacArthur C, et al. Pediatric aerodigestive foreign body injuries are complications related to timeliness of diagnosis. *Laryngoscope.* 1997;107:17-20.
4. Metrangelo S, Monetti C, Mereghini L, et al. Eight years' experience with foreign-body aspiration in children: what is really important for a timely diagnosis? *J Pediatr Surg.* 1999;34:1229-1231.

5. Fontoba JEB, Gutierrez C, Lluna J, et al. Bronchial foreign body: should bronchoscopy be performed in all patients with a choking crisis? *Pediatr Surg Int.* 1997;12:118-120.

6. King BR, King C, Coates WC. Critical procedures. In: Gausche-Hill M, Fuchs S, Yamamoto L, eds. *APLS: The Pediatric Emergency Medicine Resource.* 4th ed. Sudbury, Mass: American Academy of Pediatrics, American College of Emergency Physicians, Jones and Bartlett Publishing Co; 2004:699-700.

7. Tobias JD. Airway management for pediatric emergencies. *Pediatr Ann.* 1996;25:317-328.

8. Friedman EM. Tracheobronchial foreign bodies. *Otol Clin North Am.* 2000;33:179-185.

9. Reilly JS, Cook SP, Stool D, et al. Prevention and management of aerodigestive foreign body injuries in childhood. *Pediatr Clin North Am.* 1996;43:1403-1413.

10. Bair AE, Panacek EA, Wisner DH, et al. Cricothyrotomy: a 5-year experience at one institution. *J Emerg Med.* 2003;24:151-156.

SCENARIO #3

Airway Obstruction

Ari R. Cohen, MD, and Anne M. Stack, MD

Brief Presenting History

A 4-year-old girl with mild intermittent asthma is playing in the waiting room of the emergency department while waiting to be evaluated for a urinary tract infection. Suddenly, her mother notes that the girl is coughing and breathing noisily. She picks up the little girl and brings her to the triage nurse, who notices that the child appears scared and agitated. Another parent reports that she had just put a piece of brownie to her lips when she started coughing. She is crying and says that her throat hurts. She says that she did not eat any of the brownie.

Pediatric Assessment Triangle

Appearance: Anxious, crying

Work of Breathing: Labored with a long inspiratory phase, loud inspiratory stridor with retractions (intercostal and suprasternal)

Circulation to the Skin: Flushed with strong peripheral pulses

Initial Vital Signs

Pulse: 155

Respiratory Rate: 34

Blood Pressure: 90/40

Temperature: 37.2°C (99°F) axillary

Oxygen Saturation: 91% in room air

Physical Examination on Arrival to the Emergency Department

Airway: Loud, stridulous inspiratory sounds with each labored breath

Breathing: Dyspnea with retractions, bilateral diffuse wheezes

Circulation: Capillary refill time 2 to 3 seconds with strong central pulses

Disability: Eyes open and dilated

ASK YOURSELF

- **What is the initial assessment? What is the patient's physiologic status?**

  This young girl presents with abrupt onset of impending airway obstruction. Her anxiety is due to her narrowed airway, a sensation often referred to as "impending doom." She also has severe dyspnea, inspiratory stridor, and retractions, all signs of evolving respiratory failure.[1] The child is also highly anxious, a sign of hypoxia, but she has not yet displayed signs of altered mental status. The child is working very hard to breathe, as demonstrated by retractions and tachypnea. There are no obvious signs of cardiovascular compromise.

- **What could be causing her respiratory failure?**

  The inspiratory stridor suggests airway obstruction that is extrathoracic, most likely at the level of the vocal cords or above. The differential diagnosis of obstruction in this child includes laryngeal edema, foreign body aspiration, and infection such as epiglottitis, severe croup, bacterial tracheitis, and retrotonsillar or peritonsillar abscess.

■ **What additional history would help you establish the diagnosis?**

The rapidity of onset and lack of fever make anaphylaxis or foreign body aspiration the most likely etiologies. The presence of urticaria on the skin and of oropharyngeal swelling or angioedema would strongly suggest the diagnosis of anaphylaxis. One should remember that foreign body aspiration and anaphylaxis are not necessarily mutually exclusive. Inspiratory stridor is not an expected finding in asthma, which is a lower respiratory tract disease and usually presents with expiratory wheeze.

Additional History and Physical Examination Findings

When asked, the mother states that her daughter developed hives once before and was brought to the emergency department. She thinks that her daughter is allergic to nuts.

Past Medical History: Otherwise healthy child with no prior hospitalizations or operations

Medications: Mother has an EpiPen at home but does not carry it with her

Allergies: None known

Physical Examination: Rapidly spreading diffuse urticaria, swelling of her lips and tongue (angioedema)

ASK YOURSELF

■ **What is the most likely diagnosis?**

Anaphylaxis (with or without foreign body aspiration)

■ **What interventions are needed at this time? What complications might be expected?**

Interventions:

- Place the patient on a cardiorespiratory monitor with pulse oximetry.
- Administer 100% O_2 via face mask.
- Administer epinephrine 1:1,000 (0.01 mg/kg or 0.01 mL/kg IM; maximum dose 0.3 mL).
- Attempt to establish intravenous access.

Potential Complications:

- Incorrect dose of epinephrine could be administered; there is no effect if the 1:10,000 concentration is used.
- Route of epinephrine chosen for administration can delay the effect. The intramuscular route is now generally preferred over the subcutaneous route.[1]
- If three attempts to establish intravenous access are unsuccessful, an intraosseous needle should be placed.
- Patient could vomit because of intestinal edema with dysfunctional peristalsis.

Repeat Vital Signs

Pulse: 170

Respiratory Rate: 10

Blood Pressure: 62/25

Oxygen Saturation: 85% with 100% oxygen via face mask

Progression

The child has decreased respiratory rate with less audible stridor but worsening retractions. She becomes increasingly limp and unresponsive to painful stimuli. The skin is flushed, but perfusion worsens, with capillary refill rising to 4 seconds peripherally.

ASK YOURSELF

■ **What has happened?**

The child is no longer able to maintain patency of her narrowing airway. The effect of the first dose of epinephrine was insufficient. The drop in respiratory rate is consistent with impending respiratory arrest. The decrease in the volume of the stridor is due to decreased air movement past the obstructed airway. The patient also demonstrates signs of uncompensated shock, including hypotension, poor capillary refill, and altered mental status.

■ **What interventions are needed at this time? What complications might be expected?**

Interventions:

- Epinephrine dose should be repeated, same dose intramuscularly (or, if intravenous/intraosseous access has been established, the child can be given **epinephrine 1:10,000, 0.01 mg/kg or 0.1 mL/kg** IV slow push over 1 to 2 minutes while monitoring for arrhythmias).
- At least one large-bore intravenous line should be placed for volume resuscitation, starting with crystalloid at 20 mL/kg as a rapid bolus.
- Prepare for intubation and for a surgical airway.

Potential Complications:

- Attempt to intubate using an uncuffed 5.0 ET tube with a Miller #2 blade. This is the correct size tube as determined using the Broselow Pediatric Emergency Tape or the formula [16+(age in years)]/4. Unfortunately, the significant airway edema that has developed might make this choice unsuccessful. Visualization of landmarks may be difficult, and having ET tubes that are one and two sizes smaller than calculated is essential.
- The swelling of the larynx can make the orotracheal route impossible, requiring a surgical airway. Surgical consultation should be obtained on an emergency basis for possible emergent tracheostomy. If complete obliteration of the larynx occurs, cricothyrotomy must be performed.

Progression

A 4.0 ET tube is placed successfully and confirmed by the presence of a positive reading on end-tidal CO_2 monitoring.

Repeat Vital Signs

Pulse: 154

Blood Pressure: Unobtainable and peripheral pulses weak

Oxygen Saturation: Unobtainable; patient is wheezing but breath sounds are symmetric

ASK YOURSELF

■ **What interventions are needed at this time? What complications might be expected?**

Interventions:

- Although the respiratory failure has been treated, the systemic nature of anaphylaxis requires further management of the persistent hypotension. A repeat bolus of crystalloid 20 mL/kg is required.
- Obtain central venous access, start **epinephrine 0.1 to 1 mcg/kg/min** continuous IV infusion.
- Administer **diphenhydramine 1 mg/kg** IV and **ranitidine 1 mg/kg** IV (maximum, 50 mg).
- Administer β-agonists via nebulization for persistent wheezing.
- Administer **methylprednisolone 1 to 2 mg/kg** IV.

Potential Complications:

- Loss of intravenous access, requiring repeat doses of epinephrine via the intramuscular or endotracheal route (**1:1,000, 0.1 mg/kg, or 0.1 mL/kg** endotracheally); may be repeated every 3 to 5 minutes
- Dislodgment of ET tube with inability to reintubate due to progressive edema, requiring emergency cricothyrotomy

Progression

Patient opens her eyes, and capillary refill improves to less than 2 seconds.

Repeat Vital Signs

Pulse: 160

Respiratory Rate: Ventilated at 20

Blood Pressure: 90/33

Oxygen Saturation: 100% in 100% oxygen

ASK YOURSELF

■ **What additional complications might be expected?**

Because of the potential for a late-phase response or a biphasic reaction, deterioration due to anaphylaxis can occur even after the patient is stabilized. This is seen in up to one third of patients with severe anaphylactic reactions and often presents with bronchospasm and hypoxia. These reactions also account for up to 50% of deaths.[2,3]

Objectives of This Scenario

1. Recognize the progressive nature of this type of airway obstruction.

This patient presented with the hallmarks of an anaphylactic reaction: the abrupt nature of the respiratory distress (demonstrated by retractions and agitation) associated with the typical skin findings of angioedema and urticaria. Although cutaneous manifestations are typically the initial symptoms of a severe reaction, they can be delayed in a rapidly progressive reaction.[4] Approximately 50% of food-induced anaphylaxis cases have a quiescent interval between initial symptoms and respiratory failure.[2] In one series of fatal anaphylaxis due to food, initial symptoms developed in 3 to 30 minutes, whereas severe respiratory failure required 20 to 150 minutes to develop.[3] Although intubation is rarely necessary in anaphylaxis, those with significant airway edema should be intubated early to prevent complete obstruction.[5]

This child proceeded to develop distributive uncompensated shock with worsening tachycardia and hypotension. Vasodilation, capillary leak, increased vascular permeability, and possible direct cardiotoxic effects on the heart were the causes of cardiovascular collapse. In this scenario, the distributive shock of anaphylaxis may have decreased the relative circulating volume by up to 50%, resulting in the child's significantly low blood pressure. The heart rate increased in compensation.[6]

This case could have had a component of foreign body airway obstruction in addition to the anaphylaxis. The child does not have to consume any of the inciting antigen to have a severe reaction. The rapidity of the onset of symptoms increases the likelihood of a severe reaction, and the physician should be prepared for cardiovascular involvement. With anaphylaxis, an older child may describe a "metallic taste," tingling, or itching as the first sign, but the younger child may demonstrate only agitation or scratching at the tongue, neck, or ears. Food-induced anaphylaxis in the United States has been reported at a rate of 7.6 cases per 100,000 person-years and is estimated to cause 150 to 200 deaths per year.[7]

2. Understand the mechanisms by which anaphylaxis is mediated.

There are three different mechanisms:

- In the classic IgE-mediated mechanism, IgE antibodies formed on initial exposure to an antigen bind to the high-affinity receptors on mast cells and basophils. On re-exposure, the antigen induces bridging of the IgE molecules, leading to degranulation and release of preformed (histamine, tryptase, chymase, and heparin) and rapidly generated (prostaglandin D_2, leukotrienes, platelet-activating factor) mediators. This is the mechanism of most food- and latex-based anaphylaxis.
- Immune complexes can activate the complement cascade, resulting in the formation of anaphylatoxins (C3a and C5a), which can in turn directly trigger the release of mediators from mast cells and basophils.
- Direct release of mediators, non–IgE mediated, can be caused by certain hyperosmolar agents such as mannitol and radiocontrast material.

3. Appreciate the range of symptoms and severity of anaphylaxis.

Anaphylaxis is defined in various ways in the literature and in clinical practice. The spectrum of disease varies from simple urticaria to respiratory failure with uncompensated shock. The treatment varies depending on the severity of the reaction and attributes of the patient. A reaction confined to the skin can reasonably be treated with oral antihistamines for 48 hours. All reactions that involve "the sensation of throat pruritis or tightness, hoarseness or barky cough, difficulty swallowing, dyspnea, wheezing, cyanosis, dysrhythmia, hypotension, or change in mental status"[2] should be treated with intramuscular epinephrine. Intramuscular epinephrine should be used instead of subcutaneous epinephrine because it achieves a higher and more rapid peak concentration.[1]

Studies have shown that there may be a synergistic

effect when combining H_1 and H_2 antihistamines, and therefore intravenous diphenhydramine and intravenous cimetidine or ranitidine should be administered for severe reactions.[8] Treatment with corticosteroids for severe reactions can help ameliorate the late-phase reactions and is recommended.

Recommendations for the length of an observation period after a severe reaction vary, but a period of 8 to 24 hours seems reasonable to ensure there is no late-phase recurrence.[9] Certain populations are at higher risk of severe anaphylactic reactions: those with a history of previous anaphylactic reactions; those with a history of asthma that may be well or poorly controlled; those with allergy to peanuts, nuts, fish, or shellfish; teenaged patients; and patients on β-blockers or angiotensin-converting enzyme inhibitors.[2] Prolonged observation may be necessary for these patients.

References

1. Simons FE. Epinephrine absorption in children with a history of anaphylaxis. *J Allergy Clin Immunol.* 1998:101:33-37.
2. Sampson HA. Anaphylaxis and emergency treatment. *Pediatrics.* 2003;111:1601-1608.
3. Sampson HA, Mendelson L, Rosen JP. Fatal and near-fatal anaphylactic reactions to food in children and adolescents. *N Engl J Med.* 1992;327:380-384.
4. Kemp SF, Lockey RF. Anaphylaxis: a review of causes and mechanisms. *J Allergy Clin Immunol.* 2002;110:341-348.
5. Stenklyft PH, Cataletto ME, Lee BS. The pediatric airway in health and disease. In: Gausche-Hill M, Fuchs S, Yamamoto L, eds. *APLS: The Pediatric Emergency Medicine Resource.* 4th ed. Sudbury, Mass: American Academy of Pediatrics, American College of Emergency Physicians, Jones and Bartlett Publishing Co; 2004:69-71.
6. Fisher MM. Clinical observations on the pathophysiology and treatment of anaphylactic cardiovascular collapse. *Anaesth Intensive Care.* 1986;14:17-21.
7. Lieberman PL. *Middleton's Allergy: Principles and Practice.* 6th ed. Philadelphia, Pa: Mosby; 2003.
8. Kambam JR, Merrill WH, Smith BE. Histamine-2 receptor blocker in the treatment of protamine-related anaphylactoid reactions: two case reports. *Can J Anaesth.* 1989;36:463-465.
9. Kulick RM, Ruddy RM. In: Fleisher GR, Ludwig S, eds. *Textbook of Pediatric Emergency Medicine.* 4th ed. Philadelphia, Pa: Lippincott Williams & Wilkins; 2000:999-1015.

SCENARIO #4

Airway Obstruction

Kathlene E. Bassett, MD

Brief Presenting History

A 3-year-old child who is tracheostomy dependent presents to the emergency department via ambulance from home with severe respiratory distress of acute onset. The tracheostomy tube appears to be in place.

Pediatric Assessment Triangle

Appearance: Agitated, cyanotic

Work of Breathing: Labored respirations, retractions in all fields

Circulation to the Skin: Mottled

Initial Vital Signs

Pulse: 180

Respiratory Rate: 68

Blood Pressure: 120/80

Temperature: 37.6°C (99.7°F) axillary

ASK YOURSELF

- **What should this 3-year-old child weigh?**

  An estimated weight for a 3-year-old child is 14 kg. One can use the length-based Broselow Pediatric Emergency Tape or a pediatric table to determine weight based on age. See Appendix A. Recognize that a child with multiple medical problems might weigh less than the estimated weight because of the chronic health problems.

Physical Examination on Arrival to the Emergency Department

Airway: Tracheostomy tube appears to be in place with mucus present.

Breathing: Severe retractions, poor air movement, breath sounds significantly diminished in all fields, occasional ronchi, no wheezes

Circulation: Skin mottled and cool to the touch, delayed capillary refill of 4 seconds peripherally

Disability: Developmentally delayed, but parents believe he is not as responsive as he is normally and that he is very agitated

ASK YOURSELF

- **What is the initial assessment? What is the patient's physiologic status?**

  This child presents in severe respiratory distress of abrupt onset with cyanosis, retractions, shock, and an altered mental status. This child has impending respiratory failure with compensated shock.

- **What could be causing his distress?**

  There are several reasons a child with a tracheostomy tube can present with respiratory distress. Sudden onset of respiratory distress usually results from an obstruction of the tracheostomy tube, frequently with a mucus plug, or dislodgment of the tracheostomy tube. Respiratory distress with a gradual onset is more frequently related to pulmonary infections or reactive airways disease.[1]

■ **What additional history would help you establish the diagnosis?**

A fever and a change in the color of the tracheostomy secretions suggest an infectious etiology. A prior history of reactive airway disease would suggest an asthma exacerbation. Abrupt onset of respiratory distress is suggestive of a mucus plug or obstruction of the tracheostomy tube.

Additional History and Physical Examination Findings

This child was in a motor vehicle collision 6 months before the presentation and sustained a traumatic brain injury. He had a tracheostomy placed for chronic ventilation. He is currently ventilator dependent only at night and not oxygen dependent. His neurologic status has been steadily improving. Suctioning and repositioning of the tracheostomy tube have already been performed at home with no improvement of symptoms.

Past Medical History: Healthy prior to accident, mild reactive airways disease

Medications: Albuterol inhaler on an as-needed basis

Physical Examination: Oxygen saturation 75% with retractions and cyanosis evident; cardiac and abdominal examinations are unremarkable.

ASK YOURSELF

■ **What interventions are needed at this time?**

Start oxygen 100% O_2 by bag to tracheostomy tube

Determine if the tracheostomy tube is dislodged or obstructed. If the tube is dislodged, immediate replacement is required. If the tube is obstructed, suctioning of the tracheostomy tube is the next step.

1. Suction tracheostomy tube using 3 to 4 mL of normal saline. Repeat once if tolerated.
2. If the suction catheter will not pass through the tracheal opening, the tracheostomy tube must be changed immediately. If the tube has an inner cannula, remove it, as this may alleviate some obstruction.

Place the patient on a cardiorespiratory monitor with pulse oximetry.

Attempt intravenous access and begin fluid resuscitation with **normal saline 20 mL/kg IV.**

Repeat Vital Signs

Pulse: 170

Respiratory Rate: 70

Blood Pressure: 66/40

Oxygen Saturation: 85% on bag-valve-tracheostomy 100% oxygen

Progression

The child continues to have marked respiratory distress despite interventions. Suctioning of the tube was unsuccessful, and bag-valve-tracheostomy ventilation results in minimal air exchange.

ASK YOURSELF

■ **What is the physiologic status now?**

Impending respiratory failure and decompensated shock.

■ **What interventions are needed at this time?**

Remove complete tracheostomy tube and prepare for replacement of tube.

1. Select tracheostomy tube of same size and model as the original tube or smaller. (If not available, use an ET tube of similar caliber.)
2. Place a rolled towel under the patient's shoulders to hyperextend the neck.
3. For a cuffed tracheostomy tube, deflate the balloon with a syringe by drawing air out until the pilot balloon collapses.
4. Remove the inner cannula of the new tube, if present (many pediatric tubes do not have an inner cannula).
5. Cut the cloth or Velcro ties that hold the tube in place.

6. Remove the tracheostomy tube with a slow outward motion.
7. Gently insert the same-size tracheostomy tube with the obturator in place. Point the curve of the tube down. Never force the tube. The tube may be lubricated with water-soluble gel.
8. Securely hold the wings of the tube, remove the obturator, ventilate, and ensure proper tube placement. Then secure the tracheostomy tube.
9. If the tube cannot be inserted easily, attempt to pass a smaller tube.

Repeat fluid bolus of **normal saline 20 mL/kg IV.**

Progression

The stoma is very constricted and you are unable to advance any tracheostomy tube. The child is extremely agitated, and there is a small amount of bleeding at the stoma site.

ASK YOURSELF

■ **What interventions are needed at this time? What complications might be expected?**

Interventions:

- Call for assistance from ENT, surgery, and/or anesthesia if available.
- Pass a small, flexible oxygen tubing or ET suction catheter into the tracheal opening. Once positioned in the trachea, this oxygen tubing can serve as a stylet over which to pass the tracheal tube. Cut the oxygen tubing longer than the cannula length outside the stoma entry, and pass the tube or cannula over it into the airway.
- Attempt insertion of an ET tube into the stoma no more than 1 or 2 inches into the opening. Select an ET tube with an inner diameter that is equal to or smaller than the inner diameter of the last tracheostomy tube attempted. Note that this is a temporizing measure only; an ET tube in a stoma is not stable.
- If you are still unable to insert the cannula, prepare for RSI:
  1. Ventilate oral airway using bag-mask ventilation while covering stoma
  2. #2 Miller blade
  3. Size 4.5 ET tube
  4. **Atropine 0.1 mg/kg IV** (if succinylcholine is used)
  5. **Etomidate 0.3 mg/kg** or **midazolam 0.1 mg/kg IV**
  6. **Succinylcholine 1 to 1.5 mg/kg IV** or **rocuronium 0.6 to 1 mg/kg IV**
- End-tidal CO_2 monitor
- Secure ET tube and place NG or orogastric tube.
- Call for chest radiograph to confirm ET tube placement.
- Obtain arterial blood gases.

Potential Complications:

- RSI is unsuccessful, necessitating a surgical airway.
- Chest radiograph reveals the presence of a pneumomediastium or pneumothorax secondary to a false tracheal passage.

Progression

The patient's disposition depends on the etiology of the respiratory distress. If the tracheostomy tube was obstructed and a replacement tube results in resolution of symptoms, the patient may be discharged to home after an appropriate period of observation. If the patient receives endotracheal intubation, admission to the pediatric ICU is indicated for further treatment and work-up.

Objectives of This Scenario

1. Understand the challenges of caring for the technology-dependent child.

Technology-dependent children rely on medical devices to support bodily functions. Tracheostomy tubes, home mechanical ventilation, urologic catheters, nasogastric feeding tubes, and G-tubes are among the more common devices. These children are frequently managed in the home environment, and when problems occur that cannot be managed at home, they are brought to the emergency department, necessitating that emergency physicians have knowledge of hardware and potential complications.[2]

2. Understand the basics of tracheostomy tubes.

Modern tracheostomy tubes are plastic and are made of polyvinylchloride. They are soft, conform to the trachea, and have little tissue reactivity, causing less tracheal wall irritation than metal tubes. Plastic tubes have essentially replaced metal tracheostomy tubes, except in those children unable to tolerate plastic tubes. Many brands of tubes exist, with the most common being Shiley, Bivona, Holinger, Portex, and Berdeen. Tubes vary in luminal diameter, length, angle of curvature, and presence of inner cannulas, obturators, and cuffs. Unfortunately, tube sizes between brands are not standardized.[1,3]

Uncuffed tracheostomy tubes are more often used in the pediatric population, although older children frequently use cuffed tubes. Tube size is located on the flange or wings of the tube and refers to the inner diameter of the tube. This measurement is standardized among manufacturers, whereas the tube length and outer diameter are not. Tracheostomy tubes range in size from 00 for newborns to 7.0 for older adolescents. Inner cannulas are meant to provide a smooth surface to clear the artificial airway without losing patency. Pediatric tubes from sizes 00 to 4 typically do not have an inner cannula.[2,3]

3. Recognize problems that can occur with tracheostomy tubes and complications associated with replacement.

Mechanical obstruction of the tracheostomy tube and accidental decannulation are the most common complications of tracheostomy tubes in the pediatric age group.[1] The younger the child, the more likely these complications are. Infants have short, thick necks that make them more prone to dislodgement of the tube. Tracheostomy ties may not be snug enough to prevent decannulation. Mechanical obstruction of the cannula, often secondary to mucus plugging, usually occurs secondary to the small internal diameter of the tube in infants and children.

Accidental dislodgment of the tracheostomy tube requires immediate reinsertion of a tube the same size or smaller. If a tracheostomy tube is not available, insert an ET tube with the same diameter. Recognize that the tracheal stoma can constrict making it very difficult to insert any cannula.[4-6]

When a child presents in respiratory distress or with inadequate oxygenation or ventilation and with a tracheostomy tube in place, mechanical obstruction of the tube is most likely.[2] Oxygenation with suctioning should be immediately attempted. Normal saline, 1 to 4 mL, may be instilled into the tube in an attempt to thin secretions, followed by further suctioning. If suctioning does not provide relief of the obstruction, the physician should not hesitate to change the tracheostomy tube.

Complications are rare with replacement of a tracheostomy tube and include bleeding, creation of a false tracheal passage, pneumothorax, pneumomediastinum, and, rarely, perforation of the trachea.[2] False tracheal passages occur in tissue planes outside of the trachea and occur most frequently at 7 to 10 days after tracheostomy placement. Late complications include granuloma or stricture formation at the stoma or where the tip of the tube meets the tracheal wall.[2] An uncommon but dangerous late complication is erosion of the tracheostomy tube into the innominate artery. Bleeding from the tracheostomy frequently results from inadequate humidification but can result from granuloma formation or erosion into an artery.

4. Recognize alternatives to airway management with a tracheostomy tube.

If insertion of a tracheostomy tube is unsuccessful, attempts may be made to place a tracheostomy tube using flexible oxygen tubing as a stylet. If this method is unsuccessful, an ET tube of the same diameter or smaller may be placed into the stoma. It is important to recognize that this is only a temporizing measure. If all of these measures fail, preparations for oral or nasal endotracheal intubation should be made. Bag-mask ventilation of the oral airway while covering the tracheal stoma can be effective while preparation for intubation is made. Recognize that endotracheal intubations may be quite difficult if the tracheostomy was placed for anatomic upper airway abnormalities.

References

1. Fein JA. Approach to the care of the technologically-dependent child. In: Fleischer GR, Ludwig S, eds. *Textbook of Pediatric Emergency Medicine.* 4th ed. Philadelphia, Pa: Williams and Wilkins; 2000:1646-1648,1837.
2. Adirim TA. Children with special health care needs. In: Gausche-Hill M, Fuchs S, Yamamoto L, eds. *APLS: The Pediatric Emergency Medicine Resource.* 4th ed. Sudbury, Mass: American Academy of Pediatrics, American College of Emergency Physicians, Jones and Bartlett Publishing Co; 2004:592-607.
3. Tayal VS. Tracheostomies. *Emerg Med Clin North Am.* 1994;12:707-727.

4. King BR, King C, Coates WC. Critical procedures. In: Gausche-Hill M, Fuchs S, Yamamoto L, eds. *APLS: The Pediatric Emergency Medicine Resource*. 4th ed. Sudbury, Mass: American Academy of Pediatrics, American College of Emergency Physicians, Jones and Bartlett; 2004:699-700.

5. Krug SE. Replacement of a tracheostomy tube. In: Walsh-Sukys MC, Krug SE. *Procedures in Infants and Children*. Philadelphia, Pa: WB Saunders; 1997:56-60.

6. Kallis JM. Replacement of a tracheostomy cannula. In: Henretig FM, King C, eds. *Textbook of Pediatric Emergency Procedures*. Baltimore, Md: Williams and Wilkins; 1997:871-877.

SCENARIO #5

Respiratory Distress

Kristine Rittichier, MD

Brief Presenting History

A 2-year-old boy is brought to the emergency department by his mother who is concerned because, after having "a runny nose" for about 1 week, he suddenly began coughing a lot and developed a fever. She noticed that he also seemed to have trouble breathing.

Pediatric Assessment Triangle

Appearance: Awake, pale, lying in mother's arms, listless, ill appearance, grunting

Work of Breathing: Labored and rapid respirations, retractions in all fields, intermittent wet cough

Circulation to the Skin: Pale with perioral cyanosis, mottled lower extremities

Initial Vital Signs

Pulse: 180

Respiratory Rate: 76

Blood Pressure: 102/70

Temperature: 40.1°C (104.2°F) axillary

ASK YOURSELF

- **How much should this 2-year-old child weigh?**

  An estimated weight for a 2-year-old child is 12 kg. One can use the length-based Broselow Pediatric Emergency Tape or a pediatric table to determine weight based on age. See Appendix A.

- **What is a normal respiratory rate for a 2-year-old?**

  20 to 30 breaths per minute[1]

Physical Examination on Arrival to the Emergency Department

Airway: Patent, moving air freely with dry and tacky mucous membranes

Breathing: Grunting respirations using all accessory muscles, good breath sounds on the right with decreased breath sounds in left lower lobe, crackles and bronchial breath sounds in the left lower lobe, no wheezing on auscultation

Circulation: Pale skin, capillary refill of 4 seconds in lower extremities

Disability: Alert, looking around, but lying listlessly in mother's arms; patient allows you to examine him without complaints.

ASK YOURSELF

- **What is the initial assessment? What is the patient's physiologic status?**

  Patient presents with respiratory distress and compensated shock.

■ **What could be causing his respiratory distress?**

The physical examination findings point to a pulmonary problem. The patient has clinical findings on chest examination with decreased breath sounds, crackles, and rhonchi in the left lower lobe.[2] The differential diagnosis includes pneumonia, reactive airway disease, bronchiolitis, pneumonitis, foreign body, and congestive heart failure.

Additional History and Physical Examination Findings

Past Medical History: Bronchiolitis at age 6 months, otherwise negative

Medications: Acetaminophen

Allergies: None known

Physical Examination: Oxygen saturation 80% in room air. No evidence of trauma. Cardiac examination shows patient is tachycardic without murmur, rub, or gallop. The abdomen is not distended, and there is no hepatomegaly.

ASK YOURSELF

■ **What interventions are needed at this time? What complications might be expected?**

Interventions:

- Administer 100% O_2 via face mask for respiratory distress and hypoxia.
- Place the patient on a cardiorespiratory monitor with pulse oximetry.
- Obtain intravenous access and begin fluid resuscitation with **normal saline 20 mL/kg.**
- Draw blood for CBC, blood culture, and ABGs.
- Order portable chest radiograph.
- **Acetaminophen 15 mg/kg PR.** Because of respiratory distress this patient should be made NPO.

Potential Complications:

- Minimal improvement in oxygenation, necessitating assisted breathing
- If intravenous access not obtained, must consider alternative methods of gaining access such as an intraosseous or central venous line.

Repeat Vital Signs

Pulse: 190

Respiratory Rate: 70

Blood Pressure: 90/50

Oxygen Saturation: 89% with nonrebreather face mask

Progression

The patient's respiratory rate acutely drops to 20, pulse is 190, and he becomes much less responsive. Capillary refill remains at 4 seconds, and there are minimal breath sounds on the left.

ASK YOURSELF

■ **What is happening?**

The drop in respiratory rate indicates fatigue and impending respiratory failure. Worsening hypoxia and hypercarbia are expected, resulting in altered mental status. Worsening color and perfusion indicate a compromised circulatory status, although systolic blood pressure of 90 makes shock compensated for now.

Progression

The patient is having periods of apnea, requiring stimulation to resolve.

Laboratory Test Results

ABGs: pH 7.18, P_{CO_2} 70, P_{O_2} 130, base excess –10 on 10 L oxygen by nonrebreather mask

ASK YOURSELF

■ **What do these ABG results indicate?**

Mixed respiratory (P_{CO_2} 70) and metabolic (base excess –10) acidosis

■ What interventions are needed at this time? What complications might be expected?

Interventions:

- This patient has developed severe respiratory insufficiency and impending respiratory failure. Bag-mask ventilation with 100% O_2 should be started using cricoid pressure. Preparations should be made for RSI.
- Institute intraosseous line placement if intravenous access has not been achieved and then begin volume expansion with **20 mL/kg normal saline.**
- RSI
  1. #1 Miller blade, 4.5 ET tube (have 4.0 and 5.0 ET tubes ready)
  2. Preoxygenation
  3. Cricoid pressure
  4. Midazolam 0.1 mg/kg IV or etomidate 0.3 mg/kg IV or ketamine 2 mg/kg IV (Note: Ketamine provides bronchodilation and may be considered in this situation. Ketamine is a sialagogue. If ketamine is used, consider pretreatment with **atropine** to dry secretions.)
  5. **Rocuronium 0.6 to 1 mg/kg IV** or **succinylcholine 1 to 1.5 mg/kg IV**
- End-tidal CO_2 monitor
- Call for chest radiograph to confirm ET tube placement.
- Secure ET tube and place an NG tube.
- ABG to follow pH and Pao_2.

Potential Complications:

- Vomiting: requires suctioning, especially if cricoid pressure is not used
- Unable to visualize cords if not properly suctioned
- Lack of NG tube results in abdominal distention and impaired ventilation

■ What other complications might be expected for this patient?

- If respiratory support is not initiated, the patient could develop respiratory arrest, leading to severe hypoxia, subsequent bradycardia, and ultimately asystole.
- Mechanical ventilation can lead to barotrauma with resulting pneumothorax and/or pneumomediastinum.
- Empyema and pleural effusions can lead to worsening respiratory failure and decompensation.
- If fluid resuscitation is delayed, the patient could develop decompensated shock leading to cardiovascular collapse.
- Septic shock can result from bacteremia and overwhelming infection.

■ What disposition and additional management would be expected for this patient?

Admission to ICU for continued management of respiratory failure, dehydration, and possible septic shock. The patient must be monitored closely for the development of pleural effusion or empyema, which may require thoracentesis and/or chest tube placement.

Objectives of This Scenario

1. Recognize respiratory distress and impending respiratory failure.

Respiratory distress is present when the patient exhibits abnormal respirations, including tachypnea, bradypnea, apnea, or increased work of breathing. Respiratory failure is defined as the inability to adequately oxygenate and/or ventilate.[1] The early warning signs of respiratory failure include the use of accessory muscles, nasal flaring, grunting, cyanosis, decreased mental status, and decreased air movement on auscultation. Respiratory failure is more common in children than in adults as children tend to fatigue rapidly with acute respiratory infections.

The signs and symptoms of respiratory distress are useful for assessing the severity of illness and dictating the urgency of evaluation and therapy. Monitoring the clinical status of the patient, along with oxygen saturations via a pulse oximeter and ABG samples, will help identify impending respiratory failure.

Oxygen therapy and cardiac monitoring should be initiated immediately for patients in respiratory distress. Intubation should be considered for severe respiratory distress, hybercarbia, and acidosis.

2. Recognize signs and symptoms of pneumonia.

Pneumonia is an acute infection of the lung parenchyma. Classic signs and symptoms include fever, cough, dyspnea, rales, chest pain, and evidence of pulmonary consolidation on physical examination.[2] Viral pneumonias are commonly preceded by an upper respiratory infection. Bacterial pneumonias often have a more abrupt onset with fever, chest pain, cough, and dyspnea. Tachypnea out of proportion to the fever, often without auscultatory findings in the chest, often is a sign of pneumonia in children.

Radiographic evidence of the disease often is sought, although chest radiographic changes can lag behind the clinical presentation. Common accompanying infections include otitis media, pharyngitis, and rhinitis. Abdominal pain and/or ileus often is present.

3. Know common etiologies and treatment of pneumonia.

Most pneumonias in children are caused by viruses, with the most common etiologies being respiratory syncytial virus, human parainfluenza virus, influenza virus, and adenovirus. Viral pneumonia has its peak incidence between ages 3 and 5 years.

Bacterial pneumonias usually run a more acute and virulent course. They result in higher mortality (2 to 3 times) and morbidity rates than do viral pneumonias.[3] *Pneumococcus* is the leading cause of community-acquired bacterial pneumonia and carries a high risk of morbidity and mortality.[3-5] Other common bacterial pathogens include *Staphylococcus aureus*, *Moraxella catarrhalis*, *Haemophilus influenzae*, and *Neisseria meningitidis* in the preschool-age children and *Mycoplasma pneumoniae* and *Chlamydia pneumoniae* in school-age children and adolescents.[5]

The widespread use of the Hib vaccine has rendered *H. influenzae* serotype b an uncommon cause of pneumonia in the vaccinated population. In the same respect, there is hope that the use of the conjugated pneumococcal vaccine will have an impact on the incidence of this pneumonia in the future.

Antibiotics should be initiated in patients suspected of having a bacterial illness. Even if a viral infection is suspected, antibiotics should be strongly considered in a patient who appears toxic or who experiences respiratory distress or failure, until culture results are available. The initial choice of treatment should be based on the common etiologies for the patient's age group, immunologic status, immunization status, and, eventually, the known bacterial sensitivities.

4. Manage common complications of pneumonia.

Common complications of pneumonia include copious secretions, atelectasis, bronchospasm, wheezing, hypoxia, hypercarbia, pleural effusions, empyema, air leaks (pneumothorax, pneumomediastinum), respiratory failure, dehydration, and septic shock. Supportive measures include 100% oxygen, suctioning, nebulized β_2-agonists, and intravenous fluids. More aggressive therapies include thoracentesis with fibrinolysis,[6,7] chest tube placement, open thoracotomy, and vigorous support of shock with isotonic fluids and vasopressors as indicated.

References

1. Stenklyft PH, Cataletto ME, Lee BS. The pediatric airway in health and disease: respiratory failure. In: Gausche-Hill M, Fuchs S, Yamamoto L, eds. *APLS: The Pediatric Emergency Medicine Resource.* 4th ed. Sudbury, Mass: American Academy of Pediatrics, American College of Emergency Physicians, Jones and Bartlett Publishing Co; 2004:95.
2. Lynch T, Platt R, Gouin S, et al. Can we predict which children with clinically suspected pneumonia will have the presence of focal infiltrates on chest radiographs? *Pediatrics.* 2004;113:186-189.
3. Miller MA, Ben Ami T, Daum R. Bacterial pneumonia in neonates and older children. In: Taussig LM, Landau LI, eds. *Pediatric Respiratory Medicine.* St Louis, Mo: Mosby; 1999:595-664.
4. Tan TQ. Update on pneumococcal infections of the respiratory tract. *Semin Respir Infect.* 2002;17:3-9.
5. Gaston B. Pneumonia. *Pediatr Rev.* 2002;23:132-140.
6. Feola GP, Shaw LC, Coburn L. Management of complicated parapneumonic effusions in children. *Tech Vasc Interv Radiol.* 2003;6:197-204.
7. Ozcelik C, Inci I, Nizam O, et al. Intrapleural fibrinolytic treatment of multiloculated postpneumonic pediatric empyemas. *Ann Thorac Surg.* 2003;76:1854-1858.

SCENARIO #6

Respiratory Distress

Frank L. Overly, MD

Brief Presenting History

A 9-year-old boy presents with 6 hours of difficulty breathing and increased wheezing. Parents report that this was preceded by 2 days of cough and congestion. They have administered four albuterol nebulizer treatments at home with minimal improvement.

Pediatric Assessment Triangle

Appearance: Anxious, alert, sitting upright and calling out for his mother

Work of Breathing: Labored, with long expiratory phase, nasal flaring, and suprasternal, intercostal, and subcostal retractions

Circulation to the Skin: Extremities warm with normal color

Initial Vital Signs

Pulse: 165

Respiratory Rate: 50

Blood Pressure: 115/72

Temperature: 37.2°C (99°F) orally

Physical Examination on Arrival to the Emergency Department

Airway: Patent, moving minimal air

Breathing: Using accessory muscles, leaning forward, prolonged expiratory phase with barely audible, tight wheezes bilaterally

Circulation: Capillary refill less than 2 seconds with good pulses

Disability: Eyes open, calling for his mom, responds to questions but able to speak only two- or three-word sentences

ASK YOURSELF

- **How much should this 9-year-old boy weigh?**

  An estimated weight for a 9-year-old child is 25 kg. One can use the length-based Broselow Pediatric Emergency Tape or a pediatric table to determine weight based on age. See Appendix A.

- **What is the initial assessment? What is the patient's physiologic status?**

  This patient presents with moderate to severe respiratory distress from an asthma exacerbation.

- **What additional history and physical findings would be helpful?**

  Details concerning previous asthma exacerbations (frequency, triggers, medications, hospitalizations, ICU admissions, need for intubation) are helpful in determining the severity of this patient's condition and the historical progression of his symptoms.

  Oxygen saturation, mental status, accessory muscle use, breath sounds, peak flow (unless patient is in severe distress), and pulsus paradoxus are useful in assessing respiratory status.

■ **What is the differential diagnosis of respiratory distress in this patient?**

The patient's history, presentation, and physical findings make it most likely that this is an acute asthma exacerbation. Pneumonia is unlikely with no history of fever and diffuse wheezing instead of focal crackles. Metabolic acidosis and cardiac disease also can cause tachypnea and respiratory distress, but this patient does not have findings consistent with either of these. Metabolic acidosis can result in gasping respirations (Kussmaul breathing) to reduce the CO_2 and help raise the pH. Congestive heart failure is more common in patients with a history of heart disease and usually presents with one or more of the following: gallop rhythm, dyspnea, bilateral crackles, and hepatomegaly.

Additional History and Physical Examination Findings

He has been afebrile and eating and drinking less and has had two episodes of posttussive emesis. His sister has an URI.

Past Medical History: His asthma is usually triggered by URIs, occurring approximately five times a year. He has been hospitalized four times, once in the ICU, but never intubated. His last admission was 3 months earlier.

Medications: Albuterol inhaler or nebulizer, Flovent (fluticazone), Singulair (montelukast)

Allergies: Penicillin; response is hives.

Physical Examination: Oxygen saturation 85% in room air, peak flow is 80 L/min (less than 50% of predicted or personal best); neck supple with trachea midline, no crepitus; auscultation reveals regular rhythm, no murmurs, rubs, or gallops; abdomen is soft, with no masses or organomegaly.

ASK YOURSELF

■ **What interventions are needed at this time? What complications might be expected?**

Interventions:

- Administer 100% O_2 by face mask for respiratory distress.
- Place the patient on a cardiorespiratory monitor with pulse oximetry.
- **Albuterol 2.5 to 5 mg** and **ipratropium bromide 0.25 to 0.5 mg nebulizer** treatment.
- Obtain intravenous access and initiate fluid resuscitation with **normal saline 20 mL/kg if needed.** *Note:* Most patients with asthma are managed without an intravenous line; fluids and steroids are administered by mouth. The determination must be made as to whether the patient is able to take liquids by mouth safely or if respiratory distress necessitates intravenous access and NPO status.
- **Methylprednisolone 2 mg/kg IV** or **prednisone 2 mg/kg PO.**
- Consider **epinephrine 1:1,000, 0.1 mL/kg IM/SQ** (maximum dose 0.5 mL). *Note*: Subcutaneous epinephrine was used extensively before the widespread use of nebulized bronchodilators; it is used much less commonly now.

Potential Complications:

- Intravenous access unobtainable
- Minimal improvement in oxygen saturation with supplemental oxygen

Repeat Vital Signs

Pulse: 180

Respiratory Rate: 52

Blood Pressure: 125/78

Oxygen Saturation: 89% on 100% oxygen with nebulizer

Progression

Patient is increasingly anxious and having more difficulty breathing. Verbalizing, "I can't breathe."

ASK YOURSELF

■ **What is the physiologic status now?**

Impending respiratory failure due to status asthmaticus.

■ **What interventions are needed at this time? What complications might be expected?**

Interventions:

- If there is no intravenous line, consider **epinephrine 1:1,000, 0.1 mL/kg SQ/IM** (maximum dose 0.5 mL) or **terbutaline 0.01 mg/kg IM/SQ** (maximum dose 0.5 mg).
- Continuous **albuterol nebulizer 10 to 20 mg/hr.**
- **Terbutaline 4 to 10 mcg/kg IV bolus** over 15 to 20 minutes and **0.5 to 6.0 mcg/kg/min continuous IV infusion**

OR

- Consider **aminophylline 6 mg/kg IV bolus** and **1 mg/kg/hr continuous IV infusion** (recommended dose varies with age).
- Consider **magnesium sulfate 25 to 40 mg/kg** IV (maximum dose, **2 g**).
- Consider **heliox** (helium/oxygen mixture).
- Draw blood for ABGs, order beside chest radiograph.

Note: The point of this question is for the reader to recognize that, despite aggressive inhaled bronchodilator and corticosteroid therapy, the patient's condition has deteriorated. Therapy must at this time be accelerated to prevent respiratory failure. Please see Objectives of This Scenario for a more in-depth discussion.

Potential Complications:

Depending on the drug regimen that is selected, side effects that can be expected include vomiting, tachycardia, and increased anxiety. Aminophylline (theophylline) can result in seizures in higher doses. Magnesium can result in significant peripheral vasodilation and hypotension.

Laboratory Results

ABG: pH 7.21, Pco_2 60, Pao_2 80 on 100% oxygen

Repeat Vital Signs

Pulse: 185

Respiratory Rate: 18

Blood Pressure: 120/78

Oxygen Saturation: 89% on 100% oxygen with nebulizer

Progression

The child is no longer calling for his mom and responds only to painful stimuli. He continues to have significant retractions and expiratory wheezing, but his respiratory rate is decreasing, and he remains hypoxic on continuous albuterol.

ASK YOURSELF

■ **What do the ABG results and progression described above indicate?**

An increasing Pco_2 and low Pao_2 indicate ineffective ventilation and oxygenation and impending respiratory failure. When combined with decreasing respiratory rate and diminished level of consciousness, the diagnosis of impending respiratory failure is confirmed. It is important to always consider the clinical picture when interpreting blood gas results.

■ **When is the appropriate time to intubate a patient in status asthmaticus?**

Management of status asthmaticus is far from standardized. As mentioned, actual medications and dosages vary among institutions and care providers. Identifying status asthmaticus early and implementing aggressive therapy are the goals to prevent respiratory failure. One scoring system to predict impending respiratory failure is reviewed in Objectives of This Scenario. Most medical providers agree that depressed mental status in conjunction with other signs of respiratory failure (decreased work of breathing, increasing Pco_2, and decreasing Pao_2) are good predictors of impending respiratory failure and the need for intubation.

■ **What interventions are needed at this time? What complications might be expected?**

Interventions:

- Institute RSI.
  1. Mac blade #2, 6.0 cuffed ET tube
  2. Preoxygenation
  3. Cricoid pressure
  4. **Atropine 0.02 mg/kg IV** (if bradycardic) or **glycopyrrolate 0.04 mg/kg IV** as a drier (anti-sialagogue) for ketamine

5. **Ketamine 2 mg/kg IV** as a sedative because of its bronchodilatory effects
6. **Rocuronium 0.6 to 1 mg/kg IV** or **succinylcholine 1 to 1.5 mg/kg IV**

- End-tidal CO_2 monitor
- Call for chest radiograph to confirm ET tube placement.
- Secure ET tube and place an NG tube.

Potential Complications:

- Vomiting, requiring suctioning, especially if no cricoid pressure used
- Failed intubation if no suctioning or improper positioning
- Lack of NG tube results in abdominal distention and impaired ventilation
- If ET tube is not secured, the patient is extubated.

Progression

Patient improves gradually after the intubation is successfully completed, but he is difficult to ventilate.

Repeat Vital Signs

Pulse: 165

Respiratory Rate: Bagged ventilation

Blood Pressure: 115/70

Oxygen Saturation: 90% on 100% oxygen

ASK YOURSELF

■ What interventions are needed at this time? What complications might be expected?

Interventions:

- Bag ventilation at a reduced rate with a prolonged expiratory time
- Monitor closely for potential complications of positive-pressure ventilation in a patient with asthma: development of pneumothorax or tension pneumothorax.

Potential Complications:

- If bagging too rapidly or forcefully, oxygen saturations fall and heart rate falls as the patient develops a tension pneumothorax requiring percutaneous anterior needle decompression or chest tube placement. If not recognized and treated appropriately, bradycardia can lead to asystole.
- Hypokalemia from prolonged continuous albuterol is a potential complication.

■ What disposition and additional management would be expected for this patient?

Admit to ICU for continued β-agonist therapy and ventilatory management.

Objectives of This Scenario

1. Recognize and aggressively manage status asthmaticus.

Asthma affects 10% of American children, and the morbidity and mortality from this disease have been increasing for unknown reasons.[1-3] Status asthmaticus is a life-threatening condition from which hundreds of children die each year.[1] Individuals with a history of severe asthma exacerbations are at an increased risk for the development of status asthmaticus. The patient in this scenario has a history of multiple hospitalizations and one admission to the pediatric ICU, which should raise the level of concern. This patient presented with hypoxia, dyspnea, difficulty talking, and a peak flow less than 50% of expected. The fact that he had minimal wheeze with auscultation is indicative of severe obstruction. The amount of wheezing does not correlate with the severity of the asthma exacerbation.[4] As these patients are treated and the obstruction decreases, the degree of wheezing will actually increase.

As mentioned earlier, management of status asthmaticus is far from standardized, but practice guidelines from expert panels agree that prompt and aggressive management is essential. First-line therapy should include oxygen; nebulized bronchodilators, including an anticholinergic; and systemic corticosteroids.[5,6] Hydration status is also important in this patient population and should be assessed and treated in every case of status asthmaticus. Route of administration is determined by level of respiratory distress. Adequate hydration is important to keep secretions less viscous.[2]

As in all critically ill patients, frequent reassessment is essential. If initial interventions are not successful, terbutaline or theophylline bolus and continuous infusion, magnesium sulfate, or heliox can be used and may prevent respiratory failure.[7,8]

2. Recognize impending respiratory failure.

Predicting respiratory failure is challenging in status asthmaticus. Wood et al[9] developed a scoring system to assist in predicting which patients might need ventilatory support through mechanical ventilation. The scoring system below (Table 1) is based on signs and symptoms of airway obstruction, accessory muscle use, and cerebral function.

A score of more than 5 suggests impending respiratory failure, and a score of more than 7 is consistent with respiratory failure. Hypercarbia with an arterial Pco_2 of more than 60 is another sign of severe obstruction, although the decision to intubate a child with asthma should not depend on the results of a blood gas analysis alone. It should be based on the complete clinical picture, including mental status, work of breathing, oxygenation, and response to therapy. The patient in this case had an asthma score of more than 7 before receiving intubation. His falling respiratory rate and depressed mental status are ominous signs of respiratory failure.

3. Understand the inherent complications of intubation and ventilation of the asthmatic patient.

The decision to intubate a child with asthma can be a difficult one and is recommended only in the face of impending respiratory failure. Because asthma is a disease of the lower airways, securing the upper airway with an ET tube does not correct the underlying problem and may actually increase bronchospasm and lead to other complications. When intubating a patient who has asthma, ketamine is often chosen for sedation because of its bronchodilatory properties. Atropine or glycopyrrolate may be given before ketamine to reduce secretions.

Once the patient is intubated, the goal is to provide pressures adequate to overcome airway obstruction but low enough to prevent barotrauma. The barotrauma from positive-pressure ventilation can lead to air leaks, pneumothoraces, and pneumomediastinum. Strategies that are used to reduce barotrauma when mechanical ventilation is needed for status asthmaticus include the following.[10]

- Continued sedation and muscle relaxation are important to reduce dyssynchrony between the patient and the ventilator
- In general, the use of smaller tidal volumes and a slower-than-normal respiratory rate is recommended.
- Prolonged expiratory time reduces air trapping.
- Permissive hypercapnea, Pco_2 in the range of 40 to 90, is allowed in an attempt to reduce complications inherent to more aggressive ventilation required to normalize the Pco_2.

If barotrauma does result in a tension pneumothorax, having equipment prepared for needle decompression and/or chest tube placement will save time and possibly prevent additional morbidity.

Table 1.
Clinical Scoring System for the Diagnosis of Respiratory Failure. From: Wood DW, Downes JJ, Lecks HI. A clinical scoring system for the diagnosis of respiratory failure: preliminary report on childhood status asthmaticus. *Am J Dis Child.* 1972;123:227. Reprinted with permission.

Variable	**0**	**1**	**2**
Pao_2	70 mm Hg to 100 mm Hg in air	≤70 mm Hg in air	≤70 mm Hg in 40% oxygen
Cyanosis	None	In air	In 40% oxygen
Inspiratory breath sounds	Normal	Unequal	Decreased to absent
Accessory muscles used	None	Moderate	Maximal
Expiratory wheezing	None	Moderate	Marked
Cerebral function	Normal	Depressed or agitated	Coma

References

1. Dieckmann RA. Pediatric assessment. In: Gausche-Hill M, Fuchs S, Yamamoto L, eds. *APLS: The Pediatric Emergency Medicine Resource.* 4th ed. Sudbury, Mass: American Academy of Pediatrics, American College of Emergency Physicians, Jones and Bartlett Publishing Co; 2004:40.

2. Werner HA. Status asthmaticus in children: a review. *Chest.* 2001;199:1913-1929.

3. Hale EH. Endocrine emergencies. In: Fleisher GR, Ludwig S, eds. *Textbook of Pediatric Emergency Medicine.* 4th ed. Philadelphia, Pa: Lippincott Williams & Wilkins; 2000:999-1006.

4. McFadden ER Jr, Kiser R, DeGroot WJ. Acute bronchial asthma: relations between clinical and physiologic manifestations. *N Engl J Med.* 1973;288:221-225.

5. Murphy S, Second Expert Panel on the Management of Asthma. *Highlights of the National Asthma Education and Prevention Program Expert Panel report 2: Guidelines for the Diagnosis and Management of Asthma.* NIH publication No. 97-4051A, May 1997. Available at: http://www.nhlbi.nih.gov/guidelines/asthma/index.htm. Accessed: December 10, 2004.

6. National Asthma Education and Prevention Program Expert Panel. Executive summary. In: *NAEPP Expert Panel Report, Guidelines for the Diagnosis and Management of Asthma—Update on Selected Topics 2002.* NIH publication No. 02-5075. Available at: http://www.nhlbi.nih.gov/guidelines/asthma/asthgdln.htm. Accessed: December 10, 2004.

7. Ream RS, Loftis LL, Albers GM, et al. Efficacy of IV theophylline in children with severe status asthmaticus. *Chest.* 2001;119:1480.

8. Blitz M, Hughes R. Aerosolized magnesium sulfate for acute asthma. *Cochrane Database Syst Rev.* 2002.

9. Wood DW, Downes JJ, Lecks HI. A clinical scoring system for the diagnosis of respiratory failure: preliminary report on childhood status asthmaticus. *Am J Dis Child.* 1972;123:227-228.

10. Dworkin G, Kattan M. Mechanical ventilation for status asthmaticus in children. *J Pediatr.* 1989;114:545-549.

SCENARIO #7

Respiratory Distress

Dewesh Agrawal, MD

Brief Presenting History

A 9-day-old infant is brought to the emergency department with his parents via ambulance because he has increasing difficulty breathing. The parents report that he's also not been feeding well.

Pediatric Assessment Triangle

Appearance: Weak, pale

Work of Breathing: Tachypnea, with retractions

Circulation to the Skin: Pale, mottled, with cyanotic extremities

Initial Vital Signs

Pulse: 182

Respiratory Rate: 84

Blood Pressure: Not obtainable

Temperature: 37°C (98.6°F) rectally

Physical Examination on Arrival to the Emergency Department

Airway: Patent, moving air freely, no secretions in the mouth

Breathing: Tachypnea with moderate accessory muscle use; symmetric breath sounds with occasional crackles

ASK YOURSELF

- **Where would you best feel for the pulse on an infant?**

  The brachial and femoral arteries are the best places to feel pulses on infants. Carotid pulses are difficult to palpate in infants given their relative absence of a neck.

Circulation: Skin is mottled and cool to touch. Capillary refill time is 3 seconds centrally and 4 seconds peripherally. Femoral pulses are not palpable. Right brachial pulse is 1+/2+.

Disability: Listless, cries weakly with painful stimulation

ASK YOURSELF

- **What is the initial assessment? What is the patient's physiologic status?**

  This is an infant with a gradual onset of respiratory distress who presents with decompensated shock (diminished pulses, unobtainable blood pressure, altered mental status).

- **What is the differential diagnosis of respiratory distress and shock in this patient?**

  The differential diagnosis of respiratory distress and shock includes primary pulmonary, infectious, cardiac, hematologic, and metabolic causes. Primary pulmonary causes include severe bronchiolitis, pneumonia, and a large pneumothorax. Primary infectious causes include pulmonary infections, sepsis, and meningitis. Primary cardiac causes in infants usually are congenital heart defects with secondary congestive heart failure and cardiogenic shock due to either volume overload (overcirculation) or obstructive lesions.[1,2] Hematologic causes include extreme anemia, hemoglobin dyscrasias such as methemoglobinemia, and hypovolemia (with resultant hypovolemic shock). Primary metabolic causes in an infant include hypoglycemia and inborn errors of metabolism predisposing to metabolic acidosis (with secondary respiratory compensation and tachypnea) and hyperammonemia (which can directly stimulate the medullary respiratory center).

- **What further history would help you establish the diagnosis?**

The presence of fever at home would help establish an infectious cause of shock such as sepsis or meningitis. The presence of cough, rhinorrhea, or other signs of a respiratory tract infection would help establish an infectious cause for the respiratory distress, such as bronchiolitis or pneumonia. A history of severe diarrhea or volume loss would help establish hypovolemia as the cause of shock. A history of using well water for feeds or the use of oxidizing medications can help establish the diagnosis of methemoglobinemia. A history of significant blood loss at birth or blood type incompatibility between mother and infant would help diagnose anemia. A history of an abnormal newborn screen may help diagnose an inborn error of metabolism.

Additional History and Physical Examination Findings

The infant was fine until about 2 days ago, when parents initially noted increased respiratory rate with feeds, which has progressed into continually increased difficulty breathing. The infant is no longer able to feed because of respiratory distress. There also has been a decreased number of wet diapers. There is no history of fever, cough, or diarrhea. The child has been exclusively breastfed.

Past Medical History: Healthy full-term infant with unremarkable prenatal course and no history of birth complications or ABO incompatibility, normal newborn screen

Medications: None

Physical Examination: Anterior fontanel soft and sunken, no stridor or significant wheezing, symmetric breath sounds bilaterally with crackles, tachycardia with gallop rhythm, systolic ejection-type murmur over left precordium radiating to back, abdomen soft, hepatomegaly with liver edge palpable 4 cm below costal margin, no palpable femoral pulses but weakly palpable right brachial pulse

ASK YOURSELF

- **What is the most likely diagnosis?**

Taken together, the history of gradual onset of respiratory distress with difficulty feeding, the presentation consistent with shock, and the physical examination notable for gallop rhythm and systolic murmur radiating to back with absent lower extremity pulses strongly suggest cardiogenic shock due to critical coarctation of the aorta.

- **What interventions should be made at this time? What complications might be expected?**

Interventions:

- Administer 100% O_2 via face mask.
- Place the patient on a cardiorespiratory monitor with pulse oximetry.
- Attempt to establish intravenous access, and administer bolus of **10 mL/kg normal saline** slowly over 30 to 60 minutes. Fluid resuscitation is indicated given the history of poor feeding and decreased urine output suggesting likely dehydration. However, overaggressive fluid resuscitation can be deleterious in cardiogenic shock.[1]

Potential Complications:

- Good pulse oximetric tracing cannot be obtained in any extremity except the right upper extremity and the right ear.
- The initial attempt at intravenous access is unsuccessful; only three drops of blood is obtained.

- **Why is pulse oximetry not successful when applied to the legs or left arm?**

  Coarctation of the aorta occurs near the site of the ductus arteriosus. The blood supply to the legs, and often the left arm, is compromised compared with that of the right arm, which arises from the aorta proximal to the coarctation or ductus.

- **What should you do with the three drops of blood?**

  Perform rapid bedside glucose determination

- **What initial laboratory tests should you obtain after intravenous access is established?**

  ABGs, CBC, blood culture, electrolytes, and urinalysis/urine culture

- **What other initial studies should you obtain?**

  Chest radiography and ECG

Initial Laboratory Results

ABG (from left radial artery): pH 7.10, Pco_2 26, Po_2 45, HCO_3^- 8, base excess –21

Rapid Bedside Glucose Determination: 67 mg/dL

CBC: WBCs 14,000, hematocrit 42, platelets 348

Electrolytes: Na^+ 134 mEq/L, K^+ 4.8 mEq/L, Cl^- 102 mEq/L, HCO_3^- 8 mEq/L, BUN 12 mg/dL, creatinine 0.9 mg/dL, glucose 69 mg/dL

Urinalysis: Clear, yellow, specific gravity 1.025, otherwise negative

Initial Diagnostic Studies

Chest Radiography: Large heart with pulmonary vascular congestion

ECG: Sinus tachycardia, normal axis and intervals, voltage criteria for right ventricular hypertrophy, otherwise normal for age

ASK YOURSELF

- **Explain this patient's acid-base status.**

  This patient is acidotic (pH below 7.4). He has a primary severe metabolic acidosis (very low HCO_3^-) and a compensatory respiratory alkalosis (Pco_2 less than 40). The patient's anion gap [$Na^+ - (Cl^- + HCO_3^-)$, or $134 - 102 + 8 = 24$] is quite elevated (above 12), suggesting an anion gap metabolic acidosis. In this case, the patient most likely has lactic acidosis secondary to poor peripheral perfusion and resultant ischemia from his critical coarctation.[3]

Repeat Vital Signs (after fluid bolus)

Pulse: 190

Respiratory Rate: 88

Blood Pressure (in right upper extremity): 36/20

Oxygen Saturation: 94% in right hand, not obtainable in left foot

Progression

Despite fluid administration, patient continues with persistent hypotension and signs of cardiogenic shock with low blood pressure, obtainable only in the right upper extremity.

ASK YOURSELF

- **What interventions are needed at this time? What complications might be expected?**

  Interventions:

  - Initiate **prostaglandin E_1** therapy at **0.05 to 0.1 mcg/kg/min** (maximum dosage, 0.4 mcg/kg/min) to attempt reopening of the ductus arteriosus. If the diagnosis of a ductal-dependent lesion is suspected, prostaglandins should be started immediately without waiting for definitive diagnosis to be made, because maintenance of patency of the ductus can be a lifesaving intervention.
  - Initiate inotropic support with **dopamine at 5 to 10 mcg/kg/min** (may titrate upward to 20 mcg/kg/min).

- Attempt central venous access for continued inotropic support.
- Consider bicarbonate therapy to reverse the metabolic acidosis.
- Consult a pediatric cardiologist.

Potential Complications:

- Apnea secondary to prostaglandin E_1 therapy is common. Be prepared to intubate after initiation of prostaglandin E_1 therapy or electively intubate before initiation of therapy, especially if the patient is to be transported to another institution.
- Dopamine extravasation through peripheral intravenous line and resultant tissue necrosis

Objectives of This Scenario

1. Become familiar with the differential diagnosis of respiratory distress and shock in an infant.

This infant presented with respiratory distress and shock, which is an emergency situation that requires aggressive evaluation and resuscitation. One must be careful when evaluating neonates with respiratory distress to look beyond the pulmonary system for other potential causes. The differential diagnosis of respiratory distress and shock in an infant is quite broad, as indicated earlier.

2. Understand the presentation and pathophysiology of critical coarctation of the aorta.

About 0.8% to 1% of infants have congenital heart defects.[2,3] Coarctation of the aorta occurs in 6% to 10% of all patients with congenital heart defects.[4-6] It is a discrete narrowing of the aorta that classically occurs (in 98% of cases) just distal to the origin of the left subclavian artery at the ductus arteriosus (juxtaductal coarctation).[5-7] In the first few days of life before the patent ductus arteriosus (PDA) has closed, the PDA serves to widen the juxtaductal area of the aorta and to provide temporary relief from the obstruction. In essence, right ventricular blood is ejected through the PDA to supply the descending aorta and the lower half of the body. Congestive heart failure develops during infancy in only about 10% to 20% of patients with coarctation of the aorta. These more severe coarctations that present in infancy are referred to as *critical coarctations of the aorta*.[7]

In symptomatic infants, there is a classic triad of history of poor feeding, dyspnea, and poor weight gain. These infants present with signs of acute circulatory shock in the first few weeks of life as the ductus closes. They are usually oliguric, acidotic, and pale and in respiratory distress.[3-6] The classic sign of coarctation of the aorta is a disparity in pulsation and blood pressure in the arms and legs. A systolic ejection-type murmur often is heard along the left sternal border at intercostal spaces 3 and 4. The murmur is usually well transmitted to the left intrascapular area. On chest radiography, cardiac enlargement and pulmonary vascular congestion are noted in infants with severe coarctation. The ECG in neonates is usually normal, but it can demonstrate right or biventricular hypertrophy. Echocardiographic examination is usually diagnostic.[5-8]

In neonates with severe coarctation of the aorta, closure of the ductus arteriosus often results in hypoperfusion of the lower half of the body, acidosis, and rapid deterioration that includes shock. The obstruction presents a significant increase in afterload to the left ventricle, which may rapidly decompensate. These patients should be administered an infusion of prostaglandin E_1 to reopen the ductus and to reestablish adequate lower extremity blood flow. This helps to alleviate the acidosis and to reduce the myocardial workload.[5,7] Surgery remains the treatment of choice for critical coarctation of the aorta in the neonate; however, catheter-based balloon angioplasty with or without stenting may be considered.[4-6]

3. Recognize and manage ductal-dependent cardiac lesions and neonatal cardiogenic shock.

Congenital heart defects are generally well tolerated during fetal life. However, postnatal circulatory changes have marked effects on the clinical presentation and course of the congenital heart disease in the neonatal period. Severe obstructions to either pulmonary or systemic blood flow may be unmasked only after the first few days of life, when the ductus arteriosus begins to close.[2]

An infant with a severe obstructive left-sided cardiac lesion (critical coarctation of the aorta, critical aortic stenosis, or hypoplastic left heart syndrome) typically presents with acute illness in the newborn period. These lesions depend on a PDA for systemic blood flow. When the ductus closes, congestive heart failure, shock, acidosis, oliguria, and renal failure promptly ensue. Cardiac function is further impaired by the severe metabolic acidosis that develops in response to systemic hypoperfusion. In obstructive right-sided cardiac lesions (severe pulmonary valve stenosis or pulmonary atresia), pulmonary blood flow depends on a PDA. When the ductus closes, the resultant lack of adequate pulmonary blood flow causes severe systemic hypoxemia and secondary acidosis.[2]

When congestive heart failure and cardiogenic shock present in neonates, they are most likely secondary to obstructive congenital heart defects. Common manifestations of congestive heart failure in the neonate include (in approximate order of frequency) tachypnea, tachycardia, liver enlargement, cardiomegaly, pulmonary crackles, feeding difficulties, diaphoresis, and gallop rhythm. Because manifestations of heart failure and primary pulmonary diseases may be similar in infants, it can be difficult to recognize congestive heart failure.[1-3,9] Poor perfusion is the hallmark of congestive heart failure in infants, manifested by pallor, mottling, cyanosis, and prolonged capillary refill time.[9] Echocardiography is the best way to confirm the diagnosis of congenital heart disease.[2]

Medical management of cardiogenic shock in neonates is directed toward improving cardiac performance, augmenting peripheral perfusion, reducing acidosis, and improving oxygenation. Supplemental oxygen and slow intravenous rehydration are expected initial interventions. Inotropic support with dopamine, dobutamine, or epinephrine is frequently required as well.[1] For obstructive ductal-dependent cardiac lesions, the use of prostaglandin E_1 therapy to reopen the PDA is essential in neonates to improve oxygenation and acidosis until definitive repair can be performed.[2] The major side effect of prostaglandin E_1 is apnea. If the infant does not require intubation for the initial resuscitation, then one must be ready to intubate if the addition of prostaglandin E_1 leads to apnea. Additional adverse effects of prostaglandin E_1 include fever, hypotension, and seizure.[3]

References

1. Fitzmaurice L, Gerardi MJ. Cardiovascular system. In: Gausche-Hill M, Fuchs S, Yamamoto L, eds. *APLS: The Pediatric Emergency Medicine Resource.* 4th ed. Sudbury, Mass: American Academy of Pediatrics, American College of Emergency Physicians, Jones and Bartlett Publishing Co; 2004:136-140.
2. Lee C, Mason LJ. Pediatric cardiac emergencies. *Anesthesiol Clin North Am.* 2001;19:287-308.
3. Schamberger MS. Cardiac emergencies in children. *Pediatr Ann.* 1996;25:339-344.
4. Park MK, Troxler RG. *Pediatric Cardiology for Practitioners.* 4th ed. St. Louis, Mo: Mosby; 2002:165-172.
5. Rothman A. Coarctation of the aorta: an update. *Curr Probl Pediatr.* 1998;28:37-60.
6. Beekman RH. Coarctation of the aorta. In: Allen HD, Clark EB, Gutgesell HP, et al, eds. *Moss and Adams' Heart Disease in Infants, Children, and Adolescents.* 6th ed. Philadelphia, Pa: Lippincott Williams & Wilkins; 2001:988-1010.
7. Behrman RE, Kliegman RM, Jenson HB, eds. *Nelson Textbook of Pediatrics.* 17th ed. Philadelphia, Pa: WB Saunders; 2004:1518-1520.
8. Grover G, Silverman BK. Problems in the very early neonate. In: Fleisher GR, Ludwig S, eds. *Textbook of Pediatric Emergency Medicine.* 4th ed. Philadelphia, Pa: Lippincott Williams & Wilkins; 2000:1231-1232.
9. O'Laughlin MP. Congestive heart failure in children. *Pediatr Clin North Am.* 1999;46:263-273.

SCENARIO #8

Respiratory Distress

Mark G. Roback, MD

Brief Presenting History

A 4-year-old boy is brought to the emergency department by his mother with a history of increased trouble breathing over the past 2 days; he is much worse today. He has a history of asthma but has experienced no improvement with use of his albuterol inhaler.

Pediatric Assessment Triangle

Appearance: Pale, sleepy

Work of Breathing: Deep and labored respirations

Circulation to the Skin: Mottled and pale

Initial Vital Signs

Pulse: 160

Respiratory Rate: 54

Blood Pressure: 96/58

Temperature: 37.6°C (99.7°F) axillary

ASK YOURSELF

- **How much should this 4-year-old boy weigh?**

  An estimated weight for a 4-year-old child is 16 kg. One can use the length-based Broselow Pediatric Emergency Tape or a pediatric table to determine weight based on age. See Appendix A.

Physical Examination on Arrival to the Emergency Department

Airway: Patent, moving air freely, no secretions in the mouth

Breathing: Using all accessory muscles, deep gasping-type respirations, inspiratory and expiratory phases equally prolonged, lungs clear bilaterally without wheeze

Circulation: Skin mottled and cool to the touch, capillary refill time 3 seconds centrally and 4 seconds peripherally

ASK YOURSELF

- **Where would you best feel the central pulse in this 4-year-old patient?**

  The femoral pulse is 1+/2+. Carotid pulses may be difficult to palpate in younger children who have chubby necks.[1]

Disability: Eyes closed, patient responds to voice, pupils equal and reactive to light 4 mm to 2 mm bilaterally

ASK YOURSELF

- **What is the initial assessment? What is the patient's physiologic status?**

  This patient presents with respiratory distress, compensated shock, and altered mental status.

- **What additional history and physical findings would help to distinguish between compensated and decompensated shock?**

  History: Estimation of urine output provides an indication of renal perfusion. In this case, information about urine output could be misleading.

  Physical Examination: Assess heart rate and perfusion of the skin: color, temperature, and capillary refill time. Quality of pulses should be assessed as well as mental status. Hypotension, defined as blood pressure below the fifth percentile for age, is diagnostic of decompensated shock and has not yet occurred in this patient. Blood pressure readings within the "normal" range for age do not rule out compensated shock—hypotension is a late finding in pediatric shock.

- **What is the differential diagnosis of respiratory distress in this patient?**

  The differential diagnosis includes pulmonary, cardiac, and metabolic etiologies. The patient has a history of asthma, but physical examination findings are not consistent with an asthma exacerbation. Although this patient has no fever, cough, or crackles on physical examination that would point towards pneumonia or pneumonitis, these finding can be subtle in younger children, and these diagnoses should be considered. An oxygen saturation should be obtained in any patient with tachypnea. Hypercapnia also can cause tachypnea and would not be detected using the pulse oximeter; however, this patient's asthma is probably not sufficiently significant to make him retain CO_2, and he does not have another underlying lung disease, such as cystic fibrosis.

  Heart disease can lead to respiratory distress, but there is no history of heart disease in this patient and the physical examination has no findings typical of heart disease or failure such as gallop rhythm or murmur, crackles, hepatomegaly, or peripheral edema.

  The body compensates for a metabolic acidosis by increasing the respiratory rate and tidal volume, which results in deep, gasping respirations (Kussmaul breathing). This type of breathing increases the exhalation of CO_2, which raises the pH. It is important to note, however, that the respiratory compensation in metabolic acidosis is typically insufficient to normalize pH.

Additional History and Physical Examination Findings

The patient has experienced a 4-lb weight loss over the past 2 weeks and has been drinking and urinating more than usual. He does not have a fever, symptoms of upper respiratory infection, or complaints of pain.

Past Medical History: Asthma, otherwise negative

Medications: Albuterol inhaler as needed

Physical Examination: Oxygen saturation 98% in room air. No evidence of head trauma. The breath has a fruity odor. The abdomen is nondistended and soft but nonspecifically tender to palpation.

ASK YOURSELF

- **What interventions are needed at this time? What complications might be expected?**

  Interventions:

  - Administer 100% O_2 via face mask for respiratory distress despite adequate pulse oximeter reading
  - Place the patient on a cardiorespiratory monitor with pulse oximetry.
  - Attempt intravenous access and begin fluid resuscitation with **normal saline 20 mL/kg.**

  Potential Complications:

  - Intravenous access attempt is unsuccessful, three drops of blood is obtained.

- **What should you do with the three drops of blood?**

  Perform rapid bedside glucose determination

- **What is the differential diagnosis of altered mental status in this patient?**

  This patient presented with respiratory distress and compensated shock of unknown etiology. Respiratory distress can be associated with hypoxia or hypercapnia and result in altered mental status. The shock state and impaired perfusion to the brain also may account for the altered mental status. Inadvertent or intentional toxic ingestion is another important etiology to consider, especially when the cause is not readily apparent. Metabolic etiologies include hypoglycemia, diabetic ketoacidosis (DKA), electrolyte derangements, and inborn errors of metabolism. Infection, specifically CNS infection, is less likely in this afebrile patient, but it remains an important cause of altered mental status in pediatrics. Although there is no history of trauma, head injury and child abuse also are important causes to consider.

Repeat Vital Signs

Pulse: 152

Respiratory Rate: 16

Blood Pressure: 70/40

Oxygen Saturation: 100% on oxygen via face mask

Progression

Increasingly less responsive, respirations become agonal

ASK YOURSELF

■ What is the physiologic status now?

Impending respiratory failure and decompensated shock

Laboratory Test Results: Glucose above 500

ASK YOURSELF

■ What is the most likely diagnosis?

DKA

■ What interventions are needed at this time? What complications might be expected?

Interventions:

- Severe respiratory insufficiency and impending respiratory failure have developed in this patient. Initiate BMV with 100% oxygen using cricoid pressure. Preparations should be made for RSI.
- Attempt intraosseous line placement if attempts at intravenous access have not been successful, and institute volume expansion with **20 mL/kg normal saline.**
- RSI
  1. #2 Miller blade, 5.0 ET tube
  2. Preoxygenation
  3. Cricoid pressure
  4. **Etomidate 0.3 mg/kg IV** or **midazolam 0.1 mg/kg IV**
  5. **Rocuronium 0.6 to 1 mg/kg IV** or **succinylcholine 1 to 1.5 mg/kg IV**
- End-tidal CO_2 monitor
- Chest radiograph to confirm ET tube placement
- Secure the ET tube and place an NG tube.
- ABGs are used to follow pH; venous blood gases would be acceptable in this patient if there is no concern for hypoxia.
- **Regular insulin 0.1 units/kg/hr** IV drip
- Additional laboratory tests: Electrolytes, calcium, phosphorous, magnesium

Potential Complications:

- Vomiting requires suctioning, especially if cricoid pressure is not used.
- Inability to visualize cords if not properly suctioned
- Lack of NG tube results in abdominal distention and impaired ventilation.

■ What would you expect this patient's ABG to be, and why?

This patient's ABG is likely to demonstrate severe metabolic acidosis with a compensatory respiratory alkalosis. The results are pH 7.04, Pco_2 8, Po_2 110, base excess –14: metabolic acidosis (pH 7.04, base excess –14) with respiratory compensation (Pco_2 8).

■ Should the acidosis be treated with bicarbonate?

No. Recent studies suggest an association between bicarbonate therapy in DKA and the development of cerebral edema.[2] Bolus bicarbonate would be considered only in the case of symptomatic hyperkalemia or acidosis severe enough to result in hemodynamic instability.

■ What other complications might be expected for this patient?

- If fluid resuscitation is delayed, the patient could develop cardiovascular collapse secondary to severe hypovolemia and decompensated shock.
- Patients with DKA have a total-body potassium deficit. Initial serum potassium levels can be normal or low as a result of attempts at cellular compensation for severe metabolic acidosis. If potassium is not added to intravenous fluids, the patient could become severely hypokalemic.[3]
- Cerebral edema and increased intracranial pressure are possible.

■ What disposition and additional management would be expected for this patient?

Admission to an ICU is required for continued management of dehydration/hypovolemia, ketoacidosis, and respiratory failure and to follow closely for possible cerebral edema/increased intracranial pressure.

Objectives of This Scenario

1. Recognize respiratory distress as a presenting sign of DKA.

This patient presented with progressed signs and symptoms of ketoacidosis with Kussmaul breathing, ketotic breath, and altered mental status. After initial assessment of patent airway and adequate breathing, respiratory distress is managed with 100% oxygen. This patient has a history of reactive airway disease but, despite presenting with respiratory distress, does not have impaired air entry, an expiratory phase that is prolonged compared with the inspiratory phase, or expiratory wheezes that would be expected with a reactive airway disease exacerbation.

DKA occurs in 25% to 40% of patients with new-onset type 1 diabetes mellitus. Known diabetics experience hospital visits for DKA at a rate of 8 to 15 episodes per 100 person-years.[4]

A history of polyuria, polydypsia, and weight loss despite hyperphagia evident over a period of days to weeks supports the diagnosis of DKA. The diagnosis is confirmed with an elevated rapid glucose determination and a urinalysis with glucose and ketones. Symptoms can be precipitated by an intercurrent illness, typically a mild infection, which can confuse the picture. Abdominal pain with distention and guarding, hyperpnea, and enuresis can be mistakenly attributed to an acute abdomen, pneumonia, or a behavioral disorder. Causes of DKA in known diabetics include intercurrent illnesses (31%), omission or incorrect administration of insulin injections (69%), and, less commonly, bacterial infections (13%).[5]

2. Be able to initiate management of DKA.[3,6]

The goals of therapy in DKA are as follows:

- Correct dehydration
- Reverse acidosis and ketosis
- Restore normoglycemia and correct electrolyte abnormalities
- Avoid complications of therapy

Patients presenting in severe DKA typically are at least 10% dehydrated. Isotonic fluids are indicated in all cases, and more aggressive fluid resuscitation might be necessary to reverse hypotension. Replacing vascular volume is essential to improve tissue perfusion and reduce acidosis. An initial bolus of **10 to 20 mL/kg normal saline** or **Ringer lactate** over the first hour is typically recommended, with the remaining fluid deficit being replaced slowly over the next 48 hours using three fourths to one half normal saline. Overzealous replacement of fluids should be avoided.

A continuous infusion of **regular insulin (0.08 to 0.1 Units/kg/hr)** is usually required, along with frequent (at least every hour) glucose level determinations. Once the glucose level has fallen to approximately 250 mg/dL, dextrose should be added to the intravenous fluids.

All patients with DKA have a total-body potassium deficit; therefore, potassium, and possibly phosphate (which is almost always depleted, but which depletion is of uncertain clinical significance), should be added to intravenous fluids after the initial normal saline bolus.

As mentioned earlier, the use of sodium bicarbonate to treat acidosis in DKA can be associated with cerebral edema and is not recommended.

3. Recognize and manage cerebral edema and increased intracranial pressure.

A devastating complication of DKA is cerebral edema and increased intracranial pressure, the etiology of which is poorly understood. This complication is most likely a result of the underlying pathophysiology of DKA, degree of illness, time of presentation, and some therapeutic interventions. Glaser et al[2] found that patients with low P_{CO_2} and high BUN at the time of presentation and patients treated with bicarbonate were at an increased risk for cerebral edema.

The best treatment for increased intracranial pressure in DKA is prevention. The emergency physician must watch patients with DKA closely for changes in consciousness or responsiveness, which might signal the onset of cerebral edema and increased intracranial pressure. The fluid management of these patients must be meticulously monitored. Sodium bicarbonate should not be routinely administered. Once increased intracranial pressure is evident, therapy includes RSI, hyperventilation, and mannitol. See the section on increased intracranial pressure in the Evaluation and Management chapters.

References

1. Dieckmann RA. Pediatric assessment. In: Gausche-Hill M, Fuchs S, Yamamoto L, eds. *APLS: The Pediatric Emergency Medicine Resource.* 4th ed. Sudbury, Mass: American Academy of Pediatrics, American College of Emergency Physicians, Jones and Bartlett Publishing Co; 2004:40.
2. Glaser N, Barnett P, McCaslin I, et al. Biochemical and therapeutic factors associated with the development of cerebral edema in children with diabetic ketoacidosis. *N Engl J Med.* 2001;344:264-269.
3. Kappy MS, Bajaj L. Recognition and treatment of endocrine/metabolic emergencies in children: part I. *Adv Pediatr.* 2002;49:245-272.
4. Rewers A, Chase HP, Mackenzie T, et al. Predictors of acute complications in children with type 1 diabetes. *JAMA.* 2002;287:2511-2518.
5. Flood RG, Chiang VW. Rate and prediction of infection in children with diabetic ketoacidosis. *Am J Emerg Med.* 2001;19:270-273.
6. Hale EH. Endocrine emergencies. In: Fleisher GR, Ludwig S, eds. *Textbook of Pediatric Emergency Medicine.* 4th ed. Philadelphia, Pa: Lippincott Williams & Wilkins; 2000:1093-1098.

SCENARIO #9

Respiratory Distress

Debra L. Weiner, MD, PhD

Brief Presenting History

A 15-year-old girl presents with crampy, intermittent, abdominal pain. She is screaming with paroxysms of pain.

Pediatric Assessment Triangle

Appearance: Alert, anxious, diaphoretic, uncomfortable, obviously suffering from intermittent severe pain

Work of Breathing: Regular breathing punctuated by periods of intermittent deep respirations with prolonged expirations

Circulation to the Skin: Pink, well perfused

Initial Vital Signs

Pulse: 120

Respiratory Rate: 24

Blood Pressure: 140/88

Temperature: 38.8°C (102°F) oral

ASK YOURSELF

- **Are these vital signs normal for this patient? If not, what are normal values?**

  This girl presents with tachycardia, hypertension, tachypnea, and fever. The mean heart rate for a 15-year-old girl is 60 to 80. The range for normal systolic and diastolic blood pressures for this age is 100/60 to 140/90. Normal resting respiratory rate for this age is 12 to 16 (see Appendix A).

Physical Examination on Arrival to the Emergency Department

Airway: Patent, irregular respirations

Breathing: Breath sounds clear on both sides of chest with good air entry

Circulation: Capillary refill time less than 2 seconds

Disability: Eyes open and pupils reactive to light; when not in pain, patient responds appropriately and follows commands; when in pain, she screams and does not respond to commands.

ASK YOURSELF

- **What is the initial assessment? What is the patient's physiologic status?**

  The patient is intermittently in marked distress. She is hemodynamically stable and has intact mental status. She has no obvious respiratory distress except when in great pain.

- **What are the differential diagnoses for this patient?**

  Possibilities include gastrointestinal problems (infection/food poisoning, gastritis, ulcer, cholecystitis, pancreatitis, and constipation), genitourinary problems (renal stone), obstetric/gynecologic problems (ovarian torsion, ovarian cyst, ectopic pregnancy, spontaneous abortion, and active labor), and drug withdrawal or acute ingestion.

■ **What additional history would help you establish the diagnosis?**

Helpful elements of the initial history would include the onset, duration, location, and character of the pain. A history of similar pain, any associated symptoms, any history of recent travel, ingestions, possible food poisoning, or ill contacts should also be elicited. Finally, in this 15-year-old girl, a menstrual and sexual history would be important.

■ **Which of the differential diagnoses should be confirmed or ruled out first?**

Given that the patient is not obviously in shock or severe respiratory distress, confirming active labor is most important, particularly if labor might result in a preterm birth.

■ **What approaches should be taken to rule out pregnancy with active labor?**

The physical examination should be directed toward the following: palpation of the fundus and any fetal parts; visualization or palpation of a dilated cervix; or crowning of fetal head, buttocks, or rarely a foot. A fetal heart monitor would detect fetal heart tones. A urine pregnancy test would confirm pregnancy as well.

■ **Which other diagnoses would be essential to next address?**

Priority should be given to conditions that represent surgical emergencies such as ectopic pregnancy (this is a true surgical emergency with risk of death) and ovarian torsion (rapid surgical detorsion provides the best opportunity for salvaging the ovary).[1]

Additional History and Physical Examination Findings

The pain was of abrupt onset about 8 hours earlier. It is in the lower abdomen, radiating to the back. It has been severe, crampy, and intermittent but has gradually intensified. She has never had similar pains. She denies a sore throat, nausea, vomiting, diarrhea, urinary frequency, dysuria, hematuria, and vaginal bleeding. She denies trauma, ingestions, recent travel, and ill contacts.

Past Medical History: No major medical problems. Her last menstrual period was at least 6 or 7 months earlier. She has never been pregnant before but reports being sexually active.

Medications: None

Allergies: None known

Physical Examination: Her cervix is 10 cm dilated and 100% effaced; the head of a neonate is visible.

ASK YOURSELF

■ **What interventions are needed at this time? What complications might be expected?**

Interventions:

- Consult obstetric and neonatology services, if available.
- Set up for emergency department delivery. Although delivery in a delivery room is preferable, unless transfer to a delivery room without delivery en route is certain, the child should be delivered in the emergency department. Important supplies and equipment to have available include the following[2]:
  - Warming table or heat lamp
  - Gauze or towel, bulb syringe, suction catheters hooked up to suction source
  - Self-inflating or anesthesia bag 450 to 750 mL, in-line manometer, face mask, oxygen tubing, oxygen source, 8 French orogastric tube, 20-mL syringe
  - Towels and blankets, preferably warmed
  - ET tubes 2.5 to 4.0 French, stylet, Miller #0 and #1 laryngoscope blades, tape, end-tidal CO_2 monitor
  - Umbilical line kit, intravenous catheters 22 and 24 gauge
  - Normal saline or lactated Ringer
  - Resuscitation medications: **Epinephrine 1:10,000 IV, naloxone 0.4 or 1 mg/mL, bicarbonate 4.2% solution**

Potential Complications:

- Fetal distress
- Meconium aspiration
- Nuchal cord
- Shoulder dystocia
- Multiple gestation

■ **What factors in the maternal history make this a high-risk pregnancy, delivery, and resuscitation?**

Maternal age younger than 16 years, lack of prenatal care, prolonged rupture of membranes with possible premature rupture of membranes, hypertension (pregnancy induced or baseline), and possible infection manifested by fever

■ **What are the appropriate steps for delivery and neonatal resuscitation in this case?**

- Deliver the head.
- Suction the nose and mouth at perineum.
- Deliver the body, and keep the neonate at the level of the mother to avoid fetal-maternal or maternal-fetal transfusion resulting in anemia or polycythemia.
- Clamp and cut the cord.
- Place the infant on a warming table or under a heat lamp.
- Clear the airway, and suction mouth and nose as necessary.
- Dry the infant, and remove wet linens.
- Gently stimulate the baby.

Pediatric Assessment Triangle of Newborn Infant

Appearance: Small, obviously preterm, cyanotic, no meconium in amniotic fluid

Work of Breathing: Irregular gasping respirations with retractions

Circulation to the Skin: Cyanotic, no meconium staining

Initial Vital Signs of Newborn Infant

Pulse: 40

Respiratory Rate: 16

Blood Pressure: Not obtained

Temperature: 36°C (96.8°F) axillary

Physical Examination of Newborn Infant After Delivery

Airway: Patent, no facial deformity, palate intact

Breathing: Irregular and gasping; breath sounds coarse and wet

Circulation: Cyanotic mucous membranes and extremities

Disability: Small infant with minimal tone, no grimace, appears to be preterm with estimated gestation 29 to 31 weeks

ASK YOURSELF

■ **What is the initial assessment of the newborn? What is the newborn's physiologic status?**

Preterm newborn with respiratory distress, bradycardia, and poor perfusion.

■ **What are potential complications in infants associated with premature delivery that require intervention in the immediate perinatal period?**

Respiratory depression due to immature respiratory drive, underdeveloped respiratory musculature, and decreased lung compliance can require support ranging from oxygen alone to intubation/ventilation and treatment with surfactant.

Infection/sepsis also must be considered, especially in the face of premature rupture of membranes. Cultures of the blood and urine with empiric administration of antibiotics must be considered.[2]

■ **What is the preferred method of heart rate assessment during neonatal resuscitation?**

Cardiac auscultation or palpation of umbilical pulse.

■ **What interventions are needed at this time? What complications might be expected?**

Interventions:

- Initiation of positive-pressure ventilation (PPV) via bag-mask with 100% oxygen at 40 to 60 breaths per minute without chest compressions (or 30 breaths/min if chest compressions also are delivered). Pressure should be delivered sufficient to cause chest rise.

Potential Complications:

- Equipment failure
- Pneumothorax

Repeat Vital Signs

Pulse: 40

Respiratory Rate: 50 delivered via PPV

Blood Pressure: Not obtained

Progression

Minimal improvement in color, and mucous membranes no longer cyanotic; otherwise no significant change.

ASK YOURSELF

- **What are the indications for chest compressions during neonatal resuscitation?**

  Heart rate less than 60 despite PPV with 100% oxygen for 30 seconds.[3]

- **What are the two accepted techniques for delivering chest compressions in neonates? What are the potential complications?**

  The first technique is the *two-thumb technique*, in which hands encircle the chest and thumbs are adjacent or superimposed on the lower third of the sternum. The other is the *two-finger technique*, in which a hand is placed perpendicular to the sternum and two of the middle fingertips are placed on the lower third of the sternum. In general, the two-thumb technique is preferred.[4] The optimal initial rate is 90 compressions/min at a depth of one third the anteroposterior diameter of the chest. Ratio of compressions to breaths is 3:1, with each series of three compressions beginning during the exhalation phase of a breath.[3]

  Potential Complications:

  - Liver laceration
  - Rib fracture

Repeat Vital Signs of Newborn Infant

Pulse: 50

Respiratory Rate: 50

One-Minute Apgar Score: 3

ASK YOURSELF

How is the Apgar Score calculated?[5]

Score	0	1	2
Appearance **(color)**	Pale, blue	Peripherally blue	Pink
Pulse (heart rate)	Absent	Less than 100	Greater than 100
Grimace (response to nasal suction)	No response	Grimace	Cough or sneeze
Activity (muscle tone)	Limp	Some flexion	Active movement
Respiratory effort	Absent, irregular	Slow, weak cry	Good

Progression

Infant's color and tone are very slowly improving. The abdomen is distended.

ASK YOURSELF

- **What interventions are needed at this time?**

  The infant is not responding optimally. Heart rate remains unacceptably low, and tone is poor. Chest compressions are still required. The following are the next key steps:

  - Intubate with a #0 Miller blade and a 2.5 ET tube. The tip should be slightly above the carina; the appropriate depth can be estimated as 3 times the internal diameter of the ET tube, so in this case it is 7.5 cm.
  - Place an orogastric or NG tube to evacuate air from the stomach.
  - Obtain a chest radiograph to confirm tube placement and to evaluate lung fields.
  - Place an umbilical vein catheter. The umbilical vein is usually the most easily cannulated vessel. Alternative sites are peripheral or scalp vein. Rarely, an intraosseous line is necessary.
  - Administer **epinephrine 1:10,000 0.1 to 0.3 mL/kg IV**. Epinephrine may be given via the ET tube (can insert catheter through ET tube to ensure deep delivery); dose is **0.1 mg/kg delivered via 0.1 mL/kg of 1:1,000**), repeat every 3 to 5 minutes as needed. Administration

via ET tube should be followed by **0.5 to 1 mL of normal saline.**

Repeat Vital Signs of Newborn Infant

Pulse: 120

Respiratory Rate: 30 with assisted ventilation

Blood Pressure: 40/25

Temperature: 36°C

Progression and Disposition

The infant is pink, and the tone has improved. An evaluation for sepsis is initiated, and antibiotics are delivered. Serum glucose is checked. The child is then moved to a neonatal ICU.

Objectives of This Scenario

For a general discussion of equipment and techniques relevant to neonatal delivery and resuscitation, please refer to the section on neonatal resuscitation in the Evaluation and Management section.

1. **Recognize that two patients are involved.**

The key to this scenario is early recognition that the patient is pregnant and that delivery is imminent. Each patient should be attended to by a separate team when staff is available. Appropriate equipment for newborn delivery must be available.

2. **In the emergency delivery of the newborn, recognize the risks to the newborn due to maternal factors.**

Pregnant patients with active contractions should be transported to appropriate facilities with labor and delivery wards whenever possible. If delivery is imminent, transfer is contraindicated. The team must then assess the condition of the mother and fetus and prepare for delivery. In the absence of continuous fetal monitoring, the condition of the mother and pattern of labor are the best indicators of fetal condition. Maternal history (to determine risk factors for potential perinatal complications) should include estimated dates of confinement, maternal infection, hypertension, diabetes, medication and drug use, and complications with prior pregnancies.

Factors associated with premature delivery include:

- Maternal: age ≤16 years or ≥35 years, acute or chronic illness, abdominal trauma, poor nutrition, severe dehydration, hypertension, cigarette smoking, drug use, no prenatal care.
- Fetal: intrauterine growth retardation (IUGR), multiple gestation, infection, anomalies, demise of the fetus.
- Placental: previa, abruption, premature or prolonged rupture of membranes, placentitis.
- Uterine: cervical incompetence, uterine rupture, uterine abnormality, foreign body, chorioamnionitis, polyhydramnios.

3. **Provide emergency resuscitation of the newborn.**

Resuscitation of the newborn, as with any other pediatric patient, is based on attention to the ABCs. Radiant heat loss secondary to their large body surface area relative to mass makes newborns, especially premature newborns, particularly susceptible to hypothermia, and they must be kept dry and warm using a radiant heat source. Immediately after deliver, dry the newborn off with warm towels, clear the airway, and stimulate if the newborn is not spontaneously breathing. If the heart rate is at or above 100, if the respirations are spontaneous, and if the neonate is pink, no further intervention is necessary. If the child has central cyanosis, administer 100% free-flow oxygen. PPV is required if the child has not improved after 30 seconds. Heart rates below 60 require chest compressions. Indications for endotracheal intubation include ineffective PPV, prolonged requirement for PPV, or if an ET tube is required as a route for delivery of medications. Epinephrine (for asystole or bradycardia) and naloxone (for maternal narcotic within last 4 hours in a nonaddicted mother) may be administered via the ET tube if there is no vascular access. Bicarbonate for severe acidosis is too caustic to be administered via an ET tube and must be administered intravascularly.[3] Use of room air (21% O_2) as opposed to 100% O_2 for newborn resuscitation remains controversial.[3,6]

Factors associated with delayed response of newborn to resuscitation include the following:

- Hypoxia
- Acidosis
- Hypothermia

- Hypoglycemia
- Neurologic injury

References

1. Houry D, Abbott JT. Ovarian torsion: a fifteen-year review. *Ann Emerg Med.* 2001;38:156-159.

2. Burchfield DJ, Boychuk RB. Neonatal emergencies. In: Gausche-Hill M, Fuchs S, Yamamoto L, eds. *APLS: The Pediatric Emergency Medicine Resource.* 4th ed. Sudbury, Mass: American Academy of Pediatrics, American College of Emergency Physicians, Jones and Bartlett Publishing Co; 2004:477-493.

3. Kattwinkel J, Niermeyer S, Nadkarni V, et al. Resuscitation of the newly born infant: an advisory statement from the Pediatric Working Group of the International Liaison Committee on Resuscitation. *Resuscitation.* 1999;40:71-88.

4. Chest compressions (Lesson 4). In: Kattwinkel J, Denson S, Zaichkin J, eds. *Textbook of Neonatal Resuscitation.* Dallas, Tex: American Heart Association and American Academy of Pediatrics; 2000.

5. Apgar V. A proposal for a new method of evaluation of the newborn infant. *Curr Res Anesth Analg.* 1953;32:260-267.

6. Saugstad OD, Rootwelt T, Aalen O. Resuscitation of asphyxiated newborn infants with room air or oxygen: an international controlled trial: the Resair 2 study. *Pediatrics.* 1998;102:e1.

SCENARIO #10

Apnea

Charles G. Macias, MD, MPH

Brief Presenting History

A 4-month-old girl, who had been a 30-week premature infant, is brought to the emergency department by her parents with a 2-day history of cough, nasal congestion, and "funny" breathing with wheezing.

Pediatric Assessment Triangle

Appearance: Listless, weakly crying

Work of Breathing: Obvious distress, rapid shallow breaths

Circulation to the Skin: Pale but well perfused

Initial Vital Signs

Pulse: 178

Respiratory Rate: 68

Blood Pressure: 90/54

Temperature: 39.1°C (102.4°F) rectally

ASK YOURSELF

- **How much should this 4-month-old girl weigh?**

  An estimated weight for a 4-month-old child is 3.5 kg. One can use the length-based Broselow Pediatric Emergency Tape or a pediatric table to determine weight based on age. See Appendix A.

- **How much of this patient's tachycardia might be explained by her fever?**

  Although multiple factors can contribute to tachycardia, in children aged 2 to 12 months, each 1°C (1.84°F) rise in body temperature can cause an increase of about 10 beats/min (actually 9.6 beats/min) in pulse rate.[1] This patient's tachycardia cannot be completely explained by fever.

Physical Examination on Arrival to the Emergency Department

Airway: Secretions in mouth and nares but good air movement

Breathing: Severe intercostal retractions, nasal flaring, with abdominal excursions; coarse ronchi with scattered expiratory wheezes throughout both lung fields

Circulation: Skin not mottled; capillary refill time 2 seconds centrally

ASK YOURSELF

- **What is the initial assessment? What is the patient's physiologic status?**

  This patient is in severe respiratory distress with impending respiratory failure as demonstrated by marked tachypnea and severe intercostal retractions. At this point, there is no evidence of significant circulatory compromise.

■ What is the most likely diagnosis?

The patient's history of an upper respiratory tract infection prodrome followed by cough and wheezing is most consistent with a diagnosis of bronchiolitis. The physical examination findings of tachypnea, nasal congestion, scattered wheezing, and ronchi support this diagnosis. Although the etiology of bronchiolitis is varied, respiratory syncytial virus (RSV) is the most common virus that causes bronchiolitis in infants.[2]

■ What is the significance of "abdominal breathing?"

In the young infant, the abdominal musculature and diaphragmatic movement are used to breathe; thus, abdominal excursions along with chest wall rise may be used to clinically assess breathing. Infants can use the synergistic motion of the diaphragm and intercostal muscles to maximize the performance of these muscles to prevent the development of apnea.[3] Alternatively, paradoxical inward abdominal motion during inspiration can be a sign of respiratory distress. Paradoxical abdominal motion in the presence of dyspnea, accessory muscle use, nasal flaring, and/or grunting can herald respiratory failure.

Additional History and Physical Examination Findings

The mother states that within the past 6 hours, the child has had two episodes during which she stopped crying, her face turned blue, and her chest stopped moving. The episodes lasted 30 seconds and resolved when the mother picked up the child.

Medications: None

Allergies: None known

Physical Examination: Oxygen saturation 94% in room air

ASK YOURSELF

■ Why should the treating physician be concerned about a history of apnea?

In general, the risk factors associated with a complicated hospitalization course for children with RSV include hypoxia on admission, a history of apnea or respiratory arrest, and pulmonary consolidation.[4] Patients at risk for severe RSV disease include those with prematurity, complex congenital heart disease, chronic lung disease, neuromuscular disease, and metabolic disorders. In the emergency department presentation, the characteristics most strongly associated with more serious illness include ill appearance, oxygen saturation of less than 95%, gestational age of younger than 34 weeks, respiratory rate of 70 or greater, atelectasis on chest radiograph, and age younger than 3 months, with pulse oximetry being the single best predictor of more severe disease.[5]

■ What interventions are needed at this time?

- A determination must be made as to whether this rate of tachypnea and pattern of breathing are sustainable or whether this child is in impending respiratory failure. If breathing is deemed maintainable, then attempts to improve the airway and breathing should ensue.
- Suction thick nasal secretions.
- Administer oxygen via nasal cannula.
- Place the patient on a cardiorespiratory monitor with pulse oximetry.
- Obtain intravenous access. Children with bronchiolitis can have a marked increase in respiratory rate, thereby increasing metabolic rates and water consumption. These increases, often coupled with a history of poor feeding because of less efficient feeding and poor breathing and swallowing coordination, can manifest with clinical evidence of dehydration, necessitating intravenous hydration.[2,6] If the patient's decreased fluid intake, increased work of breathing, and increased metabolic rate are profound, then the child with bronchiolitis can present in hypovolemic shock. Moreover, it is essential to establish intravenous access when there is the potential for impending respiratory failure.

Repeat Vital Signs

Pulse: 60

Respiratory Rate: 0

Oxygen Saturation: 70%

Progression

The patient has become apneic.

ASK YOURSELF

- **What interventions are needed at this time? What complications might be expected?**

Interventions:

- Stimulate the infant with tactile stimulation.
  - If *unresponsive*, more definitive airway management intervention must ensue.
  - If *responsive*, a trial of β-agonist with a nebulized mask treatment with **albuterol (0.25 mL**, which is equivalent to 2.5 mg) or nebulized **epinephrine 0.5 mL of 1:1,000** while continuing oxygen delivery can cause sufficient bronchodilation and stimulation to improve the patient's breathing.

Potential Complications:

- The patient can continue to have persistent episodes of apnea, which suggests a more central mechanism of apnea. In this instance, bronchodilatory effects of β-agonist therapy alone will not resolve the patient's airway and breathing compromise, and a definitive airway must be established (BMV and endotracheal intubation).
- The patient may respond to stimulation but can continue to have marked retractions and wheezing, indicating an escalation of respiratory distress. A trial of nebulized **epinephrine** may be attempted (**0.5 mL of 1:1,000**) while continuing oxygen delivery. See "Objectives of This Scenario" for a discussion of the use of albuterol and epinephrine in the management of bronchiolitis.

Repeat Vital Signs

Pulse: 90

Respiratory Rate: 78

Oxygen Saturation: 86% in oxygen via face mask

Progression

The patient is responsive to stimuli but has marked tachypnea and retractions. Despite prior attempts at nebulized therapy, she continues to have a rising respiratory rate with decreasing oxygen saturation.

ASK YOURSELF

- **What interventions are needed at this time? What complications might be expected?**

Interventions:

- Assist breathing with BMV and 100% oxygen. Prepare for RSI.
- RSI
  1. #0 Miller blade, 3.5 ET tube
  2. Cricoid pressure
  3. **Midazolam 0.1 mg/kg IV** or **etomidate 0.3 mg/kg/IV**
  4. **Rocuronium 0.6 to 1 mg/kg** IV (*Note:* other muscle relaxants [succinylcholine or vecuronium] may be used, but if the patient is apneic with minimal response, a muscle relaxant may not be required.)
  5. Confirm ET tube placement with end-tidal CO_2 monitor, chest radiograph
  6. Secure ET tube, place an NG tube.

Potential Complications:

- Inability to visualize the vocal cords due to marked secretions; suction will be critical to the success of the procedure.
- Bradycardia if atropine is not used
- Vomiting if cricoid pressure is not applied

Repeat Vital Signs

Pulse: 145

Oxygen saturation: 99% postintubation

ASK YOURSELF

- **What disposition and additional management would be expected for this patient?**

  Admission to the pediatric ICU for ongoing ventilatory support.

Objectives of This Scenario

1. Recognize respiratory distress and impending respiratory failure.

The signs and symptoms of respiratory distress are varied, depending primarily on the patient's age and time of presentation within the progression to respiratory failure. Older children may complain of shortness of breath, chest pain, or air hunger, which a preverbal child may be unable to communicate and manifest only as "fussiness."

An infant younger than 4 months is an obligate nose breather; therefore, upper respiratory tract infections can cause significant compromise. The physical examination is of paramount importance. Attention should be given to the degree of tachypnea (initial mechanism for preserving minute ventilation), adequacy of tidal volume (by observing chest rise or abdominal excursion), and presence of bilateral breath sounds (assessing symmetry and air movement), nasal flaring, retractions (subcostal, intercostal, supraclavicular), accessory use of neck muscles, head bobbing, and changes in inspiratory/expiratory ratio.

Progression from respiratory distress to respiratory failure can be evident by clinical findings of decreased or absent breath sounds, severe retractions, use of accessory muscles, cyanosis (excluding patients with cyanotic congenital heart disease), poor muscle tone, grunting, weak cough or gag, and eventual depression of mental status and response to pain.

Physiologic findings of Pao_2 of less than 60 mm Hg in 60% oxygen (excluding patients with cyanotic heart disease), $Paco_2$ of greater than 60 mm Hg and rising, vital capacity of less than 15 mL/kg, and maximum inspiratory force (pressure) greater than –20 cm H_2O have historically been used to determine which patients should be intubated. However, no absolute blood gas values define respiratory failure; the diagnosis of respiratory failure is based primarily on **clinical parameters**, and radiographs or laboratory studies should not delay a decision to secure an airway or to assist ventilations.

2. Manage acutely a patient with apnea and respiratory failure.

Management goals for the treatment of respiratory failure and apnea are the same: restoration of adequate oxygenation and ventilation. The potential of the airway to allow airflow to the lungs should be maximized (ie, perform basic airway positioning maneuvers). Oxygen should be delivered in the highest concentration possible to maximize tissue oxygenation, and humidification should be added as soon as practical. Noninvasive pulse oximetry should be monitored continuously, as should end-tidal CO_2 if available. An ABG analysis can serve as a more accurate analysis of ventilation and oxygenation.

The apneic child is only minutes from profound hypoxemia, cardiovascular collapse, and irreparable CNS damage. Any child with a definite history of apnea must be managed with caution in a hospital setting with sufficient resources and staff to provide respiratory resuscitation. Although stimulation can provide temporary resolution of apnea, more aggressive management is usually necessary; assisted ventilation must be provided if spontaneous ventilation is inadequate (BMV or endotracheal intubation). Once endotracheal intubation has occurred, one should assess chest-wall rise, symmetry of breath sounds, absence of gastric breath sounds (in the older child), oxygen saturation by pulse oximetry, end-tidal CO_2, and chest radiography to confirm proper tube placement.

3. Recognize the association of apnea with bronchiolitis.

Although no precise definition for *bronchiolitis* has been universally accepted, it may be thought of as a wheezing-associated illness in early life preceded by signs and symptoms of an upper respiratory tract infection. In the northern hemisphere, it is a seasonal disease with peak activity during the winter months and lasting, most frequently, into the spring. Serious cases occur most commonly in infants younger than 1 year, especially in those younger than 1 to 3 months. Any number of viruses (parainfluenza, influenza type A, adenovirus, rhinovirus) may cause bronchiolitis, but the pathology and epidemiology in this patient are closely affiliated to those of RSV, the most common cause of bronchiolitis.[2]

Apnea is the most frequent complication of RSV infection in young infants, occurring in about 18% of hospitalized infants; those at highest risk for apnea are extremely young (<6 weeks) or premature (gestational age of ≤32 weeks at birth).[7-9]

The prognosis is good because apnea is usually of short duration and does not tend to recur with subsequent respiratory infections. Apnea typically appears only in the initial phase of illness. Severe complications can occur in children of any age with underlying cardiac or pulmonary disease or in those who are immunocompromised.

4. Understand the role of nebulized therapies in treating bronchiolitis.

The use of β_2-agonists such as nebulized **albuterol** may help in treating the hyperreactive airways that can accompany bronchiolitis. Several double-blind placebo-controlled trials have shown a clinical response to nebulized albuterol, but it is important to note that the response is not universal and the efficacy data in controlled trials are conflicting. Because the potential for clinically significant improvement exists, any child with bronchiolitis who presents in distress should receive consideration for a trial of β-agonist therapy, with subsequent therapy guided by his or her response to that trial.[10,11] Nebulized anticholinergic agents do not appear to be useful in the patient with bronchiolitis. The literature regarding the use of nebulized **epinephrine** appears to suggest a potential short-term benefit of epinephrine over albuterol among outpatients, but there may be a limited impact on length of hospital stay and the inpatient population.[12-14] More large multicenter trials are required to support the routine use and delineate the best role of epinephrine among the outpatient and emergency department populations.

Additional Comments

The use of steroids (either systemic or inhaled) in the acute management of bronchiolitis in most studies has demonstrated no appreciable short- or long-term benefits.[15,16] However, there is emerging controversy in that recent literature has suggested there may be some benefit from the use of oral dexamethasone in the initial 4 hours of therapy. As is the case with epinephrine, more large multicenter clinical trials will help delineate the role of steroid use.[17]

References

1. Hanna CM, Greenes DS. How much tachycardia in infants can be attributed to fever? *Ann Emerg Med.* 2004;43:699-705.
2. Ngai P, Bye MR. Bronchiolitis. *Pediatr Ann.* 2002;31:90-97.
3. Lopes JM, Muller NL, Bryan MH, et al. Synergistic behavior of inspiratory muscles after diaphragmatic fatigue in the newborn. *J Appl Physiol.* 1981;51:547-551.
4. Wang EE, Law BJ, Stephens D. Pediatric Investigators Collaborative Network on Infections in Canada (PICNIC) prospective study of risk factors and outcomes in patients hospitalized with respiratory syncytial viral lower respiratory tract infection. *J Pediatr.* 1995;126:212-219.
5. Shaw KN, Bell LM, Sherman NH. Outpatient assessment of infants with bronchiolitis. *Am J Dis Child.* 1991;145:151-155.
6. Pinnington LL, Smith CM, Ellis RE, et al. Feeding efficiency and respiratory integration in infants with acute viral bronchiolitis. *J Pediatr.* 2000;137:523-526.
7. Welliver JR, Welliver RC. Bronchiolitis. *Pediatr Rev.* 1993;14:134-139.
8. Church NR, Anas NG, Hall CB, et al. Respiratory syncytial virus-related apnea in infants: demographics and outcome. *Am J Dis Child.* 1984;138:247-250.
9. Meert K, Heidemann S, Abella B, et al. Does prematurity alter the course of respiratory syncytial virus infection? *Crit Care Med.* 1990;18:1357-1359.
10. Staat MA. Respiratory syncytial virus infections in children. *Semin Respir Infect.* 2002;17:15-20.
11. Kellner JD, Ohlsson A, Gadomski AM, et al. Efficacy of bronchodilator therapy in bronchiolitis. A meta-analysis. *Arch Pediatr Adolesc Med.* 1996;150:1166-1172.
12. Menon K, Sutcliffe T, Klassen TP. A randomized trial comparing the efficacy of epinephrine with salbutamol in the treatment of acute bronchiolitis. *J Pediatr.* 1995;126:1004-1007.
13. Wainwright C, Altamirano L, Cheney M, et al. A multicenter, randomized, double-blind, controlled trial of nebulized epinephrine in infants with acute bronchiolitis. *N Engl J Med.* 2003;349:27-35.
14. Hartling L, Wiebe N, Russell K, et al. A meta-analysis of randomized controlled trials evaluating the efficacy of epinephrine for the treatment of acute viral bronchiolitis. *Arch Pediatr Adolesc Med.* 2003;157:957-964.
15. Roosevelt G, Sheehan K, Grupp-Phelan J, et al. Dexamethasone in bronchiolitis: a randomised controlled trial. *Lancet.* 1996;348:292-295.
16. Berger I, Argaman Z, Schwartz S, et al. Efficacy of corticosteroids in acute bronchiolitis: short term and long term followup. *Pediatr Pulmon.* 1998;26:162.
17. Schuh S, Coates AL, Binnie R, et al. Efficacy of oral dexamethasone in outpatients with acute bronchiolitis. *J Pediatr.* 2002;140:27-32.

SCENARIO #11

Apnea

Karen Gruskin, MD

Brief Presenting History

A somnolent 14-year-old boy is found alone in an examining room in the emergency department after fracture reduction. The pulse oximeter alarm is beeping, and the reading is 83%.

Pediatric Assessment Triangle

Appearance: Pale and not moving, lying in bed with eyes closed

Work of Breathing: Shallow with poor effort

Circulation to the Skin: Perioral cyanosis, cool extremities

Initial Vital Signs

Pulse: 60

Respiratory Rate: 8

Blood Pressure: 60/30

Temperature: 37.5°C (99.5°F) oral

Weight Given in Chart: 50 kg

Physical Examination on Arrival to the Emergency Department

Airway: Patent, no evidence of obstruction

Breathing: Shallow respirations, clear breath sounds

Circulation: Capillary refill time 2 to 3 seconds with diminished pulses

Disability: Pinpoint pupils, withdraws to pain

His right arm is in a long arm cast. Peripheral intravenous catheter in the left antecubital fossa has blood backed up in the tubing.

ASK YOURSELF

■ What is the initial assessment? What is the patient's physiologic status?

This patient has hypoventilation, hypoxia, and hypotension indicative of respiratory insufficiency and impending respiratory failure with decompensated shock.

■ What interventions are needed at this time? What complications might be expected?

Interventions:

- The first priority is to assess the airway while providing open airway positioning and suction as needed.
- Provide oxygen.
- Stimulate the patient (sternal rub) in an attempt to increase respiratory rate.
- If unsuccessful in increasing respiratory rate, provide positive pressure ventilations via bag-mask with 100% O_2.
- Apply cricoid pressure.
- Patient should be placed on a cardiorespiratory monitor if not already done.
- Check intravenous line for patency and re-establish if occluded or infiltrated.

- Initiate **20 mL/kg bolus of normal saline** to address shock.

Potential Complications:

- Vomiting, especially if cricoid pressure not used
- Unable to deliver oxygen because of an equipment failure
- Unable to establish intravenous access

Progression

With BMV, the oxygen saturation improves to 100%.

ASK YOURSELF

■ What could be causing the patient's hypoventilation and desaturations?

Shallow respirations and diminished rate are most consistent with a central cause of hypoxia such as a brain or brain stem injury, an intentional ingestion, or, as in this case, hypoventilation caused by drugs administered.

■ What additional history would help you establish the diagnosis?

It would be imperative to determine which narcotic and/or sedation drugs were provided for pain therapy and fracture reduction in this patient and in what doses (in mg/kg) they were provided. It would also be important to determine the extent of the patient's injuries—specifically, whether there was an associated head injury or suspicion of significant blood loss. Finally, it would be important to determine if the patient had an underlying history of substance abuse or depression such that he may be a chronic abuser of benzodiazepines and/or narcotics.

Additional History and Physical Examination Findings

The patient injured his arm by falling on an outstretched hand at a skateboard park. The fall was witnessed. There was no head trauma, no loss of consciousness, and no other injuries. The patient received fentanyl 2 mcg/kg IV for pain on arrival to the emergency department. Twenty minutes later, midazolam 0.1 mg/kg and fentanyl 2 mcg/kg IV were administered for the reduction of his fracture. Because of inadequate sedation, he received additional midazolam 0.1 mg/kg IV two additional times over the next 10 minutes.

Past Medical History: No significant past medical or psychiatric history; no history of substance abuse

Medications: No routine medications

Allergies: Rash following use of penicillin

Physical Examination: No evidence of trauma other than the casted extremity; pupils are pinpoint and minimally responsive; no evidence of vomitus

ASK YOURSELF

■ What is the most likely diagnosis?

The history of onset of hypoventilation with pinpoint pupils after procedural sedation and analgesia with fentanyl and midazolam is most consistent with an iatrogenic drug overdose. In general, once a fracture reduction is completed, a patient must be monitored closely. Peak drug effects may not, as of yet, have occurred, and with cessation of noxious stimulus, a patient's drive to breathe can diminish. An unrecognized head injury in a patient being treated for an extremity fracture must always be considered.

Progression

The patient has no respiratory effort but is pink with an oxygen saturation of 100% with BMV.

ASK YOURSELF

■ What interventions are needed at this time? What complications might be expected?

Interventions:

- Continue BMV with cricoid pressure, repositioning, and suctioning as necessary to maintain a patent airway.
- Give **naloxone 2 mg IV** and **flumazenil 0.2 mg IV** to reverse oversedation with narcotic and benzodiazepine, respectively. Both may be given intramuscularly if intravenous access has not been reestablished.
- Continue fluid bolus.

Potential Complications:

- Unable to provide adequate saturations despite BMV with 100% O_2; check face mask fit and oxygen source, reposition, and confirm airway patency.
- Patient vomits secondary to BMV if cricoid pressure is not used.

Repeat Vital Signs

Pulse: 100

Respiratory Rate: 18

Blood Pressure: 102/68

Oxygen Saturation: 98% with face mask oxygen

Progression

Patient initially is awake and breathing after naloxone and flumazenil administration but, after 15 minutes, is again somnolent, and respiratory rate has fallen to 6. Oxygen saturation is 85% and falling.

ASK YOURSELF

- **What has happened now?**

  The effects of the naloxone and flumazenil can wear off, causing the patient's respiratory rate to again decrease and the patient to become unresponsive. If the airway is not properly secured and respiratory effort followed closely, progressive respiratory failure can develop.

- **What interventions are needed at this time?**
  - Repeat **naloxone 2 mg IV** every 2 to 3 minutes to a maximum cumulative dose of 10 mg and **flumazenil 0.2 mg IV** every 1 to 3 minutes to a maximum cumulative dose of 1 mg.
  - Continue to support breathing with BMV and 100% O_2 as needed.

Progression

After a second round of naloxone and flumazenil, the patient's pulse rate increases to 120, the patient develops spontaneous respirations, and the blood pressure increases to 120/80. The patient opens his eyes.

ASK YOURSELF

- **What additional complications might be expected for this patient?**
  - As the effect of the narcotic is antagonized by the naloxone and flumazenil, the patient can become progressively agitated, increasing the risk for aspiration and possible barotrauma.
  - The effects of the naloxone and flumazenil can wear off, causing the patient to again become unresponsive and apneic.
  - Additionally, in this scenario full reversal doses of naloxone were used; should the patient require pain medication for his initial injury, narcotics will not be effective until the effect of the naloxone wears off over the next 4 to 6 hours. It would have been possible to use smaller doses of naloxone for partial reversal; however, most fractures after reduction and casting do not require narcotic analgesia, and this patient was profoundly sedated.

Objectives of This Scenario

1. Recognize apnea as a presentation of drug overdose.

The triad of coma, pinpoint pupils, and depressed respirations in a patient receiving intravenous narcotics for an orthopedic procedure should be considered a narcotic overdose until proved otherwise. The administration of a benzodiazepine can further heighten the respiratory suppressive effects of a narcotic.[1-8]

2. Recognize and manage respiratory insufficiency and failure.

The initial depressed respiratory drive should be managed with 100% oxygen and ventilation assisted by BMV as needed. Most often, BMV assistance for several minutes until the effects of naloxone and flumazenil are apparent is sufficient. However, intubation may be necessary in a drug overdose in which the respiratory drive and airway protective reflexes are depressed for a prolonged period of time, such as is seen in massive narcotic and/or benzodiazepine overdoses or in the face of longer-acting agents such as barbiturates. Patients with an initial good response to naloxone and/or flumazenil may require additional doses to prevent relapse into somnolence and respiratory depression.[1-8]

3. Manage overdoses of narcotics and benzodiazepines with specific antidotes.

Narcotic overdoses may be treated with **naloxone 0.1 mg/kg IV/IM** or **0.2 to 1 mg/kg dose diluted in 3 to 5 mL normal saline via ET tube** (maximum doses: approximately 1 mg for a young child and 2 mg for school-age and older children). Repeat every 2 to 5 minutes as needed up to a total dose of 10 mg.[1,2,7,8] Be aware that naloxone can precipitate an abstinence syndrome in patients with chronic narcotic use. Symptoms of narcotic withdrawal include lacrimation, rhinorrhea, yawning, nausea, vomiting, diarrhea, restlessness/combativeness, and extreme anxiety.

Benzodiazepine overdoses may be treated with **flumazenil 0.01 mg/kg** (maximum dose of 0.2 mg) every 1 to 3 minutes to a usual total dose maximum of 1 mg. Flumazenil is contraindicated for patients receiving benzodiazepine as therapy for a seizure disorder, as well as after acute tricyclic antidepressant overdoses. If frequent repeated doses are necessary, both drugs can be administered as continuous infusions.[1,2,7,8]

References

1. American Academy of Pediatrics Committee on Drugs. Guidelines for monitoring and management of pediatric patients during and after sedation for diagnostic and therapeutic procedures. *Pediatrics.* 1992;89:1110-1115.
2. Sacchetti A, Schafermeyer R, Geradi M, Pediatric Committee of the American College of Emergency Physicians. Pediatric analgesia and sedation. *Ann Emerg Med.* 1994;23:237-250; erratum in *Ann Emerg Med.* 1994;24:540.
3. American College of Emergency Physicans. Use of pediatric sedation and analgesia. *Ann Emerg Med.* 1997;29:834-835.
4. American Society of Anesthesiologists. Practice guidelines for sedation and analgesia by non-anesthesiologists. *Anesthesiology.* 1996;84:459-471.
5. American Society of Anesthesiologists Task Force on Sedation and Analgesia by Non-Anesthesiologists. Practice guidelines for sedation and analgesia by non-anesthesiologists. *Anesthesiology.* 2002;96:1004-1017.
6. Green SM, Krauss B. Procedural sedation terminology: moving beyond "conscious sedation." *Ann Emerg Med.* 2002;39:433-435.
7. Krauss BS, Shannon M, Damian FJ, et al. *Guidelines for Pediatric Sedation.* Dallas, Tex: American College of Emergency Physicians; 1995.
8. Krauss B, Brustowicz RB, eds. *Pediatric Procedural Sedation and Analgesia.* Philadelphia, Pa: Lippincott Williams & Wilkin; 1999:189-199.

SCENARIO #12

Apnea

Joe E. Wathen, MD

Brief Presenting History

A 9-month-old boy is brought in with a 2-day history of vomiting and diarrhea. Today, the mother noticed that her infant was listless and was not drinking. There is no report of the infant having a fever.

Pediatric Assessment Triangle

Appearance: Listless, pale, poorly responsive

Work of Breathing: Shallow breathing

Circulation to the Skin: Mottled

Initial Vital Signs

Pulse: 170

Respiratory Rate: 30

Blood Pressure: 76/40

Temperature: 36.3°C (97.3°F) rectal

Weight: 8.2 kg

Physical Examination on Arrival to the Emergency Department

Airway: Patent, moving air freely, no secretions in the mouth

Breathing: Shallow breathing with an episode of apnea of about 20 seconds responding to stimulation; no accessory muscle use, lungs clear bilaterally without wheezes

Circulation: Skin mottled and cool to touch, capillary refill time of 3 seconds centrally and 4 seconds peripherally

Disability: Eyes closed, responsive only to painful stimuli, pupils equal and reactive to light 4 mm to 2 mm bilaterally

ASK YOURSELF

- **What is the initial assessment? What is the patient's physiologic status?**

  This child presents with shallow respirations and an apneic episode, which signal impending respiratory failure. In addition, the patient displays compensated shock (tachycardia, delayed distal perfusion, low end of normal blood pressure) and altered mental status.

- **How is apnea defined?**

  Apnea in children is defined as a respiratory pause longer than 10 to 20 seconds.[1-3] Associated findings that are of concern include pallor, mottling, cyanosis, desaturations, bradycardia, and altered mental status. In young infants, periodic breathing can occur normally and should be differentiated from apnea. Periodic breathing consists of short respiratory pauses (5 to 10 seconds) followed by episodes of increased respiratory rate and should not be associated with other findings. Apnea can be either central or obstructive. Central apnea is marked by absence of respiratory effort; obstructive apnea occurs when airflow ceases even though respiratory effort continues.

■ **What is the differential diagnosis of apnea in this patient?**

Among pulmonary etiologies, respiratory syncytial virus is one of the most likely causes. This virus is common, especially during winter outbreaks of bronchiolitis and in those with premature birth and young age.[4,5] It can be responsible for apnea even in patients with minimal or no respiratory symptoms. Pertussis infections also can cause apnea.[6] Nasopharyngeal washes can be sent to the laboratory to test for these infectious agents. Other respiratory infections such as severe pneumonia with or without effusion can progress to the point of causing significant hypoxia, ineffective ventilation (CO_2 retention), and respiratory failure. This patient has not had prior respiratory symptoms. There are no significant physical examination findings to indicate a respiratory etiology. Although significant hypoxia seems unlikely in this patient on the basis of the physical examination, oxygen saturation should be determined on all patients to rule out hypoxia-induced apnea.

Infectious diseases such as meningitis and sepsis represent life-threatening causes of apnea in infants. The presence of either hyperthermia or hypothermia suggests this etiology. Meningitis even in the absence of fever must be included in the differential.

Metabolic abnormalities can cause apnea in infants. Blood glucose levels should be promptly assessed in these infants, because hypoglycemia can be present with a variety of underlying systemic conditions. Other electrolyte abnormalities also can exist, and a serum electrolyte panel that includes calcium should be obtained. Acid-base abnormalities should be considered. Inborn errors of metabolism also can be present.

Seizure activity may present with just apnea in infants. Traumatic brain injury (ie, shaken baby syndrome), intracranial mass, hydrocephalus, and infantile botulism also can present with apnea.

Other differential diagnoses include arrhythmias secondary to an ingestion or caused by an underlying condition such as prolonged QTc, gastroesophageal reflux, severe anemia, or sudden infant death syndrome (SIDS). The diagnosis of SIDS is a diagnosis of exclusion; SIDS is more common in younger infants and is associated with smoke exposure and prone sleep positioning.[7-9]

Additional History and Physical Examination Findings

The patient had initially been given a home oral rehydration therapy consisting of diluted formula and a sport drink, and then the mother was advised to use bicarbonate water, which she made using one spoonful of baking soda to one cup of water. Despite this therapy, the child became progressively more lethargic and continued to have vomiting and diarrhea. There was no history of trauma, upper respiratory infection symptoms, or other neurologic findings.

Past Medical History: No prior illnesses, term infant

Family History: Sibling had gastrointestinal symptoms a week earlier

Medications: None

Allergies: None known

Physical Examination: Head atraumatic and normocephalic; pupils 3 mm and reactive; dry mucous membranes and decreased skin turgor; breath sounds, when present, are clear; patient has now had five episodes of apnea with oxygen desaturations to the 50s; abdomen soft, nondistended with hypoactive bowel sounds

ASK YOURSELF

■ **What interventions are needed at this time? What complications might be expected?**

Interventions:

- Administer 100% O_2 by face mask or BMV for respiratory insufficiency
- Place the patient on a cardiorespiratory monitor with pulse oximetry.
- Attempt intravenous access and begin fluid resuscitation with **normal saline 20 mL/kg.**
- Immediate laboratory tests: Rapid glucose and bedside hematocrit if available
- Additional laboratory tests: CBC, blood culture, serum electrolyte panel, calcium, phosphorus, blood gases

Potential Complications:

- Difficulties in maintaining adequate oxygen saturations with BMV
- Intravenous access unobtainable

■ What should be done with the airway?

The airway should be repositioned and suctioned. Chest wall rise with BMV also should be assessed, and preparations should be made for endotracheal intubation.

■ What interventions are needed at this time? What complications might be expected?

Interventions:

- This patient displays recurrent apnea and is at risk for complete respiratory failure. If left untreated he will progress to severe hypoxia, bradycardia, asystole, and death. BMV with 100% oxygen should be provided with cricoid pressure. Preparations should be made for RSI.
- Place intraosseous line if intravenous access has not been achieved, and institute volume expansion with **20 mL/kg normal saline.**
- RSI
  1. #1 Miller blade
  2. Size 4.0 ET tube
  3. Preoxygenate
  4. Cricoid pressure
  5. **Atropine 0.02 mg/kg IV/IO** (minimum, 0.1 mg) is recommended to block reflex bradycardia.
  6. If signs of head trauma and/or increased intracranial pressure are present, premedicate with **lidocaine 1 mg/kg IV/IO.**
  7. **Etomidate 0.3 mg/kg IV/IO** or **midazolam 0.1 mg/kg IV/IO**
  8. **Fentanyl 1 to 2 mcg/kg IV/IO**; consider holding if not hemodynamically stable
  9. **Rocuronium 0.6 to 1 mg/kg IV/IO** or **succinylcholine 1 to 1.5 mg/kg IV/IO**
- End-tidal CO_2 monitor
- Call for chest radiograph to confirm ET tube placement.
- Secure ET tube and place an NG tube.

Potential Complications

- Vomiting requires suctioning, especially if cricoid pressure is not used.
- Inability to visualize cords if not properly suctioned
- Lack of NG tube results in abdominal distention and impaired ventilation.

■ What should be done now?

Reassess ABCs.

■ What additional information do you need?

Laboratory test results for additional testing done previously.

Repeat Vital Signs

Pulse: 152

Respiratory Rate: 40 (bagged)

Blood Pressure: 80/40

Oxygen Saturation: 100%

Laboratory Test Results

Venous blood gases (before intubation): pH 7.7, P_{CO_2} 31, P_{O_2} 28, HCO_3 40, base excess 19.7

Serum electrolyte panel: Sodium 151, potassium 1.5, chloride 77, bicarbonate >40, BUN 28, glucose 100

Hematocrit 36

ASK YOURSELF

■ What is the metabolic abnormality?

This patient has a hypernatremic, hypokalemic, metabolic alkalosis. The base excess is a positive 19.7, which represents a significant metabolic alkalosis. In most clinical situations in which there is an ill child, an acidotic condition is more common and a negative number is seen for the base excess.

■ Why does this patient experience apnea?

This patient has apnea due to the metabolic abnormalities mentioned, primarily the metabolic alkalosis and significant hypokalemia. The body will compensate for the metabolic alkalosis by generating a respiratory acidosis through hypoventilation. To compensate for hypokalemia, a cellular influx of hydrogen ions occurs in exchange for potassium, which results in increased serum bicarbonate levels and worsening of the metabolic alkalosis.

■ What interventions are needed at this time?

- Venous access, if not already obtained
- Continue rehydration (intravenous/intraosseous); begin with normal saline.
- Treat severe hypokalemia with intravenous potassium.
- Additional laboratory tests: Follow ABGs/VBGs and serum electrolytes.

■ What intravenous fluids could you use after initial normal saline bolus, if the patient is now euvolemic?

Intravenous fluids could be switched to D_5 **0.25 normal saline with 40 mEq/L KCl.**

■ What other complications might be expected for this patient?

- If fluid resuscitation is delayed, the patient could develop cardiovascular collapse and arrest secondary to severe hypovolemia and decompensated shock.
- Intraosseous lines are excellent for initial access because fluids, medications, and blood may be given through them; however, they can infiltrate. Peripheral or central lines should be established as soon as possible, allowing for the discontinuation and removal of the intraosseous line. When intravenous or intraosseous access is not achieved or in cases of dehydration with less severe metabolic abnormalities, oral rehydration or rehydration using an NG tube is an effective and frequently more desirable treatment option.

■ What disposition and additional management would be expected for this patient?

The patient may be sent to the ICU for continued management of dehydration/hypovolemia, ventilatory support, and correction of the metabolic abnormalities. Extubation can occur once the metabolic abnormality is corrected and the normal drive to breathe returns.

Objectives of This Scenario

1. Recognize a significant apneic event or apparent life-threatening event.

Nonsignificant events include periodic breathing (discussed earlier), brief choking episodes, and breath-holding episodes. Breath-holding episodes are classified as either pallid or cyanotic events that can lead to syncope and seizure activity.[10] A preceding event that causes the child to become upset is an important historical question. The patient, however, in this scenario presents with apneic breathing. A significant apneic episode may occur at home and not be witnessed by the initial treating physician. Separating significant events from those that are not significant can be difficult. Apparent life-threatening events are suddenly occurring symptoms that appear frightening to the infant's care provider; symptoms can include breathing abnormality, color change, or alteration in muscle tone or mental status.[1,3] Resuscitation often is attempted. Such patients are typically admitted to the hospital for diagnostic workup. However, the overall rate of either positive emergency department diagnostic evaluations or significant medical interventions for infants presenting with apparent life-threatening events remains low.[11] In addition, despite hospitalization and extensive work-up, as many as 40% of these patients are discharged without a diagnosis.

2. Initiate management of apnea.

The initial priority is to resuscitate the patient, providing adequate oxygenation and ventilation. Airway positioning should occur to maximize the airflow. Blow-by oxygen and suctioning may be sufficient. If not, CPAP or BMV can be used. In the event of persistent apnea or ineffective ventilation or oxygenation, intubation and mechanical ventilation are indicated. After initial resuscitation and stabilization, the next priority is to identify life-threatening conditions; these include hypoxia, septic shock, hypoglycemia, arrhythmias, and head trauma.

3. Evaluate the infant/child with an apneic event.

The differential diagnosis of apnea is extensive and age dependent. Therefore, the evaluation can be tailored for each patient depending on the detailed history and physical examination. Laboratory tests may include a CBC with differential, electrolytes, glucose, BUN, calcium, pulse oximetry and ABG or VBG, ECG, and nasal wash for RSV/pertussis. Initial radiographic evaluation includes a chest radiograph to look for pneumonia/pneumonitis or cardiomegaly.

Apnea of infancy represents a nonspecific response to a variety of clinical conditions. This phenomenon keeps the evaluation of infants wide, with initial exclusion of life-threatening etiologies such as certain infectious processes and traumatic brain injuries. Lumbar punctures should be performed on any infant with suspicion of meningitis. Choanal atresia or stenosis can contribute to obstructive apnea; passage of a nasogastric tube can elucidate these conditions.

Gastroesophageal reflux has been reported in up to 26% of cases of apparent life-threatening events and can trigger either central or obstructive apnea secondary to laryngospasm.[12] Inpatient evaluation may include a pH esophageal probe, barium swallow, and a pneumogram to evaluate for gastroesophageal reflux with associated aspiration and laryngospasm.

Electroencephalography needs to be considered to diagnosis epilepsy because apnea or an apparent life-threatening event can be the first manifestation of a seizure disorder.[13] However, a normal EEG recorded between events does not exclude seizure as the etiology of apnea or apparent life-threatening events.

Because traumatic brain injury can occur without external signs of trauma and has been reported to be found in about 3% of infants with apparent life-threatening events, head CT scanning along with dilated ophthalmoscopic examination should be considered in those infants with concerning physical examination findings or with no apparent cause for the apnea or apparent life-threatening events.[14,15] Other forms of child abuse also have been associated with apparent life-threatening events and require a high index of suspicion to illuminate (ie, intentional smothering, intentional poisoning, and Munchausen syndrome by proxy).[16]

References

1. Torey SB. Apnea. In: Fleisher GR, Ludwig S, eds. *Textbook of Pediatric Emergency Medicine.* 4th ed. Philadelphia, Pa: Lippincott Williams & Wilkins; 2000:147-151.
2. Burchfield DJ, Boychuk RB. Neonatal emergencies. In: Gausche-Hill M, Fuchs S, Yamamoto L, eds. *APLS: The Pediatric Emergency Medicine Resource.* 4th ed. Sudbury, Mass: American Academy of Pediatrics, American College of Emergency Physicians, Jones and Bartlett Publishing Co; 2004:477-493 .
3. Berman S. Apnea and sudden infant death syndrome. In: Berman S, ed. *Pediatric Decision Making.* 4th ed. Philadelphia, Pa: Mosby; 2003:734-737.
4. Bruhn FW, Mokrohisky ST, McIntosh K. Apnea associated with respiratory syncytial virus infection in young infants. *J Pediatr.* 1977;90:382-386.
5. Church NR, Anas NG, Hall CB, et al. Respiratory syncytial virus-related apnea in infants. Demographics and outcome. *Am J Dis Child.* 1984;138:247-250.
6. Jenkinson D. Natural course of 500 consecutive cases of whooping cough: a general practice population study. *BMJ.* 1995;310:299-302.
7. Positioning and sudden infant death syndrome (SIDS): update. American Academy of Pediatrics Task Force on Infant Positioning and SIDS. *Pediatrics.* 1996;98:1216-1218.
8. Jeffery HE, Megevand A, Page H. Why the prone position is a risk factor for sudden infant death syndrome. *Pediatrics.* 1999;104:263-269.
9. Anderson HR, Cook DG. Passive smoking and sudden infant death syndrome: review of the epidemiological evidence. *Thorax.* 1997;52:1003-1009.
10. Breningstall GN. Breath-holding spells. *Pediatr Neurol.* 1996;14:91-97.
11. De Piero AD, Teach SJ, Chamberlain JM. ED evaluation of infants after an apparent life-threatening event. *Am J Emerg Med.* 2004;22:83-86.
12. Davies F, Gupta R. Apparent life threatening events in infants presenting to an emergency department. *Emerg Med J.* 2002;19:11-16.
13. Nunes ML, Appel CC, da Costa JC. Apparent life-threatening episodes as the first manifestation of epilepsy. *Clin Pediatr (Phila).* 2003;42:19-22.
14. Altman RL, Brand DA, Forman S, et al. Abusive head injury as a cause of apparent life-threatening events in infancy. *Arch Pediatr Adolesc Med.* 2003;157:1011-1015.
15. Pitetti RD, Maffei F, Chang K, et al. Prevalence of retinal hemorrhages and child abuse in children who present with an apparent life-threatening event. *Pediatrics.* 2002;110:557-562.
16. Meadow R. Suffocation, recurrent apnea, and sudden death. *J Pediatr.* 1990;117:351.

SCENARIO #13

Shock

Stanley H. Inkelis, MD

Brief Presenting History

A 4-month-old boy is brought in to the emergency department by paramedics because his parents said he was becoming poorly responsive today. He has a history of vomiting and diarrhea for 1 day, and now he has a glassy-eyed stare and rapid breathing.

Pediatric Assessment Triangle

Appearance: Pale, poor eye contact

Work of Breathing: Rapid, deep respirations

Circulation to the Skin: Mottled

Initial Vital Signs

Pulse: 190

Respiratory Rate: 50

Blood Pressure: 64/38

Temperature: 38.9°C (102°F) rectal

Physical Examination on Arrival to the Emergency Department

Airway: Open, good air movement

Breathing: Rapid, deep, even; no retractions, stridor, wheezing, crackles, or decreased breath sounds

Circulation: Tachycardia, thready pulse stronger centrally than peripherally; capillary refill time at forearm of 5 seconds; extremities cool

Disability: Eyes open but gaze not fixed; responds only to very painful stimuli with a whimper; pupils respond equally to light

ASK YOURSELF

- **What is the initial assessment? What is the patient's physiologic status?**

  This child presents with altered mental status, tachypnea (Kussmaul respirations), and decompensated shock.

- **What is the cause of this child's decompensated shock?**

  The child's history of vomiting and diarrhea (acute gastroenteritis), rapid, deep breathing, and mental status changes suggests that he is severely dehydrated and that shock is due to hypovolemia. Severe dehydration is associated with a decreased intravascular volume (hypovolemia) and shock (hypovolemic shock). Other causes of hypovolemic shock such as insensible water loss, urinary loss, and blood loss are very unlikely in this child. Septic shock should be considered because of fever, ill appearance, and young age. Because the patient's compensatory mechanisms are unable to support his perfusion, resulting in hypotension, he is in a physiologic state of decompensated shock.[1]

■ **What additional history and physical examination findings would help you establish the diagnosis?**

History: The frequency of the vomiting and diarrhea, as well as the quantity (large or small amounts) and quality (watery, bloody, mucous), is helpful in establishing the amount of water loss (dehydration) and the potential etiology. Ascertaining the current frequency of urination compared with the child's normal urine output also is helpful in determining the degree of dehydration.

Physical Examination: The child's fontanel should be assessed to determine whether it is sunken. The eyes should be assessed for tearing and to determine whether they are sunken. Skin should be assessed for color (mottling), temperature, turgor, and capillary refill time. Peripheral and central pulses should be palpated, and the quality determined.

Additional History and Physical Examination Findings

The child was seen the previous day because he had vomiting and diarrhea. The parents were told that he had acute gastroenteritis and that he was well hydrated. They were given oral rehydration instructions, as well as instructions to return if there were signs of dehydration. The child weighed 11 kg on that visit. The vomiting and diarrhea persisted; the child was unable to keep down fluids and vomited after every feeding. He had approximately 10 large-volume bowel movements with no blood or mucus since his prior visit.

Past Medical History: Healthy, with no previous significant illness

Medications: None

Immunizations: Up to date, including the four-month pneumococcal conjugate vaccines

Physical Examination: Oxygen saturation 90% on room air; anterior fontanel sunken; no tears and eyes are sunken; mucous membranes very dry; skin retracts very slowly when pinched ("tenting" of the skin); current weight 9.3 kg

ASK YOURSELF

■ **What interventions are needed at this time?**

- Administer 100% O_2 via face mask.
- Place the patient on a cardiorespiratory monitor with pulse oximetry.
- Attempt to establish intravenous access.
- Fluid resuscitation with **normal saline 20 mL/kg** as a rapid bolus
- Obtain blood for rapid glucose determination, electrolytes, and VBG analysis, and obtain urine for a urinalysis.

■ **What should you do if intravenous attempts are unsuccessful?**

Because this child is in decompensated shock, if intravenous access is unsuccessful after 90 seconds, prepare to start an intraosseous line. Placement of a central venous line is another alternative, but an intraosseous line is preferable in this case of decompensated shock because it can be placed more quickly.

■ **Where should the intraosseous needle be placed?**

The intraosseous needle should be inserted in the proximal tibia, on the medial side, 1 to 2 cm below and away from the tibial tuberosity, in the center of the flat part of the bone. Other potential sites are the distal femur, 1 to 2 cm proximal to the superior border of the patella and slightly medial or lateral to the anterior ridge, and the distal tibia, 1 to 2 cm proximal to the medial malleolus in the center of the bone.[2]

■ **How do you confirm that the needle is in the marrow space?**

If there is a sudden decrease in resistance and the needle remains upright without support, you are most likely in the marrow space. If marrow is aspirated, you have confirmed placement. Otherwise, easy infusion of fluid into the marrow space without extravasation in the soft tissues confirms placement.

■ **What are the potential complications of intraosseous line placement?**

Fracture, infection (cellulitis or osteomyelitis), and compartment syndrome[2]

Repeat Vital Signs

Pulse: 180

Respiratory Rate: 46

Blood Pressure: 76/52

Temperature: 38.5°C (101.3°F)

Oxygen Saturation: 100% in face mask oxygen

Progression

The child's mental status is unchanged. Respirations continue to be rapid and deep, and capillary refill at the forearm is 4 seconds.

ASK YOURSELF

- **What is the physiologic status now?**

  The child continues to demonstrate inadequate perfusion and remains in hypovolemic shock after the first fluid bolus. However, his blood pressure has normalized, because his compensatory mechanisms of reduction in vagal tone and increase in heart rate and contractility, triggered by catecholamine release, are no longer overwhelmed. Consequently, he is no longer in a physiologic state of decompensated shock but has reverted to a physiologic state of compensated shock.[1]

- **What interventions are needed at this time?**

  Fluid resuscitation should continue with a second rapid bolus of **normal saline 20 mL/kg.**

Laboratory Test Results: Rapid glucose determination, 25; other laboratory test results pending

ASK YOURSELF

- **What interventions are needed at this time?**

  Correct the hypoglycemia as quickly as possible with **glucose (dextrose) 0.5 g/kg** IV/IO infusion (may give as 2 mL/kg of D_{25} or as 5 mL/kg of D_{10}). (*Note:* A helpful way of remembering how much dextrose to infuse so that you are always giving 0.5 g/kg is to multiply the number of mL/kg by the percentage of dextrose [D%] so that the product equals 50.) Because the hypoglycemia is likely to persist, D_{10} at 1.5 times maintenance rate should be continued until the catabolic state is reversed.[3]

Laboratory Test Results: WBC count 14,400, hemoglobin 16, hematocrit 48, platelets 324,000, Na^+ 135, K^+ 3.5, Cl^- 104, HCO_3^- 6, BUN 50, creatinine 1.8, glucose 28, Ca^{2+} 10.2

VBG analysis: pH 7.05, P_{CO_2} 13, P_{O_2} 50, base excess –12

Urine could not be obtained.

ASK YOURSELF

- **What is the anion gap? How would you interpret the laboratory results?**

  The anion gap is the difference between the serum sodium and the sum of the serum chloride plus serum bicarbonate [$Na^+ - (Cl^- + HCO_3^-)$]. HCO_3^- of 6 is very low, and the anion gap is elevated (25); both are consistent with a metabolic acidosis. The VBG confirms metabolic acidosis (pH 7.05, base excess –12) with respiratory compensation (P_{CO_2} 13).

- **What is the differential diagnosis of an elevated anion gap metabolic acidosis, and what is the cause in this patient?**

  MUDPILES is a useful mnemonic for the causes of elevated anion gap metabolic acidosis.

M	methanol
U	uremia
D	diabetes mellitus
P	paraldehyde
I	iron, isoniazid
L	lactic acidosis
E	ethanol, ethylene glycol
S	salicylates, starvation

  Given that this child is in decompensated hypovolemic shock with poor perfusion to his vital organs, he develops anaerobic metabolism and accumulates lactic acid, resulting in lactic acidosis. This is the explanation for his metabolic acidosis.[4]

Repeat Vital Signs

Pulse: 176

Respiratory Rate: 44

Blood Pressure: 78/56

Temperature: 38.5°C (101.3°F)

Oxygen Saturation: 100% in face mask oxygen

Progression

The child is making some eye contact with his parents; his respirations are still rapid but not as deep as earlier. Capillary refill at the forearm is 3 seconds. He produces urine.

ASK YOURSELF

■ What is the physiologic status now?

The child remains in compensated hypovolemic shock, but he is improving.

■ What interventions are needed now?

Continue fluid resuscitation with a third rapid bolus of **normal saline 20 mL/kg.**

Repeat Vital Signs

Pulse: 140

Respiratory Rate: 30

Blood Pressure: 80/58

Temperature: 38.3°C (100.9°F)

Oxygen Saturation: 100% in face mask oxygen

Progression

The child is interacting with his parents, responding appropriately to pain and breathing much less rapidly and deeply. His fontanel and eyes are less sunken, and his skin turgor is improving. Capillary refill is 2 seconds.

ASK YOURSELF

■ What has happened?

The patient's clinical status has improved greatly. He is still dehydrated but is responding to the rapid restoration of his intravascular volume. He is no longer in shock.

■ Is there a need for further intervention?

The child will need to continue to receive intravenous fluids. These are infused according to maintenance and replacement needs and should be started immediately after the boluses are infused. If you need to make a decision about how much fluid to give hourly, you may start by giving 1.5 to 2 times maintenance fluids. Once you have time to calculate replacement fluids, the child should be on a more precise hourly rate. It is also important to recheck the serum glucose level; patients frequently require more than one bolus of dextrose to treat hypoglycemia.

■ What additional complications might be expected for this patient?

- If fluid resuscitation is delayed, progressive organ failure will continue and result in cardiovascular collapse and cardiopulmonary arrest.
- If fluid losses are greater than fluid input, multiple sites of intravenous access may be needed or an intraosseous or a central line may be placed to improve the circulatory state.
- Hypotension may be refractory to fluid resuscitation. The child may require vasopressor support if he does not respond to fluid resuscitation.
- The child may potentially revert to his state of hypovolemic shock if he is not monitored carefully. Frequent reassessment helps determine additional therapy. Reassess, reassess, reassess!
- If hypoglycemia is not recognized and glucose is not given, the child may seize from this deficit and/or develop irreversible CNS injury.

■ What disposition and additional management would be expected for this patient?

This child requires continued monitoring and management of his severe dehydration and hypovolemia in a hospital setting. Maintenance and replacement fluids should be continued to return him to his normal state of hydration; then he must demonstrate the ability to maintain his hydration orally.

Objectives of This Scenario

1. Recognize the signs and symptoms of severe dehydration.

The patient in this scenario presented with a history of vomiting and diarrhea in conjunction with Kussmaul breathing, tachycardia, hypotension, thready pulse, prolonged capillary refill, absent tearing, dry mucous membranes, sunken eyes and fontanel, and decreased urine output. None of the patient's signs and symptoms alone predicts the diagnosis of dehydration, but the constellation of findings associated with the history points to the diagnosis of severe dehydration. One study demonstrated that clinically important dehydration could be diagnosed if a child had at least 3 of 10 common findings associated with dehydration and suggested that, to diagnose severe (>10%) dehydration, a child should have 6 or 7 of these findings.[5] The authors also identified a subset of clinical indicators—abnormal general appearance, capillary refill greater than 2 seconds, dry mucous membranes, and absent tears—that may be the most reliable predictors of dehydration. In their study, the presence of two of these findings suggested 5% dehydration, and the presence of three or more was associated with at least 10% dehydration.

2. Recognize the signs and symptoms of hypovolemic shock.

The child's altered mental status associated with tachycardia, pulse stronger centrally than peripherally, cool extremities, prolonged capillary refill, and hypotension all are suggestive of inadequate tissue perfusion. When tissue perfusion is inadequate to meet the metabolic needs of vital organs, as in this child, the patient is in shock. Given that this child experienced severe water loss from vomiting and diarrhea, he has a decreased circulating volume (hypovolemia) and is in hypovolemic shock.[1,4,6]

3. Manage severe dehydration and hypovolemic shock.

The goals of therapy in patients with severe dehydration and hypovolemic shock are to 1) correct dehydration and 2) reverse hypovolemic shock and restore an euvolemic condition.

Patients with severe dehydration are at least 10% volume depleted. Rapid aggressive fluid resuscitation is essential in improving outcome.[4,6] The administration of normal saline or lactated Ringer solution boluses of 20 mL/kg as rapidly as possible up to 60 mL/kg decreases morbidity and mortality in patients in shock.[4,6] After the initial rapid fluid resuscitation and restoration of euvolemia, maintenance and replacement fluids should be started immediately.

The volume of maintenance fluids over 24 hours is calculated according to the child's weight: for the first 10 kg, 100 mL/kg; for 11 to 20 kg, 50 mL/kg; and for more than 20 kg, 20 mL/kg. Another way of doing this calculation is as follows: for children weighing less than 10 kg, give 100 mL/kg/24 hr; for children 11 to 20 kg, 1,000 mL plus 50 mL/kg/24 hr for every 1 kg over 10 kg; and for children heavier than 20 kg, 1,500 mL plus 20 mL/kg/24 hr for every 1 kg over 20 kg. To calculate the hourly maintenance fluid requirements, divide the total by 24 or use the "4-2-1" rule. The latter rule is based on the above calculations and provides a quick hourly calculation as follows: for the first 10 kg, give 4 mL/kg/hr; for the next 10 kg, 2 mL/kg/hr; and for every 1 kg above 20 kg, 1 mL/kg/hr. In this child, who weighs 11 kg (ideal body weight), his maintenance fluid requirement would be 1,000 mL (first 10 kg) and 50 mL (for the additional 1 kg), for a total of 1,050 mL/24 hr, which equals 44 mL/hr. If you use the "4-2-1" rule, the hourly rate will be 40 mL (first 10 kg) and 2 mL (for the additional 1 kg), for a total of 42 mL/hr.

The calculation of replacement fluids is based on the severity (percentage) of dehydration. This percentage is most accurately determined if recent weights are available. The percentage of dehydration is equivalent to the percentage of body weight lost. The child in this scenario has lost 1.7 kg, or 15% of his body weight. He is therefore 15% dehydrated.

If the previous weight is not available, the severity of dehydration is estimated by the clinical findings of the history and physical examination. In this child with marked clinical findings of severe dehydration and hypovolemic shock, we can estimate that he is at least 15% dehydrated (equivalent to a 15% weight loss). Based on these clinical findings, he has an approximately 1.7-L (kg) deficit (15% × 11 kg = ≈1.7 kg). Half of the fluid deficit (850 mL) is given over the first 8 hours, and the remainder is given over the next 16 hours.[7] This child would receive 350 mL of a maintenance fluid over the first 8 hours and 850 mL of replacement fluid (total 1,200 mL). Over the next 16 hours, he would receive 700 mL of maintenance fluid and 850 mL of replacement fluid (total 1,550 mL). Potassium should be added to the intravenous solution once the child urinates.

The patient has isotonic (serum sodium 130 to 150 mEq/L) dehydration. If one calculates the maintenance and replacement caloric and sodium needs of children with isotonic dehydration, D_5 0.45% normal saline is the appropriate stock solution to use after the initial resuscitation bolus of normal saline. The maintenance and replacement fluid management of hypotonic and hypertonic dehydration are beyond the scope of this scenario and are discussed elsewhere.[8]

4. Recognize hypoglycemia in seriously ill children.

Hypoglycemia is common in children with severe diarrhea[9] and in children requiring resuscitative care.[10] There are no good predictors of hypoglycemia in patients with diarrhea and dehydration or in seriously ill patients who require resuscitative care.[10,11] Because greater morbidity and mortality are associated with hypoglycemia, routine rapid glucose testing is recommended in seriously ill children with dehydration or requiring resuscitation. To remember to obtain a rapid glucose test, the mnemonic ABCS (with the S indicating "sugar") has been suggested.[10]

References

1. Fitzmaurice L, Gerardi MJ. Cardiovascular system. In: Gausche-Hill M, Fuchs S, Yamamoto L, eds. *APLS: The Pediatric Emergency Medicine Resource.* 4th ed. Sudbury, Mass: American Academy of Pediatrics, American College of Emergency Physicians, Jones and Bartlett Publishing Co; 2004:106-145.
2. King BR, King C, Coates WC. Critical procedures: vascular access. In: Gausche-Hill M, Fuchs S, Yamamoto L, eds. *APLS: The Pediatric Emergency Medicine Resource.* 4th ed. Sudbury, Mass: American Academy of Pediatrics, American College of Emergency Physicians, Jones and Bartlett Publishing Co; 2004:736-738.
3. Glaser N, Enns GM, Kuppermann N. Metabolic disease. In: Gausche-Hill M, Fuchs S, Yamamoto L, eds. *APLS: The Pediatric Emergency Medicine Resource.* 4th ed. Sudbury, Mass: American Academy of Pediatrics, American College of Emergency Physicians, Jones and Bartlett Publishing Co; 2004:186-207.
4. Tobias J. Shock in children: the first 60 minutes. *Pediatr Ann.* 1996;25:330-338.
5. Gorelick MH, Shaw KN, Murphy KO. Validity and reliability of clinical signs in the diagnosis of dehydration in children. *Pediatrics.* 1997;99:E6. Available at: http://www.pediatrics.org/cgi/content/full/99/5/e6. Accessed August 23, 2004.
6. Thomas JT, Corcillo JA. Hypovolemic shock in pediatric patients. *New Horizons.* 1998;6:120-129.
7. Shaw KN. Dehydration. In Fleisher GR, Ludwig S, eds. *Textbook of Pediatric Emergency Medicine.* 4th ed. Philadelphia, Pa: Lippincott; 2000:197-201.
8. Greenbaum LA. Deficit therapy. In: Behrman RE, Kliegman RM, Jenson HB, eds. *Nelson Textbook of Pediatrics.* 17th ed. Philadelphia, Pa: WB Saunders; 2004:245-249.
9. Bennish ML, Azad AK, Rahman O, et al. Hypoglycemia during diarrhea in childhood. *N Engl J Med.* 1990;322:1357-1363.
10. Losek JD. Hypoglycemia and the ABC'S (sugar) of pediatric resuscitation. *Ann Emerg Med.* 2000;35:43-46.
11. Reid S, McQuillan S, Losek J. Hypoglycemia complicating dehydration due to acute gastroenteritis. *Clin Pediatr.* 2003;42:641-646.

SCENARIO #14

Shock

William Tsai, MD

Brief Presenting History

A 12-month-old boy is brought to the emergency department because he has a fever, fast breathing, and bluish discoloration around the lips.

Pediatric Assessment Triangle

Appearance: Sleepy, does not maintain eye contact

Work of Breathing: Tachypneic, with mild retractions

Circulation to the Skin: Some slight perioral bluish discoloration and mottling of the extremities

Initial Vital Signs

Pulse: 150

Respiratory Rate: 32

Blood Pressure: 100/35

Temperature: 39.5°C (103.1°F) rectal

Oxygenation Saturation: 96% in room air

ASK YOURSELF

- **How much should this 12-month-old boy weigh?**

  The 50th percentile weight for a 12-month-old child is 10 kg. Alternatively, one can use the length-based Broselow Pediatric Emergency Tape or a pediatric table to determine weight based on age. (See Appendix A.)

Physical Examination on Arrival to the Emergency Department

Airway: Patent

Breathing: Tachypneic with symmetric breath sounds and moderate intercostal and subcostal retractions; good air entry bilaterally; no stridor or wheezing

Circulation: Capillary refill about 3 seconds with 3+ palpable peripheral pulses

Disability: Eyes open to stimulation, but child appears sleepy; cries shrilly when moved even slightly

ASK YOURSELF

- **What is the initial assessment? What is the patient's physiologic status?**

  This child presents with tachypnea, fever, and extreme irritability. Despite the tachypnea, he has clear breath sounds and no evidence of obstruction anywhere in the large or small airways. Nonetheless, he has respiratory distress and a depressed mental status. The tachycardia and wide pulse pressure with the alteration in mental status are highly suggestive of early decompensated shock.

- **What could be causing this constellation of symptoms?**

  The fever suggests an infectious cause. Other causes of tachypnea include agitation, lower respiratory tract disease, and metabolic acidosis with respiratory compensation.

■ **What additional history would help you establish the diagnosis?**

Careful documentation of the preceding illness is important. The type and duration of symptoms, the course of fever, and the presence or absence of a history of asthma or wheezing are important to note. The sequence of symptoms during the course of illness can be useful in formulating a differential diagnosis in a child with fever, tachypnea, and irritability. A review of systems should note the presence of upper respiratory infection symptoms, diarrhea, vomiting, poor oral intake, and decreased urine output.

Additional History and Physical Examination Findings

This child has been ill for about 3 days. The illness began as an upper respiratory infection manifested by coughing, rhinorrhea, and mild fussiness. The fever has been present for 2 days beginning with a temperature of 38.5°C that reached as high as 39°C today. He has also become more irritable and more difficult to console. His mother noted a bluish discoloration around his lips for the past half-day and the presence of fast breathing for the past several hours. The mother denies the child has a history of vomiting or diarrhea. He has had poor oral intake for the past 3 days and fewer wet diapers than usual.

Past Medical History: Healthy child with no history of respiratory problems

Medications: None

Physical Examination: This ill-appearing child is tachypneic, and there are moderate intercostal and subcostal retractions. Of note, the breath sounds are clear bilaterally with no evidence of wheezing or crackles. His capillary refill is now 3 to 4 seconds in his hands and feet. There is a slight discoloration of his skin periorally. He has a bulging fontanel and responds only to painful stimuli.

ASK YOURSELF

■ **What is the differential diagnosis?**

The progression of this febrile illness suggests a serious bacterial infection with evolving septic shock. In the setting of a febrile illness and an ill-appearing child, the formulation of an accurate differential diagnosis is essential. Fever in a child may cause irritability, tachypnea, and tachycardia due to an increase in basal metabolic rate. The presence of fever, retractions, and tachypnea suggests a lower respiratory tract infection such as bronchiolitis or pneumonia. Meningitis can manifest as fever and irritability. Nuchal rigidity is not always present. Alternatively, the etiology of tachypnea can be secondary to metabolic acidosis with an attempt by the child to compensate by hyperventilating. Common causes of metabolic acidosis are dehydration, diarrhea, and sepsis.

■ **What interventions are needed at this time?**

- Administer 100% O_2 via face mask for respiratory distress despite adequate pulse oximetry reading.
- Place the patient on a cardiorespiratory monitor with pulse oximetry.
- Place an intravenous catheter and draw blood samples for CBC, blood culture, and rapid glucose determination.
- Administer a bolus of **normal saline 20 mL/kg** IV over 10 to 20 minutes.
- Catheterize bladder for urinalysis and urine culture samples.
- Administer antipyretics to reduce fever; this may help eliminate fever as the cause of the child's irritability and tachypnea.
- Administer empiric intravenous broad-spectrum antibiotics. A lumbar puncture that is performed before antibiotics are administered is always desirable when meningitis is suspected, but it is not mandatory, particularly in an unstable patient. Antibiotics should never be withheld or delayed in this situation.

Repeat Vital Signs

Pulse: 165

Respiratory Rate: 40

Blood Pressure: 65/35

Temperature: 38°C (100.4°F)

Oxygen Saturation: 94% in room air

Progression

The child does not respond to attempts at intravenous access. He now arouses minimally to all painful stimuli. The declining blood pressure has been noted. Perioral discoloration has become obvious perioral cyanosis. The child's pulses are now barely palpable in his extremities, and his extremities are cool.

ASK YOURSELF

■ What has happened?

The child has developed further depressed mental status, hypotension, and diminished pulses. The differential diagnosis is now limited to the different forms of shock: hypovolemic, septic, hemorrhagic, anaphylactic, cardiogenic, and neurogenic. This case scenario suggests septic or hypovolemic shock.

■ What is the physiologic status of this patient?

This child has respiratory distress with impending respiratory failure, decompensated shock, and depressed mental status.

■ What interventions are needed at this time?

- Administer a second bolus of **normal saline 20 mL/kg**.
- Administer **ceftriaxone 100 mg/kg** and **vancomycin 20 mg/kg**. Vancomycin is required because of the suspicion of meningitis and the increasing prevalence of penicillin-resistant strains of *Streptococcus pneumoniae.*
- Continue supplemental oxygen while preparing to manage the airway and assist breathing.
- Perform an ABG analysis.

Repeat Vital Signs

Pulse: 165

Respiratory Rate: 40

Blood Pressure: 75/40

Temperature: 38°C (100.4°F) rectal

Oxygen saturation: 98% on 100% O_2 via face mask

Progression

ABG: pH 7.15, Pco_2 25, Po_2 195, HCO_3^- 6, base deficit –12; blood glucose 180

ASK YOURSELF

■ What is your interpretation of the arterial blood gas results?

Severe metabolic acidosis with respiratory compensation

■ What interventions are needed at this time? What complications might be expected?

Interventions:

- Intubate the child to protect his airway, diminish his work of breathing, and maximize oxygen delivery.
- RSI as follows:
  1. #1 Miller blade, 4.0 ET tube
  2. Preoxygenation
  3. Cricoid pressure
  4. **Atropine 0.02 mg/kg** IV
  5. **Etomidate 0.3 mg/kg** IV (preferred over thiopental because the patient is hypotensive)
  6. **Succinylcholine 1 to 1.5 mg/kg** IV or **rocuronium 0.6 to 1 mg/kg** IV
- End-tidal CO_2 monitor to verify intubation of the trachea
- Chest radiograph to confirm ET tube placement
- Secure ET tube and place NG tube.
- Repeat ABG analysis.
- Continued fluid boluses to support perfusion. After **40 to 60 mL/kg of crystalloid**, consider colloid.

Potential Complications:

- Endotracheal intubation, although indicated, can result in further hypotension and bradycardia, which can progress to cardiac arrest (especially if thiopental is used).
- Vomiting, especially if cricoid pressure is not used
- Loss of intravenous access, which necessitates intraosseous placement

Progression

Intubation is performed.

Repeat Vital Signs

Pulse: 60

Respiratory Rate: 25 with bagging

Blood Pressure: Unobtainable; pulses not palpable

Pulse Oximetry: Unobtainable

ECG Monitor:

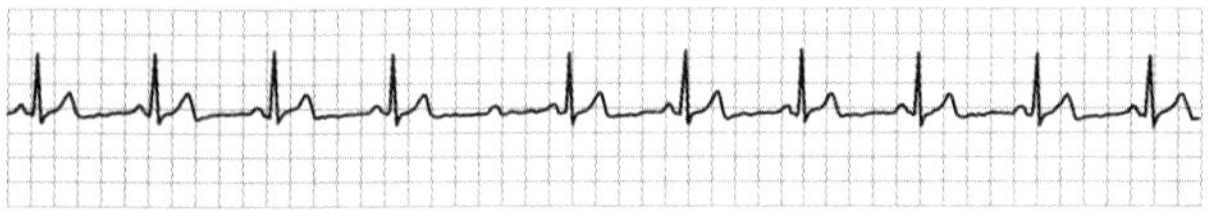

ASK YOURSELF

- **What interventions are needed at this time? What complications might be expected?**

Interventions:

- Initiate algorithm for bradycardia ("Evaluation and Management: Circulation," Figure 2).
- Begin chest compressions at rate of 100.
- If intravenous access not obtained by this point, obtain intraosseous access.
- Administer **epinephrine 1:10,000 (0.1 mL/kg) IV/IO** with saline flush.
- Repeat fluid bolus of **20 mL/kg normal saline.**
- Check placement of the ET tube.
- Consider administration of **sodium bicarbonate 0.5 to 1 mEq/kg IV.**

Potential Complications:

- Failure to verify tube position, with either intubation of esophagus with auscultation of breath sounds over stomach or intubation of right main stem bronchus
- Bagging with excessive pressure can impede venous return and result in further hypotension. In addition, it can cause a pneumothorax.

Progression

Pulses return after a single dose of intravenous epinephrine and second 20-mL/kg bolus of normal saline. Monitor now reveals sinus tachycardia.

Repeat Vital Signs

Pulse: 180

Respiratory Rate: Ventilated at 30

Blood Pressure: 65/35

Oxygen Saturation: 100%

ASK YOURSELF

- **What interventions are needed at this time?**
  - Aggressive **isotonic fluid** administration to a total of **60 to 80 mL/kg**. Beyond that, colloid should be considered.
  - Because of the persistent hypotension, begin a cardiac pressor medication. **Dopamine** is a good initial agent, starting at **10 mcg/kg/min.**
  - Draw blood samples for CBC, electrolytes, BUN, creatinine, glucose, type and screen, prothrombin time/partial thromboplastin time, and evaluation for evidence of disseminated intravascular coagulation.
  - Place central venous catheter and an arterial catheter.
  - After stabilization, perform lumbar puncture to evaluate for meningitis. Strongly consider starting empiric **dexamethasone, 0.6 mg/kg,** to ameliorate long-term neurologic complications of presumed bacterial meningitis.
  - Admit to a pediatric ICU.

Objectives of This Scenario

1. Recognize the clinical signs and symptoms of septic shock.

This patient presented with signs of sepsis and compensated shock that quickly progressed to decompensated septic shock. Sepsis and septic shock result from the body's complex response to infection and begins with a systemic inflammatory response mediated by cytokine release, which can lead quickly to organ dysfunction and death.[1] Findings of fever, tachycardia, and tachypnea and signs of poor perfusion and shock with an elevated WBC count all suggest sepsis with or without meningitis.

In children with sepsis, fever is usually present, although hypothermia can occur, especially in infants, and portends a poor prognosis. Patients have symptoms ranging from irritability to coma. In the early stages of sepsis, tachycardia increases cardiac output to maintain organ perfusion. Patients can initially be flushed and have bounding pulses and brisk capillary refill—"warm shock." As sepsis progresses, patients increase their systemic vascular resistance and become vasoconstricted, as manifested by cool, mottled skin with diminished pulses and prolonged capillary refill time. Tachypnea results from increased oxygen demands as well as an attempt to compensate for metabolic acidosis.

The definition of *decompensated shock* is the presence of hypotension (systolic blood pressure less than 5th percentile for age).[2] Some sign of organ hypoperfusion such as mottled, cool extremities with markedly prolonged capillary refill time, oliguria, or altered mental status also must be present. Hypotension is a late finding in pediatric shock and signifies impending cardiovascular collapse. The patient in this case scenario presented with all of the necessary features for the diagnosis of septic shock.[3]

2. Know the differential diagnosis of fever and tachypnea.

Fever and tachypnea are common signs in acute care pediatrics. Tachypnea is frequently due to fever and the coincident increase in basal metabolic rate, or it can be due to an agitated or crying child. Tachypnea can be a compensatory response to the metabolic acidosis associated with septic shock. Pneumonia, bronchiolitis, and asthma can present in this fashion, but the presence of bilaterally clear lung fields without any evidence of wheeze or crackles points away from these diagnoses. Myocarditis and ensuing cardiogenic shock can present with fever, tachycardia, and tachypnea.[4] However, these patients would be expected to have signs of cardiogenic shock such as a gallop rhythm or murmur, crackles in the lungs, hepatomegaly, or peripheral edema. In patients who have fever, tachypnea, and a clinical suspicion for sepsis or septic shock, an ABG analysis can help to diagnose a metabolic acidosis, but history and physical examination findings and an elevated or a very low WBC count combined with response to therapy are usually sufficient to confirm the diagnosis.

3. Be able to manage septic shock.

Management of sepsis and septic shock involves prompt recognition and aggressive treatment with early goal-directed therapy. In patients with sepsis, an example of distributive shock, vasodilation and capillary leak result in a relative hypovolemic state. Cardiac dysfunction with impaired ejection fraction is common in septic shock as well. Once intravenous access is obtained, treatment with isotonic crystalloid and the administration of broad-spectrum antibiotics are the essential elements of initial therapy.[5] Antimicrobial coverage should be chosen based on the resistance patterns of the Gram-positive and Gram-negative organisms present in that community. Typically, as noted earlier, empiric therapy should include a third-generation cephalosporin and vancomycin for coverage of penicillin-resistant *Streptococcus pneumoniae*.[6] If bacterial meningitis is high on the differential diagnosis, the clinician should consider the administration of dexamethasone prior to or with the administration of the first dose of antibiotic. This therapy may limit the neurologic sequelae in children and adults and may have a mortality benefit.[7] After initial fluid therapy (usually 40 mL/kg of isotonic crystalloid), if hypotension persists, ionotropic agents such as dopamine or epinephrine should be started.

Patients with severe metabolic acidosis due to septic shock, such as the patient in this case scenario, should be intubated to reduce oxygen consumption due to work of breathing and to maximize oxygen delivery.[8]

References

1. Zimmerman J. Sepsis/septic shock. In: Fuhrman BP, Zimmerman JJ, eds. *Pediatric Critical Care.* 2nd ed. St Louis, Mo: Mosby Inc; 1998:1088-1100.
2. Zaritsky AL, Nadkarni VM, Hickey RW, et al, eds. *PALS Provider Manual.* Dallas, Tex: American Academy of Pediatrics and American Heart Association; 2002:30.
3. Levy MM, Fink MP, Marshall JC, et al. 2001 SCCM/ESICM/ACCP/ATS/SIS International Sepsis Definitions Conference. *Crit Care Med.* 2003;31:1250-1256.
4. Press S, Lipkind RS. Acute myocarditis in infants. Initial presentation. *Clin Pediatr.* 1990;29:73-76.
5. Carcillo JA, Davis AL, Zaritsky A. Role of early fluid resuscitation in pediatric septic shock. *JAMA.* 1991;266:1242-1245.
6. Avner JR, Sharieff GQ. Medical emergencies. In: Gausche-Hill M, Fuchs S, Yamamoto L, eds. *APLS: The Pediatric Emergency Medicine Resource.* 4th ed. Sudbury, Mass: American Academy of Pediatrics, American College of Emergency Physicians, Jones and Bartlett Publishing Co; 2004:447-472.
7. van de Beek D, de Gans J, McIntyre P, et al. Corticosteroids in acute bacterial meningitis. The Cochrane Database of Systematic Reviews; 2005.
8. Fitzmaurice L, Gerardi MJ. Cardiovascular system. In: Gausche-Hill M, Fuchs S, Yamamoto L, eds. *APLS: The Pediatric Emergency Medicine Resource.* 4th ed. Sudbury, Mass: American Academy of Pediatrics, American College of Emergency Physicians, Jones and Bartlett Publishing Co; 2004:107-140.

SCENARIO #15

Shock

Anne M. Stack, MD

Brief Presenting History

A 16-month-old girl awakes from her afternoon nap with fever, fussiness, and lethargy. She refuses to drink, and her mother brings her into the emergency department for evaluation.

Pediatric Assessment Triangle

Appearance: Pale with decreased activity

Work of Breathing: Increased respiratory rate and grunting

Circulation to the Skin: Mottled

Initial Vital Signs

Pulse: 190

Respiratory Rate: 36

Blood Pressure: 87/33

Temperature: 38.8°C (101.8°F) rectal

Physical Examination on Arrival to the Emergency Department

Airway: Patent, moving air freely

Breathing: Hyperpneic with some grunting; clear and equal breath sounds

Circulation: Skin mottled, extremities cool to touch and trunk warm; capillary refill time 3 seconds centrally, 4 seconds peripherally, peripheral pulses are 1+

Disability: Alert and anxious, cries when disturbed, moves all extremities

ASK YOURSELF

- **What is the initial assessment? What is the patient's physiologic status?**

  This child presents febrile and in compensated shock manifested by significant tachycardia, hyperpnea, and poor perfusion. The blood pressure is within normal limits for age, but low blood pressure is a late finding in pediatric shock.

- **What additional physical findings would help distinguish between compensated and decompensated shock?**

  Altered mental status would demonstrate failure to provide sufficient blood and nutrients to the brain. As shock advances, tachypnea and hyperpnea can change to bradypnea. Assessment of the quality of peripheral pulses also is helpful. Systolic blood pressure is preserved until the late stages of shock in children, because of their ability to use increased heart rate to maintain cardiac output. A widening pulse pressure, indicating low systemic vascular resistance, can be a clue that decompensated shock is imminent.[1]

- **Why is this child hyperpneic?**

  Patients in shock are unable to provide sufficient blood nutrients and oxygen to satisfy the needs of the tissues. This leads to metabolic acidosis. Hyperpnea (or deep respirations) is the body's attempt to correct the metabolic acidosis by exhaling CO_2.[1]

Additional History and Physical Examination Findings

The patient appeared well to her mother in the morning except that she was a little less playful than usual. On arrival at the hospital, the mother notices a fine purple rash on the child's face, chest, and extremities. The mother runs a small day care center in her home.

Past Medical History: The patient has a history of recurrent ear infections and is otherwise healthy.

Medications: None

Allergies: None known

Immunizations: Up to date

Physical Examination: Oxygen saturation on an earlobe is 97% in room air; diffuse, nonblanching, petechial and purpuric rash most notable on the extremities

ASK YOURSELF

■ What is the most likely diagnosis?

The onset of fever and petechiae/purpura in an ill-appearing child most likely represents bacterial sepsis, possibly meningococcemia or other bacteremia with disseminated intravascular coagulation.[2,3] The child is in distributive shock.

■ What interventions are needed at this time? What complications might be expected?

Interventions:

- At this point, the child's ability to maintain her airway should be evaluated. She is still in compensated shock, and her mental status is not altered. Breathing is tachypneic and hyperpneic, but her respirations are not slowing.
- Administer 100% O_2 via face mask.
- Place the patient on a cardiorespiratory monitor with pulse oximetry.
- Attempt to establish intravenous access and begin fluid resuscitation with normal saline 20 mL/kg.
- Laboratory tests: rapid glucose determination, blood culture, CBC, ABG, prothrombin time/partial thromboplastin time, fibrinogen, d-dimer, specimen to blood bank for type and hold, electrolytes, calcium
- Administer **ceftriaxone 100 mg/kg** IV/IO.
- Place Foley catheter, and send urine for urinalysis and culture.
- Attempt to obtain central intravenous access.
- All medical personnel must observe strict respiratory precautions.

Potential Complications:

- Intravenous access unobtainable due to poor peripheral perfusion. Because fluid resuscitation and antibiotic therapy are critical, the next attempts should be to establish intraosseous access.

Progression

A rapid glucose determination is 25 mg/dL.

ASK YOURSELF

■ Why is the child hypoglycemic?

Either hyperglycemia or hypoglycemia can occur in severe stress states in children. Plasma insulin levels and glucose utilization are increased in shock.[4]

■ What interventions are needed at this time? What complications might be expected?

Interventions:

- Administer **$D_{25}W$ 2 to 4 mL/kg** IV/IO push (0.5 to 1 g/kg).
- Repeat rapid glucose determination.

Potential Complication:

- Failure to suspect and correct hypoglycemia results in seizure.

Laboratory Test Results: ABG analysis: pH 7.18, Pco_2 30, Po_2 145, base excess –9.

Repeat Vital Signs

(After the first administration of 20 mL/kg normal saline)

Pulse: 188

Blood Pressure: 61/28

Respiratory Rate: 18; respirations slow

Oxygen Saturation: 91% with increased grunting

Mental Status: Altered, with markedly increased somnolence and loss of muscle tone

Rash: Worsening

Capillary Refill: Greater than 4 seconds

ASK YOURSELF

■ **What interventions should be made at this time? What complications might be expected?**

Interventions:

- Decompensated shock has developed, and the child is in impending respiratory failure. Preparations should be made for RSI.
- Continue attempts to obtain vascular access at a second site and continue volume expansion with a second 20 mL/kg normal saline bolus
- RSI
  1. #2 Miller blade, 4.5 ET tube
  2. Preoxygenation
  3. Cricoid pressure
  4. Consider **atropine 0.02 mg/kg** IV (mandatory before succinylcholine)
  5. **Etomidate 0.3 mg/kg** IV or **midazolam 0.1 mg/kg** IV
  6. **Rocuronium 0.6 to 1 mg/kg** IV is probably the preferred paralytic due to its cardiovascular stability.
- End-tidal CO_2 monitor
- Chest radiograph to confirm ET tube placement
- Secure ET tube and place NG tube.
- Consider placement of arterial monitoring catheter.
- Reassess perfusion after second 20 mL/kg normal saline bolus; consider third **20 mL/kg normal saline** bolus.
- Begin **dopamine 5 to 10 mcg/kg/min** infusion; titrate up as blood pressure requires.

Potential Complications:

- Vomiting: requires suctioning, especially if cricoid pressure not used during intubation
- Vomitus in airway, inability to visualize cords
- ET tube dislodged (moved during taping or ineffective taping)
- Failure to provide adequate fluid resuscitation can result in cardiorespiratory arrest secondary to severe hypovolemia and uncompensated shock.

Repeat Vital Signs

Pulse: 160

Blood Pressure: 88/48

Respiratory Rate: Ventilated at 30

Oxygen Saturation: 100% on 100% O_2

ASK YOURSELF

■ **What disposition and additional management would be expected for this patient?**

Admission to pediatric ICU for continued management of septic shock; central venous pressure monitoring; early goal-directed therapy

Objectives of This Scenario

1. Recognize fever and petechiae/purpura as a medical emergency.

This patient presented with an ill appearance and with fever and petechiae. Although petechiae can be a common exanthem in febrile children, one comprehensive study of all children presenting to a pediatric emergency department with fever and petechiae showed that 11.3% who were ill-appearing had serious invasive bacteremia.[2] Antibiotics should not be delayed. Caregivers should be careful to observe respiratory precautions.

2. Recognize compensated shock and the transition to decompensated shock.

Shock is defined as failure of the circulation to provide sufficient nutrients and oxygen to fulfill needs of the tissues. Early signs can be subtle, and one must have a high index of suspicion to make the diagnosis. For example, the patient can present slightly tachycardic for age or with a widened pulse pressure with preserved systolic blood pressure. Compensated shock can be described by the Pediatric Assessment Triangle findings of appearance: alert, anxious; work of breathing: tachypnea or hyperpnea; and circulation: tachycardia, flushed warm or cool extremities. Progression to decompensated shock is marked by the development of hypotension together with an alteration in mental status, continued tachypnea or ominous slowing of the respiratory rate, and tachycardia or bradycardia, absent peripheral pulses, and/or mottled or cyanotic skin.[1]

3. Initiate early goal-directed therapy for patients presenting in septic shock.

Evidence suggests that the low cardiac output state of septic shock is associated with high mortality rates.[5] Recent literature emphasizes early initiation of goal-directed therapy, which requires careful and quantitative monitoring of physiologic responses to therapeutic interventions.[6] Fluid resuscitation should begin as soon as shock is recognized. In addition to aggressive fluid resuscitation, the use of vasopressors and inotropic drugs to attain and maintain normal cardiac index constitutes the current strategies of goal-directed therapy, particularly in the adult population. Up to 60 mL/kg of fluid in the form of isotonic crystalloid and blood to achieve a hematocrit of 30% or greater can be necessary. Inotropic medications (dopamine and/or dobutamine) should be used when appropriate fluid resuscitation fails to restore adequate organ perfusion.[6]

References

1. Dieckmann RA. Pediatric assessment. In: Gausche-Hill M, Fuchs S, Yamamoto L, eds. *APLS: The Pediatric Emergency Medicine Resource.* 4th ed. Sudbury, Mass: American Academy of Pediatrics, American College of Emergency Physicians, Jones and Bartlett Publishing Co; 2004:40.
2. Mandl KD, Stack AM, Fleisher GR. Incidence of bacteremia in infants and children with fever and petechiae. *J Pediatr.* 1997;131:398-404.
3. Hale EH. Endocrine emergencies. In: Fleisher GR, Ludwig S, eds. *Textbook of Pediatric Emergency Medicine.* 4th ed. Philadelphia, Pa: Lippincott Williams & Wilkins; 2000:1093-1098.
4. Naylor JM, Kronfeld DS. In vivo studies of hypoglycemia and lactic acidosis in endotoxic shock. *Am J Physiol.* 1985;248;E309-E316.
5. Saladino RA. Management of septic shock in the pediatric emergency department in 2004. *Clin Pediatr Emerg Med.* 2004;5:20-27.
6. Dellinger RP, Carlet JM, Masur H, et al. Surviving Sepsis Campaign guidelines for management of severe sepsis and septic shock. *Crit Care Med.* 2004;32:858-873.

SCENARIO #16

Shock

Leticia Manning Ryan, MD

Brief Presenting History

A 2-year-old boy is brought in by his mother. He was found lying on her bedroom floor, vomiting blood.

Pediatric Assessment Triangle

Appearance: Pale, decreased activity, ill-appearing; poorly responsive

Work of Breathing: Respirations are not labored, but rate is increased.

Circulation to the Skin: Extremities cool; capillary refill 3 to 4 seconds in extremities

Initial Vital Signs

Pulse: 184

Respiratory Rate: 44

Blood Pressure: 85/39

Temperature: 38.2°C (100.8°F) rectal

Physical Examination on Arrival to Emergency Department

Airway: Patent; small amount of bloody vomitus present in and around mouth

Breathing: Breath sounds symmetric and clear without crackles, ronchi, or wheezes

Circulation: Heart tones significant for tachycardia; capillary refill 3 to 4 seconds in hands and feet; central pulses 2+ and peripheral pulses 1+

Disability: Poorly responsive to voice; eyes open; pupils 4 mm, symmetric, and reactive; movement of all extremities in response to pain

ASK YOURSELF

- **How much should this 2-year-old weigh?**

  An estimated weight for a 2-year-old is 13 kg. One can use the length-based Broselow Pediatric Emergency Tape or a pediatric table to determine weight based on age. See Appendix A.

- **What is the initial assessment? What is this patient's physiologic status?**

  This child presents with hematemesis, compensated shock, and altered mental status.

- **What are the different forms of shock?**

  Hypovolemic shock is the most common type of shock seen in infants and children. Shock of this type results from a decrease in intravascular volume. Common causes include dehydration and blood loss. Cardiogenic shock is a state of poor myocardial function and contractility that is often associated with an underlying congenital heart condition but also can occur with an acquired heart condition such as myocarditis. Distributive shock is caused by inappropriate vasodilation with a maldistribution of blood flow and increased vascular capacity. Etiologies include sepsis, anaphylaxis, and spinal cord injury. Septic shock, a form of distributive shock, has components of hypovolemia, cardiac dysfunction, and maldistribution of blood flow.[1]

■ What additional history would help you establish the diagnosis?

A recent history of recurrent vomiting followed by hematemesis would suggest Mallory-Weiss syndrome. A history of prior abdominal surgery, abdominal pain, trauma, NSAID use, or lower gastrointestinal bleeding would support an intra-abdominal etiology. Abrupt onset in a previously well child suggests a toxic ingestion or an esophageal foreign body. The presence of fever, recent illness, or recent travel would help identify infection and an associated coagulopathy. A history of liver disease or jaundice would support hepatic failure. The presence of a known bleeding disorder or a recent history of bleeding/bruising supports a hematologic disorder.

Additional History and Physical Examination Findings

The child had been previously well. After playing in the kitchen unsupervised while the mother was feeding his newborn sister, he was found lying on the floor vomiting a large amount of blood. An empty pill bottle was on the floor. The mother did not bring the bottle with her but says that they were "prenatal vitamins."

Past Medical History: Healthy child with no known underlying hematologic problems

Medications: None

Allergies: None known

Physical Examination: No signs of external trauma; sclera anicteric; abdomen distended, diffusely tender in epigastrium; no hepatomegaly; rectal examination reveals bright red blood in the rectum, tone normal, stool strongly heme positive

ASK YOURSELF

■ What is the most likely diagnosis?

The abrupt onset of the symptoms in an unsupervised child with access to an iron-containing medication strongly suggests an iron ingestion. Maternal pregnancy or recent birth of a sibling are major risk factors for iron poisoning in young children, and the period immediately after delivery is associated with the greatest risk.[2]

■ What interventions are needed at this time? What complications might be expected?

Interventions:

- Position airway; suction airway as needed.
- 100% O_2 by face mask
- Prepare for RSI because the patient's airway must be secured because of his depressed sensorium, need for gastric decontamination, and potential hemodynamic instability. Thiopental should be avoided in this case of nascent shock.
- Place the patient on a cardiorespiratory monitor with pulse oximetry.
- Attempt to establish intravenous access.
- Send blood for CBC, blood glucose, electrolytes, BUN, liver function tests, serum iron, type and crossmatch, and toxicology screen.
- Begin **normal saline bolus 20 mL/kg IV.**
- Consider call to blood bank for O-negative blood.
- Place NG tube (instead of larger-bore orogastric tube) to attempt gastric lavage and whole-bowel irrigation (only after airway is secured)
- Obtain abdominal radiograph to corroborate ingestion.

Potential Complications:

- Vomiting, especially if cricoid pressure is not used, suction not available, or gastric tube not placed
- Inability to obtain venous access necessitating intraosseous or central venous line placement

Initial Laboratory Findings

Rapid blood glucose 120; ABG analysis: pH 7.18, P_{CO_2} 30, P_{O_2} 280

Repeat Vital Signs

Pulse: 180

Respiratory Rate: 25

Blood Pressure: Not obtainable

Pulse oximeter not functioning

Progression

Patient is increasingly somnolent and unresponsive to painful stimulation; he is exhibiting minimal respiratory effort. Capillary refill in extremities is greater than 4 seconds.

ASK YOURSELF

- **What is the physiologic status now?**

  Impending respiratory failure and decompensated shock marked by loss of blood pressure.

- **What interventions are needed at this time? What complications might be expected?**

  Interventions:

  - BMV with 100% O_2
  - RSI:
    1. #2 Miller (straight) blade
    2. 4.5 uncuffed ET tube
    3. Preoxygenate
    4. Cricoid pressure
    5. **Atropine 0.02 mg/kg IV** (if **succinylcholine** is used)
    6. **Etomidate 0.3 mg/kg IV** or **midazolam 0.1 mg/kg IV**
    7. **Rocuronium 0.6 to 1 mg/kg IV** or **vecuronium 0.1 to 0.2 mg/kg IV**
    8. Pulse oximeter
    9. End-tidal CO_2 monitor
    10. Secure ET tube
    11. Chest radiograph to confirm ET tube position
  - Continue volume resuscitation.
    1. Repeat normal **saline bolus 20 mL/kg IV.**
    2. Consider transfusion with unmatched O-negative blood.
  - Consider **sodium bicarbonate 1 mEq/kg IV** for pronounced metabolic acidosis.

  Potential Complications:

  - Vomiting, especially if cricoid pressure not used, suction not available, or gastric tube not placed
  - Inability to visualize airway if not properly positioned, laryngoscope light not functioning, or copious hematemesis
  - Right mainstem intubation if tube position not verified
  - ET tube dislodged if not secured with tape

Repeat Vital Signs

Pulse: 180 (sinus tachycardia)

Blood Pressure: 90/60

Capillary Refill: 3 seconds in hands and feet

Laboratory Tests and Radiographs

Blood glucose 180 mg/dL; hematocrit 30%; WBC count 25,000; ABGs: pH 7.20, P_{CO_2} 30, P_{O_2} 220. Chest radiograph reveals tip of ET tube 2 cm above carina; abdominal radiograph reveals radiopaque objects in stomach and small bowel.

ASK YOURSELF

- **What interventions are needed at this time? What complications might be expected?**

  Interventions:

  - Consider gastric lavage. (Recognize that gastric lavage has little benefit at 1 hour or more after ingestion despite the fact that this patient has radiologic evidence of ingested material in the stomach, probably concretions.[3])
  - Initiate whole-bowel irrigation with polyethylene glycol electrolyte lavage solution.
  - Begin chelation therapy with **deferoxamine 15 mg/kg/hr IV.**
  - Repeat abdominal radiograph after gastric lavage.

  Possible Complications:

  - Bradycardia and arrest caused by hypoxia or acidosis if airway not secured

- Seizure caused by hypoxia or acidosis requiring **lorazepam 0.1 mg/kg IV**
- Coagulopathy caused by hepatic toxicity requiring fresh frozen plasma
- Potential exists for acute onset of shock, seizures, sepsis, and profound hepatic toxicity and failure.

Objectives of This Scenario

1. Recognize the presentation of hemorrhagic shock.

Shock is a syndrome of inadequate end-organ perfusion requiring oxygen and aggressive intravascular fluid resuscitation. The patient has tachycardia and poor skin perfusion, which are initial signs of shock in pediatric patients, but also displays later signs such as compromised blood pressure, the hallmark of decompensated shock.

2. Manage gastrointestinal hemorrhage and hypovolemia.

Hypovolemic shock in pediatric patients is treated initially with isotonic crystalloid at 20 mL/kg by rapid IV bolus. If reassessment reveals ongoing compromised perfusion, the 20-mL/kg bolus is repeated. Patients refractory to this aggressive therapy should be considered for transfusion of unmatched O-negative blood followed by cross-matched blood as time allows. Close attention should be paid to ongoing losses. Perfusion should be reassessed after each fluid bolus.

3. Manage the complications of iron ingestion.[3-7]

Although serum irons levels are useful, toxicity from iron overdose remains a clinical diagnosis. Ingested iron acts directly on the gastrointestinal mucosa causing necrosis of the stomach and intestines and subsequent hemorrhage. Liver injury results from the presence of free iron in the circulation.

The first priority in management is maintaining airway, breathing, and circulation as well as obtaining intravascular access. Patients in shock should be supported with aggressive fluid resuscitation with intravenous isotonic crystalloid and blood transfusions if indicated.

Rapid gut decontamination is a high priority. This may be accomplished by gastric lavage and whole-bowel irrigation; endoscopy should be considered if repeat abdominal films reveal persistent iron pills fragments. Gastric lavage has little benefit more than 1 hour after ingestion or in the presence of pill concretions. Whole-bowel irrigation is considered the technique of choice in large ingestions but should be used cautiously in patients with active gastrointestinal bleeding or ileus. Gastroscopy and gastrostomy have been performed with massive overdoses. Iron is not adsorbed to charcoal. Intragastric complexing with bicarbonate, phosphate, or deferoxamine is ineffective and can be dangerous.

In severe ingestions (presence of symptoms or serum iron concentration >350 mcg/dL), iron chelation is accomplished using deferoxamine 15 mg/kg/hr IV to enhance the excretion of iron. A change in urine color to a pinkish-orange (vin rose) indicates the presence of an iron-deferoxamine complex. When this complex is present, significant serum iron levels are suggested; however, absence of this color change does not rule out toxicity.

Also, severe iron intoxication can result in profound metabolic acidosis requiring sodium bicarbonate intravenously. Additional clinical manifestations requiring intervention include hypoglycemia or hyperglycemia, anemia, and colloid loss due to gastrointestinal hemorrhage, hepatic failure, and associated coagulopathy.

References

1. Fitzmaurice L, Gerardi MJ. Cardiovascular system. In: Gausche-Hill M, Fuchs S, Yamamoto L, eds. *APLS: The Pediatric Emergency Medicine Resource.* 4th ed. Sudbury, Mass: American Academy of Pediatrics, American College of Emergency Physicians, Jones and Bartlett Publishing Co; 2004:137-140.
2. Juurlink DN, Tenebein M. Iron poisoning in young children: association with the birth of a sibling. *CMAJ.* 2003;168:1539-1542.
3. Erickson TB. Toxicology: ingestions and smoke inhalation. In: Gausche-Hill M, Fuchs S, Yamamoto L, eds. *APLS: The Pediatric Emergency Medicine Resource.* 4th ed. Sudbury, Mass: American Academy of Pediatrics, American College of Emergency Physicians, Jones and Bartlett Publishing Co; 2004:249-251.
4. Osterhoudt KC, Shannon M, Henretig FM. Toxicologic emergencies: iron. In: Fleisher GR, Ludwig S, eds. *Textbook of Pediatric Emergency Medicine.* 4th ed. Philadelphia, Pa: Lippincott Williams and Wilkins; 2000:914-917.
5. Baranwal AK, Singhi SC. Acute iron poisoning: management guidelines. *Indian Pediatr.* 2003;40:534-540.
6. Singhi SC, Baranwal AK, M J. Acute iron poisoning: clinical picture, intensive care needs and outcome. *Indian Pediatr.* 2003;40:1177-1182.
7. Fine JS. Iron poisoning. *Curr Probl Pediatr.* 2000;30:71-90.

SCENARIO #17

Shock

Joshua Nagler, MD, and Richard G. Bachur, MD

Brief Presenting History

A 7-year-old boy is brought to the emergency department by his father after the child became short of breath during a soccer game today. He had complained of chest and abdominal pain the previous night.

Pediatric Assessment Triangle

Appearance: Awake and alert, anxious

Work of Breathing: Tachypneic, mild subcostal retractions

Circulation to the Skin: Pale, delayed capillary refill

Initial Vital Signs

Pulse: 145

Respiratory Rate: 36

Blood Pressure: 86/66

Temperature: 38.3°C (100.9°F) axillary

Physical Examination on Arrival to the Emergency Department

Airway: Patent, normal voice

Breathing: Tachypneic, good aeration, crackles and rales at the bases bilaterally, subcostal retractions

Circulation: Tachycardic, strong distal pulses, capillary refill 2 to 3 seconds, extremities cool

Disability: Awake, alert, cooperative

ASK YOURSELF

- **What is the initial assessment? What is the patient's physiologic status?**

  This child presents in respiratory distress with signs of compensated shock.

- **What is the differential diagnosis of respiratory distress in this patient?**

  Tachypnea and increased work of breathing in a patient with bilateral rales could be caused by either primary pulmonary or primary cardiac disease. Fever, chest pain, and abdominal pain could also be consistent with either etiology. Leading diagnoses at this point include pneumonia and CHF.

- **What additional history and physical examination findings would help you establish the diagnosis?**

  With regard to the history, cough by itself is nonspecific, although production of purulent sputum would be more consistent with a pulmonary infection. Chest pain also can occur with both pulmonary and cardiac disease, although the quality and timing of the pain, along with any positional nature or pleuritic component, can sometimes help differentiate the etiology.

  With regard to the physical examination, hepatomegaly, jugular venous distention, and edema, if present, are consistent with CHF. A new murmur, gallop, or rub might suggest endocarditis, myocarditis, or pericarditis, respectively. Pulsus paradoxus, muffled heart sounds, and jugular venous distention often are seen with pericarditis.

Additional History and Physical Examination Findings

The patient was seen 1 week earlier for a febrile illness, diagnosed as a viral syndrome. He has had several days of progressive shortness of breath, limiting his activity. He has no cough. His abdominal pain is on his right side, and his chest pain is worse when he lies back.

Past Medical History: Negative

Medications: None

Allergies: None known

Physical Examination: Oxygen saturation 92% in room air; no jugular venous distention; gallop rhythm present without murmur or rub; liver mildly enlarged and tender

ASK YOURSELF

■ **What is the most likely diagnosis?**

The constellation of fever, chest pain, gallop rhythm, rales, and hepatomegaly are most consistent with myocarditis.

■ **What interventions are needed at this time? What are the potential complications?**

Interventions:

- Administer supplemental oxygen.
- Place the patient on a cardiorespiratory monitor with pulse oximetry.
- Attempt intravenous access.
- Obtain chest radiograph and electrocardiogram.
- Consider echocardiogram to evaluate cardiac function.
- Administer **furosemide 1 mg/kg** IV. Use with caution if there is any concern of decreased intravascular volume.

Potential Complications:

- Inability to obtain intravenous access
- Failure to administer supplemental oxygen or placing the patient in a supine position, both of which can worsen respiratory distress.
- Aggressive intravenous hydration, which also can worsen respiratory distress.

Repeat Vital Signs

Pulse: 125

Respiratory Rate: 30

Blood Pressure: 92/64

Oxygen Saturation: 97% via face mask

Chest Radiography: Moderate cardiomegaly with increased pulmonary vascular markings and interstitial fluid at bases

Electrocardiography: Decreased QRS voltages, nonspecific ST-T wave abnormalities in precordial leads

Progression

Patient suddenly complains of palpitations and increasing chest pain, and then he becomes pale and unresponsive.

ASK YOURSELF

■ **What other information do you need immediately?**

Heart rate, presence or absence of central pulses, and cardiac rhythm on monitor

ECG Monitor:

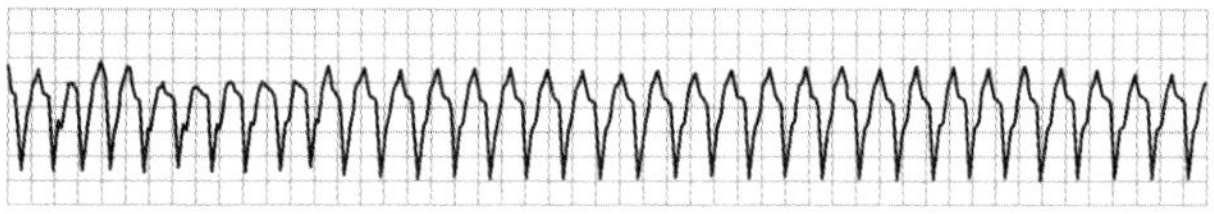

Physical Examination

Airway: Patent

Breathing: Respiratory rate decreases abruptly with increased rales and retractions.

Circulation: Absent brachial and femoral pulses, capillary refill greater than 4 seconds

Disability: Unarousable

ASK YOURSELF

■ **What interventions should be made at this time? What complications might be expected?**

Interventions:

- Initiate algorithm for pulseless arrest ("Evaluation and Management: Circulation," Figure 1).
- Begin ventilation and oxygenation with BMV and chest compressions at a rate of 100 until a defibrillator is available and charged.
- Defibrillation should be first priority. However, be sure to initiate CPR while preparing the defibrillation equipment.
- Place intraosseous line if intravenous access has not been obtained.
- Prepare for intubation.
  1. #2 Miller blade, 6.0 ET tube
  2. Cricoid pressure
  3. Unresponsive patient in arrest may be intubated without premedication.
- Defibrillate up to three times at 2 J/kg, 4 J/kg, and 4 J/kg if VT persists. Check rhythm and pulse after each shock.
- Continue compressions as long as pulses are absent and VT continues.
- Administer **epinephrine 0.01 mg/kg** IV, **0.1 mg/kg** via ET tube.
- Defibrillate at 4 J/kg within 30 to 60 seconds of epinephrine administration. Check rhythm and pulse.
- Continue compressions if patient remains pulseless.
- **Amiodarone 5 mg/kg** IV/IO or **lidocaine 1 mg/kg** IV/IO/ET.
- Defibrillate at 4 J/kg within 30 to 60 seconds of medication. Check rhythm and pulse.
- Check for pulse after any change in rhythm.

Potential Complications:

- Vomiting can occur during BMV if not applying cricoid pressure.
- Multiple issues can arise with the defibrillator: not available, pads/gel not available, wrong size paddles on unit, unit in synchronized mode, battery power insufficient.
- Another provider touching patient during defibrillation becomes unresponsive.

■ **During RSI in a patient with cardiac disease, what medications would be most appropriate?**

Etomidate is the most cardiovascularly stable sedative agent. Fentanyl and midazolam also might be considered. In patients with dysrhythmias possibly secondary to electrolyte abnormalities, including hyperkalemia, nondepolarizing neuromuscular blocking agents (rocuronium and vecuronium) may be safer than succinylcholine. (*Note:* Any medications [sedatives] that could further compromise cardiac output must be administered with extreme caution.)

Progression

Return of sinus rhythm after amiodarone and fifth shock; weak distal pulses

Repeat Vital Signs

Pulse: 170

Respiratory Rate: 30 (by assisted ventilation)

Blood Pressure: 62/42

Oxygen Saturation: 100%

ASK YOURSELF

■ **What additional complications might be expected for this patient?**

Patients with myocarditis are at risk for continued dysrhythmias. The use of inotropic agents, although it is necessary, can increase this risk. The combination of myocardial disease and further myocyte injury secondary to repeated defibrillation puts this patient at high risk of ongoing cardiogenic shock.

Objectives of This Scenario

1. Recognize signs and symptoms of CHF in children.[1,2]

CHF in previously healthy children is rare. In addition, many presenting signs and symptoms are nonspecific. Therefore, it is easy to overlook this diagnosis. Clinical presentation varies with age and severity. In infants, signs and symptoms commonly include tachypnea, tachycardia, poor feeding or sweating with feeds, and failure to thrive. Hepatomegaly and gallop rhythm are frequently noted on examination. Wheezing is the predominant pulmonary finding, so it can be difficult to differentiate from bronchiolitis. Older children often present with exercise intolerance and fatigue; many have abdominal pain. Tachycardia and tachypnea are common, often with crackles, rales, or wheezing. Jugular venous distention is easier to appreciate in older children than in infants. Signs and symptoms in adolescents are similar to those in adults and include fatigue, dyspnea on exertion, orthopnea, and gastrointestinal symptoms. Basilar crackles, rales, and peripheral edema occur frequently, and a gallop rhythm with or without an associated holosystolic murmur may be heard. Patients of all ages typically have a large cardiac silhouette on chest radiography, but echocardiography may be necessary to differentiate an enlarged heart from a pericardial effusion or an enlarged thymus.

2. Institute the initial management of acute CHF.

CHF is one of the few acute presentations in pediatrics for which empiric intravenous fluids can be detrimental. This highlights the importance of frequent reevaluation after therapeutic interventions. Immediate management of CHF includes elevation of the head of the bed (cardiac chair or infant seat if available) and administration of supplemental oxygen.[3] Diuretics can be used to treat pulmonary edema secondary to CHF, although this should be done with caution in any patient who might be intravascularly compromised. Inotropic agents also are used to treat acute CHF, although again they should be used carefully, particularly in patients with myocarditis who are very sensitive to the arrhythmogenic properties of these agents.[1] When using digoxin, for example, it is recommended to use one half the usual starting dose.[3] For patients in cardiogenic shock, dobutamine may be advantageous because it has inotropic properties but does not increase systemic vascular resistance.[4]

3. Recognize clinical presentations of myocarditis and treatment options.

There is a wide spectrum of clinical presentations for patients with myocarditis. Many with mild disease are thought to have subclinical symptoms and never seek medical care. Patients can be completely asymptomatic but have physical examination findings, ECG changes, or arrhythmias that lead to the diagnosis. Others present with signs and symptoms of heart failure as described earlier. Often, these patients are thought to have subacute or chronic myocarditis, clinically indistinguishable from a dilated cardiomyopathy. In the acute setting, additional symptoms can include preceding flu-like illness, fever, chest pain (often worse when supine), abdominal pain, and malaise.[5] There is no single diagnostic test for myocarditis. Creatine kinase-MB and troponin levels are frequently elevated, although normal levels do not exclude the diagnosis. Chest radiography usually shows cardiomegaly. ECG findings are common. One study found that in children with biopsy-proven myocarditis, 100% had ST-T changes and 80% had low QRS voltages.[6] Diagnosis can be made by endomyocardial biopsy, although sensitivity is only 35% to 60% depending on what is chosen as the gold standard.[1] Echocardiography is useful to confirm and quantify the degree of cardiac dysfunction. Adenovirus and enterovirus are the most common causative agents, although many known viral agents have been isolated.[7] Treatment is supportive. Patients require monitoring for and treatment of arrhythmias and CHF, usually in an ICU setting. Although some studies have suggested benefits from the use of intravenous immunoglobulin and/or immunosuppression, there are insufficient data from large-scale trials to uniformly support these therapies.[5] Most patients recover spontaneously, with a median time to return of normal ventricular function of 2 to 3 months.[6,8]

4. Manage the child with ventricular tachycardia.

Ventricular tachycardia is rare in children. It occurs most commonly in children with congenital heart disease, particularly those with prior cardiac surgery or catheterization. Other causes include myocarditis, cardiomyopathies, electrolyte and metabolic disturbances, cardiac tumors, drugs, and prolonged QT syndrome.[9] It is important to identify and to treat reversible causes whenever possible. There is some evidence to suggest that amiodarone should be the first-line treatment for stable VT with adequate perfusion.[10] Other treatment options include lidocaine, procainamide, and synchronized electrical cardioversion. Pulseless VT is treated with rapid electrical defibrillation. There is no clear evidence to support amiodarone over lidocaine in the pulseless VT algorithm for children.[10] Finally, for out-of-hospital arrests, automatic external defibrillators (AEDs) may be available. Although previous recommendations did not support the use of AEDs in children younger than 8 years, recently published guidelines now allow for their use in children aged 1 to 8 years and recommend their use for children with documented pulseless VT or ventricular fibrillation.[11]

References

1. Bernstein D. Heart failure and diseases of the myocardium. In: Behrman RE, Kliegman RM, Jenson HB, eds. *Nelson Textbook of Pediatrics.* 17th ed. Philadelphia, Pa: WB Saunders; 2004:1430-1436,1440-1444.
2. Kay JD, Colan SD, Graham TP Jr. Congestive heart failure in pediatric patients. *Am Heart J.* 2001;142:923-928.
3. Park MK. Congestive heart failure. In: *Pediatric Cardiology for Practitioners.* 4th ed. St Louis, Mo: Mosby; 2002.
4. Giroir BP, Levin DL, Perkin RM. Shock. In: Levin DL, Morriss FC. eds. *Essentials of Pediatric Intensive Care.* 2nd ed. New York, NY: Churchill Livingstone; 1997:280-301.
5. Feldman AM, McNamara D. Myocarditis. *N Engl J Med.* 2000;343:1388-1398.
6. Lee KJ, McCrindle BW, Bohn DJ, et al. Clinical outcomes of acute myocarditis in childhood. *Heart.* 1999;82:226-233.
7. Bowles NE, Ni J, Kearney DL, et al. Detection of viruses in myocardial tissues by PCR: evidence of adenovirus as a common cause of myocarditis in children and adults. *J Am Coll Cardiol.* 2003;42:466-472.
8. Fuse K, Kodama M, Okura Y, et al. Predictors of disease course in patients with acute myocarditis. *Circulation.* 2000;102:2829-2835.
9. Gewitz MH, Vetter VL. Cardiac emergencies. In: Fleisher GR, Ludwig S, eds. *Textbook of Pediatric Emergency Medicine.* 4th ed. Philadelphia, Pa: Lippincott Williams and Wilkins; 2000:659-700.
10. Guidelines 2000 for Cardiopulmonary Resuscitation and Emergency Cardiovascular Care. Part 10: Pediatric advanced life support. The American Heart Association in collaboration with the International Liaison Committee on Resuscitation. *Circulation.* 2000;102(suppl I):I-291–I-342.
11. Samson RA, Berg RA, Bingham R, Pediatric Advanced Life Support Task Force, International Liaison Committee on Resuscitation for the American Heart Association, European Resuscitation Council. Use of automated external defibrillators for children: an update—an advisory statement from the Pediatric Advanced Life Support Task Force, International Liaison Committee on Resuscitation. *Pediatrics.* 2003;112:163-168.

SCENARIO #18

Shock

Dewesh Agrawal, MD

Brief Presenting History

A 19-day-old infant is brought to the emergency department via ambulance after his parents found him having a seizure in his crib.

Pediatric Assessment Triangle

Appearance: Actively seizing (generalized and symmetric tonic-clonic activity)

Work of Breathing: Tachypneic, labored respirations

Circulation to the Skin: Pale, mottled, circumoral and peripheral cyanosis

Initial Vital Signs

Pulse: 192

Respiratory Rate: 74

Blood Pressure: Not obtainable

Temperature: 37.6°C (99.7°F) rectal

Oxygen Saturation: 72% in room air

ASK YOURSELF

- **How much should this 19-day-old infant weigh?**

  An estimated weight for a 19-day-old child is 3 kg. One can use the length-based Broselow Pediatric Emergency Tape or a pediatric table to determine weight based on age. (See Appendix A.)

Physical Examination on Arrival to the Emergency Department

Airway: Upper airway obstructive sounds with snoring and gurgling respirations

ASK YOURSELF

- **What needs to be done emergently to manage this child's airway?**

  This child's airway is not patent. This patient requires emergent airway repositioning, that is, manual airway-opening maneuvers such as the head tilt-chin lift or the jaw-thrust maneuver (if trauma is suspected). The mouth and nose should be suctioned and oxygen applied. After these maneuvers are performed, this patient's obstructive airway sounds and work of breathing diminish.

Breathing: Tachypnea, good aeration with clear breath sounds bilaterally

Circulation: Mottled skin; capillary refill time 4 to 5 seconds; weakly palpable femoral pulses

Disability: Actively seizing, unresponsive

ASK YOURSELF

- **What is the initial assessment? What is the patient's physiologic status?**

  The child has active seizure activity with decompensated shock. Respiratory distress has resolved with above treatment.

■ **What is the differential diagnosis of seizures in a neonate?**

The differential diagnosis of neonatal seizures is quite broad. Common causes include sepsis, CNS infections, disseminated herpes simplex, trauma, intracranial hemorrhage, inborn errors of metabolism, other metabolic causes (hypoglycemia, hyponatremia, hypocalcemia, hypomagnesemia, or hyperphosphatemia), drug withdrawal, congenital CNS anomalies, hypoxic-ischemic encephalopathy, febrile seizures, toxicologic causes, and hypertension.[1]

■ **What interventions are needed at this time? What complications might be expected?**

Interventions:

- Administer 100% O_2 via face mask.
- Continue to assess ventilation and support as needed.
- Place the patient on a cardiorespiratory monitor with pulse oximetry.
- Attempt to establish intravenous access.
- Provide antiepileptic therapy with **lorazepam 0.1 mg/kg** IV/IO or **diazepam 0.3 mg/kg** IV/IO or (if no intravenous/intraosseous access) **diazepam 0.5 mg/kg** PR
- Administer intravenous fluid bolus of **normal saline 20 mL/kg**

Potential Complications:

- Unsuccessful intravenous attempts requiring intraosseous line placement
- Continued status epilepticus refractory to initial dose of lorazepam or diazepam necessitating repeat dosing of lorazepam or diazepam followed by **phenobarbital 20 mg/kg** IV/IO

■ **Initial attempt at intravenous access is unsuccessful, and three drops of blood are obtained. What should you do with the three drops of blood?**

Rapid bedside glucose determination (value is 22)

■ **How should the hypoglycemia be treated?**

Rapid glucose infusion of 0.5 to 1 g/kg with a dextrose solution: **$D_{10}W$ 5 to 10 mL/kg** (*Note:* because of the high solute load and subsequent potential for deleterious fluid shifts, $D_{25}W$ is typically not administered in the first month of life).

■ **What initial laboratory tests would you obtain after intravenous access is established in this neonate with status epilepticus?**

Keeping the differential diagnoses in mind, initial laboratory workup should include ABG analysis, CBC, blood culture, and electrolytes.

Initial Laboratory Results (before dextrose administration)

ABG analysis: pH 7.08, Pco_2 27, Po_2 54, HCO_3^- 7

Serum electrolytes: Na^+ 122, K^+ 7.4, Cl^- 91, HCO_3^- 7, BUN 16, creatinine 0.4, glucose 24, Ca^{2+} 9.3, Mg^{2+} 2.0, phosphorus 4.4

CBC: WBC count 18,000 (differential 62% polys, 28% lymphs, 9% monos), hematocrit 41%, platelets 278,000

Additional History and Physical Examination Findings

The infant was fine until a few days ago, when the parents noted decreased oral intake. The infant has vomited a few times, has been sleepy, and has not waked up for feeds. There have been fewer than normal wet diapers. The child has no history of fever, upper respiratory tract infection symptoms, or diarrhea, and he has been exclusively breastfed.

Past Medical History: Healthy full-term male infant with unremarkable prenatal course except for amniocentesis that revealed 46,XX karyotype; midwife-assisted uncomplicated home vaginal delivery; noted to have genital hypoplasia at birth but deemed male (outpatient pediatric urology consultation pending)

Medications: None

Physical Examination: Non-dysmorphic-appearing infant, normocephalic, atraumatic skull, anterior fontanel open flat and depressed, pupils equally round and reactive to light, clear but shallow respirations, tachycardia, no murmurs, weakly palpable femoral pulses, abdomen soft, no organomegaly, no vesicular rash or oral lesions, decreased skin turgor, cool and mottled extremities, ambiguous genitalia with abnormal microphallus-like structure with presumed hypospadius, hyperpigmented scrotal structure with lack of palpable testes

Progression

Generalized and symmetric tonic-clonic seizure briefly terminates after antiepileptic therapy and dextrose administration but has now resumed.

Repeat Vital Signs

Pulse: 188

Respiratory Rate: 66

Blood Pressure: Not obtainable

Oxygen Saturation: 94%

ASK YOURSELF

■ **What interventions are needed at this time? What complications might be expected?**

Interventions:

- Continue 100% O_2 via face mask.
- Continue to assess ventilation, and support as needed.
- Administer hypertonic saline to partially correct symptomatic hyponatremia (6 mL/kg of 3% saline is expected to raise serum sodium by 5 mEq/L).[2,3]
- Because of **potassium 7.4 mEq/L**, obtain electrocardiogram (once seizure resolves).

Potential Complications:

- Airway obstruction requiring airway repositioning
- Respiratory arrest requiring RSI
- If succinylcholine is used for RSI, then pulseless ventricular tachycardia or ventricular fibrillation develops secondary to significant hyperkalemia.

Progression

Seizure resolves after administration of hypertonic saline.

Electrocardiography: Sinus tachycardia at 180, tented/peaked T waves diffusely

ASK YOURSELF

■ **What interventions are needed at this time? What complications might be expected?**

Interventions:

- Hyperkalemia resulting in electrocardiographic changes should be treated emergently with **calcium chloride 10% (0.2 mL/kg IV)** or **calcium gluconate 10% (0.5 to 1 mL/kg IV)** to reverse the membrane destabilizing effects of hyperkalemia. Insulin and glucose also may be considered.
- In addition, systemic alkalinization with **sodium bicarbonate (1 mEq/kg IV)** should be considered, given this patient's severe metabolic acidosis and hyperkalemia.

Potential Complications:

- Loss of peripheral intravenous access if sodium bicarbonate is given in the same intravenous line as calcium chloride with lack of adequate flush. Calcium chloride and sodium bicarbonate react to form calcium carbonate, which can precipitate out (as chalk) and obstruct the intravenous line.

Progression

Electrocardiographic changes associated with hyperkalemia resolve after calcium and sodium bicarbonate therapy.

Repeat Vital Signs and Assessment

Pulse: 178

Respiratory Rate: 64

Blood Pressure: Not obtainable

Patient still appears to be in shock with signs of poor perfusion and weakly palpable central pulses.

ASK YOURSELF

- **What is the most likely etiology for this infant's metabolic derangements with subsequent seizures and decompensated shock?**

This patient has acute adrenal insufficiency secondary to congenital adrenal hyperplasia. The following all serve as valuable clues in making this diagnosis: 1) the presentation of poor feeding, lethargy, and shock; 2) the characteristic metabolic derangements (hyponatremia, hyperkalemia, acidosis, and hypoglycemia); and 3) the physical examination notable for abnormal genitalia with hyperpigmentation. Lack of cortisol results in hypoglycemia and hypotension with secondary lactic acidosis secondary to poor perfusion. Lack of aldosterone results in renal salt wasting, hyponatremia, hypovolemia, and type IV (hyperkalemic) renal tubular acidosis. This infant's hyponatremia and hypoglycemia likely both precipitated his seizure. This infant is genetically a female (given the amniocentesis karyotype of 46,XX). However, the excess adrenal androgens observed with severe cases of neonatal congenital adrenal hyperplasia can result in virilization of a female infant, resulting in ambiguous genitalia and assignment of male phenotype at birth.[4-8]

- **What interventions are needed at this time?**
    - Once acute adrenal insufficiency secondary to congenital adrenal hyperplasia is recognized, stress-dose steroids should be administered (**hydrocortisone 25 mg** IV).
    - Repeat intravenous fluid bolus of **normal saline 20 mL/kg** if signs of poor perfusion continue.
    - Persistent hypotension can necessitate inotropic support.
    - Serum should be drawn for determination of an adrenal steroid profile before the administration of replacement steroid therapy if possible.

Objectives of This Scenario

1. Be familiar with the differential diagnosis of adrenal insufficiency presenting as shock in an infant.

Because most of the symptoms of adrenal insufficiency are nonspecific, other more common diagnoses must be considered. In infants, adrenal insufficiency might be confused with other illnesses that similarly present with lethargy, poor weight gain, tachycardia, and shock. These include infectious causes (eg, sepsis with secondary septic shock), congenital heart disease (with secondary cardiogenic shock), other metabolic disorders (eg, inborn errors of metabolism), hematologic disorders (eg, methemoglobinemia or severe anemia), and neurologic disease (eg, infantile botulism or head injury from child abuse). The presence of hyponatremia, hyperkalemia, acidosis, and hypoglycemia, as well as ambiguous genitalia (often but not always present) and hyperpigmentation, will help to differentiate congenital adrenal hyperplasia from these other possibilities.[4]

2. Emergently manage hyperkalemia in infants.

With significant hyperkalemia (K^+ >7 mEq/L), peaked (or tented) T waves, loss of P waves, and progressive widening of the QRS complex can be seen on the ECG. Symptomatic hyperkalemia or hyperkalemia resulting in ECG changes should be treated with **calcium chloride 10% (0.2 mL/kg IV)** or **calcium gluconate 10% (0.5 to 1 mL/kg IV)** to reverse the membrane-destabilizing effects of hyperkalemia. Movement of potassium from the extracellular space into cells is enhanced by several mechanisms, including alkalinization (with **sodium bicarbonate 1 mEq/kg IV**), use of a combination of **glucose (0.5 to 1 g/kg = 2 to 4 mL/kg $D_{25}W$** or **5 to 10 mL/kg $D_{10}W$ IV)** and **insulin (0.1 units/kg IV)**, and use of **albuterol** aerosol. Insulin and glucose must be used with extreme caution in this instance because hypoglycemia can result. Likewise, albuterol should be used with caution, as its β-adrenergic effect can promote arrhythmias. Net gastrointestinal excretion of potassium can be achieved by administering **Kayexalate (sodium polystyrene sulfonate) 1 g/kg** PO/PR. Hemodialysis is useful in extreme cases and for long-term treatment of hyperkalemia associated with renal failure.[9,10]

3. Recognize and manage the emergent neonatal complications of congenital adrenal hyperplasia.

Congenital adrenal hyperplasia, which includes several different disorders with varying genotypes and phenotypes, is the leading cause of adrenal insufficiency in infants, affecting 1 in 10,000 to 20,000 infants.[5,7] The clinical manifestations and metabolic derangement result from lack of adequate production of cortisol and aldosterone.[4,5]

Infants with adrenal insufficiency typically present with poor feeding (and resultant poor weight gain), vomiting, and lethargy. On physical examination, these infants can be hypotensive and tachycardic. Depending on the degree of virilization, female infants can manifest ambiguous genitalia, but male infants usually have normal-appearing genitalia. Due to the high concentration of adrenocorticotropic hormone, infants of both sexes can be hyperpigmented, particularly in the genitalia. Hyperkalemia and acidosis predispose these patients to cardiac arrhythmias.[4-8]

Laboratory evaluation in patients with primary adrenal insufficiency typically reveals hyponatremia, hyperkalemia, metabolic acidosis, and hypoglycemia secondary to the deficiency of aldosterone and cortisol. BUN and creatinine values can be elevated secondary to dehydration.[4-7]

Acute adrenal insufficiency with secondary shock is treated with fluid resuscitation, administration of glucose to correct hypoglycemia, and administration of stress-dose glucocorticoids. An initial fluid bolus of 20 mL/kg of normal saline should be given and repeated as necessary to restore perfusion. After correcting the hypoglycemia, a continuous infusion of dextrose (either D_5 or D_{10}) should be started. Intravenous hydrocortisone should be administered immediately (25 mg for infants, 50 mg for children younger than 4 years, and 100 mg for children older than 4 years). Symptomatic hyperkalemia also should be treated as discussed previously.[4,11]

References

1. Burchfield DJ, Boychuk RB. Neonatal emergencies. In: Gausche-Hill M, Fuchs S, Yamamoto L, eds. *APLS: The Pediatric Emergency Medicine Resource.* 4th ed. Sudbury, Mass: American Academy of Pediatrics, American College of Emergency Physicians, Jones and Bartlett Publishing Co; 2004:477-493.

2. Lauriat SM, Berl T. The hyponatremic patient: practical focus on therapy. *J Am Soc Nephrol.* 1997;8:1599-1607.

3. Sarnaik AP, Meert K, Hackbarth R, et al. Management of hyponatremic seizures in children with hypertonic saline: a safe and effective strategy. *Crit Care Med.* 1991;19:758-762.

4. Glaser N, Enns GM, Kuppermann N. Metabolic disease. In: Gausche-Hill M, Fuchs S, Yamamoto L, eds. *APLS: The Pediatric Emergency Medicine Resource.* 4th ed. Sudbury, Mass: American Academy of Pediatrics, American College of Emergency Physicians, Jones and Bartlett Publishing Co; 2004:194-196.

5. Speiser PW, White PC. Congenital adrenal hyperplasia. *N Engl J Med.* 2003;349:776-788.

6. Pang S. Congenital adrenal hyperplasia. *Endocrinol Metab Clin North Am.* 1997;26:853-891.

7. Behrman RE, Kliegman RM, Jenson HB, eds. *Nelson Textbook of Pediatrics.* 17th ed. Philadelphia, Pa: WB Saunders; 2004:1909-1916.

8. Larsen PR, Kronenberg HM, Melmed S, et al, eds. *Williams Textbook of Endocrinology.* 10th ed. Philadelphia, Pa: WB Saunders; 2003:532-538.

9. Gaffar M. Diagnosis and treatment of hyperkalemia. *Resid Staff Physician.* 2003;49:18-21.

10. Cronan K, Norman ME. Renal and electrolyte emergencies. In: Fleisher GR, Ludwig S, eds. *Textbook of Pediatric Emergency Medicine.* 4th ed. Philadelphia, Pa: Lippincott Williams and Wilkins; 2000:820-822.

11. Hale DE. Endocrine emergencies. In: Fleisher GR, Ludwig S, eds. *Textbook of Pediatric Emergency Medicine.* 4th ed. Philadelphia, Pa: Lippincott Williams and Wilkins; 2000:1103-1105.

SCENARIO #19

Shock

Mark G. Roddy, MD

Brief Presenting History

An 8-month-old girl is brought in with her mother via ambulance from home after the child became decreasingly responsive and very pale. The mother says the child has had some vomiting and has not been eating well for the past 12 hours.

Pediatric Assessment Triangle

Appearance: Pale, moaning, agitated, inconsolable

Work of Breathing: Grunting and tachypneic with mild subcostal retractions

Circulation to the Skin: Pale throughout, with mottled appearance of extremities

Initial Vital Signs

Pulse: 190

Respiratory Rate: 40

Blood Pressure: 55/40

Temperature: 37°C (98.6°F) rectal

Oxygen Saturation: 98% in room air

ASK YOURSELF

- **How much should this 8-month-old child weigh?**

  An estimated weight for an 8-month-old is 9 kg. One can use the length-based Broselow Pediatric Emergency Tape or a pediatric table to determine weight based on age. See Appendix A. (The 50th percentile for a 1-year-old boy is 10 kg.)

Physical Examination on Arrival to the Emergency Department

Airway: Patent, vomitus in mouth and on chin

Breathing: Mild intercostal and subcostal retractions, symmetric and normal breath sounds bilaterally, no wheezes, rhonchi, or rales

Circulation: Normal heart sounds, capillary refill of 3 seconds in hands and feet, rapid and faint peripheral pulses

Disability: Eyes closed, moaning, agitated, responds to voice moving extremities purposefully

ASK YOURSELF

- **What is the initial assessment? What is the patient's physiologic status?**

  This child presents in respiratory distress with altered mental status and decompensated shock.

- **What history, vital signs, and physical examination findings would help you distinguish compensated from decompensated shock?**

  In terms of history, a parental report of urine output and number of episodes of emesis can indicate the amount of fluid loss and dehydration.

In addition, reports of mental status, activity, speech, and behavior are all indicative of CNS perfusion status. Critical elements of the physical examination include an assessment of mental status, heart rate, and skin perfusion, with particular attention to color, temperature, capillary refill time, and quality of pulses. Blood pressure below the 5th percentile for age indicates hypotension.

In general, compensated shock consists of evidence of poor end-organ perfusion with the presence of a blood pressure within normal limits for age. Signs of early or compensated shock include tachycardia, tachypnea, mild respiratory distress, delayed or fast capillary refill, and cutaneous vasodilation. Hypotension is diagnostic of decompensated shock in this patient. Other signs consistent with decompensated shock include worsening tachypnea, tachycardia, and perfusion. Mental status changes can progress from irritability to confusion and nonresponsiveness. *Note:* Children can maintain a normal blood pressure with up to 25% volume loss, so hypotension in this patient requires immediate intervention.

■ What is the most important first step in the resuscitation of this patient?

As always, focus on the ABCs. First ensure that the airway is patent and that the patient is able to oxygenate and ventilate. If this patient cannot do this on her own, BMV with a reservoir delivering 100% oxygen should be used to oxygenate and ventilate the patient. Two large-bore peripheral intravenous lines should be placed in a timely fashion.

■ How should this patient be fluid resuscitated?

If intravenous access cannot be obtained, an intraosseous line should be placed on the flat, medial surface of the proximal tibia, 1 to 2 cm below the tibial tuberosity.[1] An isotonic crystalloid (lactated Ringer or normal saline) bolus of 20 mL/kg is then given as quickly as possible. After reassessment, if the patient's perfusion and blood pressure do not respond to the initial fluid bolus, an additional 20 mL/kg of isotonic crystalloid bolus may be given. If perfusion and blood pressure do not respond to 40 to 60 mL/kg of intravenous fluids, colloid (blood products) should be considered for further volume expansion.

■ What is the differential diagnosis of decompensated shock in this patient?

Hypovolemia (decreased circulating blood volume) must be considered This patient has a history of multiple days of vomiting, which may have led to significant water and electrolyte losses. Other causes of hypovolemia include severe diarrhea, trauma with associated blood loss, peritonitis, and increased capillary permeability leading to capillary leak.

Sepsis, anaphylaxis, spinal cord injury, and barbiturate overdose can cause a distributive shock,[1] in which vasodilation leads to an increase in vascular capacity and a functional hypovolemia.

Cardiogenic shock is distinguished from the other forms of shock by associated signs of congestive heart failure such as rales in the lung bases or cardiac gallops on auscultation, palpation of hepatomegaly, and observation of jugular venous distention.

Additional History and Physical Examination Findings

The mother reports that the patient fell over the edge of a box 3 days earlier. She ate formula and finger foods normally until 12 hours earlier, when she began to have bilious emesis with blood streaks after several episodes of vomiting. She has had normal urine and stool output.

Past Medical History: Full-term, normal spontaneous vaginal delivery; no significant underlying illnesses

Medications: None

Immunizations: Up to date

Allergies: None known

Physical Examination: Mental status continues to deteriorate: eyes remain closed to verbal stimulation, extremities withdraw to pain, and patient continues to groan. Secondary survey reveals normal pupils and bruises on chin, pinna of right ear, and sternum. Abdomen is distended with no bowel sounds auscultated and diffuse tenderness and guarding. Rectal examination is heme-negative.

ASK YOURSELF

■ What interventions are needed at this time? What complications might be expected?

Interventions:

- Administer 100% O_2 via face mask.
- Place the patient on a cardiorespiratory monitor with pulse oximetry.
- Given the possibility of trauma, cervical spine precautions should be instituted.
- Intravenous or intraosseous access and fluid resuscitation with second bolus of **isotonic fluid 20 mL/kg**
- RSI: the patient has become unresponsive in the presence of decompensated shock; at this time, a definitive airway is needed for adequate resuscitation.
  1. #1 Miller blade and 4.0 ET tube
  2. Preoxygenation
  3. Cricoid pressure
  4. **Midazolam 0.1 mg/kg** IV or **etomidate 0.3 mg/kg** IV
  5. **Rocuronium 0.6 to 1 mg/kg** IV or **succinylcholine 1 to 1.5 mg/kg** IV

  In the presence of shock, thiopental and other drugs such as fentanyl that can aggravate hypotension should be avoided.
- Check tube placement by listening for breath sounds in axillae and by end-tidal CO_2 monitor
- Perform chest radiograph to confirm ET tube placement
- Secure ET tube and place NG tube for abdominal decompression.

Potential Complications:

- Inability to obtain rapid intravenous access requires that an intraosseous line be placed immediately.
- Emesis during intubation attempt: maintain cricoid pressure throughout intubation attempt and have suctioning equipment available before intubation.
- Inability to place ET tube. Stop attempt, suction, place NG tube, and use BMV with cricoid pressure.

■ What is the differential diagnosis of altered mental status in this patient?

This patient presents with vomiting, hypotension, and mild respiratory distress. Respiratory distress can lead to hypoxia or hypercapnea, resulting in altered mental status. However, she has normal breath sounds and oxygenation and a significant history of vomiting, so the respiratory distress is likely secondary to metabolic derangements such as metabolic acidosis. There is also a history of minor abdominal trauma, and bruises are found in multiple locations on the patient, so head injury and other sources of trauma must be considered as possible causes. Numerous ingestions can obviously also cause altered mental status. Finally, infection must always be considered as a cause of altered mental status in any pediatric patient, particularly one with a history of vomiting.

■ Which laboratory and radiologic studies are warranted for this patient?

Because of the broad differential diagnosis that includes metabolic acidosis, ingestion, infection, and trauma as possible causes of this patient's condition, baseline laboratory tests should include an ABG analysis, CBC, blood culture, electrolytes, kidney and liver function tests, amylase, coagulation studies, type and cross match, urinalysis, and urine drug screen.

Given the possibility of head trauma and blunt abdominal trauma based on the history and physical examination of this patient, a basic trauma series consisting of cervical spine, chest, and pelvic radiographs should be obtained. Abdominal films are rarely a useful tool in the evaluation of blunt abdominal trauma. A head CT without contrast should be obtained as soon as the patient is hemodynamically stable, because bruises on the chin and ear and altered mental status indicate the possibility of occult head trauma. In addition, with a history of guarding, absent bowel sounds, and vomiting, an abdominal CT with intravenous contrast with or without oral contrast (whether oral contrast is used in the CT evaluation of blunt abdominal trauma depends on the institution) should be performed if the patient can maintain hemodynamic stability after intravenous fluid replacement. Almost all solid organ injuries and about 96% of hollow viscous injuries requiring laparotomy can be identified on CT.[2]

The focused assessment with sonography for trauma (FAST) examination has become a standard screening test at many adult trauma centers for blunt abdominal trauma. Despite its advantages of speed, cost, and noninvasiveness, the role of FAST in evaluating pediatric trauma has not been defined. Children who remain hemodynamically unstable after fluid resuscitation currently undergo laparotomy. Most of those who are hemodynamically stable are managed nonoperatively; a knowledge of specific solid organ injuries is required for prediction of outcome and for management decisions. Because hollow viscous injury is much more common in children than adults because of their poorly developed abdominal muscles, more protuberant abdomen, and more compliant chest wall and because CT is recognized as superior to FAST in identifying hollow viscous rupture, the exact role of FAST in evaluating children has yet to be determined.[2]

■ What potential complications might develop for this patient during resuscitation?

- Patients with significantly altered mental status may not be able to protect their airways. Failure to obtain a definitive airway can result in an inability to oxygenate and ventilate the patient.
- In decompensated shock, if intravenous fluid resuscitation is delayed by numerous unsuccessful attempts to establish intravenous or intraosseous access, the patient could progress to cardiovascular arrest secondary to hypovolemia and acidosis. Careful reevaluation of the patient after fluid boluses to ensure proper perfusion and maintenance of hemodynamic stability is of paramount importance.
- In-line cervical spine immobilization must be maintained in any patient with a possible traumatic neck injury.

■ What is the role of diagnostic peritoneal lavage in the evaluation of pediatric blunt abdominal trauma?

Historically, diagnostic peritoneal lavage has been used to identify patients with intra-abdominal injury that may require laparotomy. However, the results of this procedure are nonspecific (do not identify specific organ injury) and are falsely positive in a high percentage of patients. In addition, diagnostic peritoneal lavage carries a significant risk of bladder, bowel, and vessel perforation.[2] With the development of high-speed CT scanners and the fact that most patients with blunt abdominal trauma do not require surgery, the use of diagnostic peritoneal lavage has diminished dramatically. Hemodynamically unstable patients go directly to the operating room for exploratory laparotomy; stable patients undergo abdominal CT scanning for a more definitive diagnosis.

Repeat Vital Signs (postintubation)

Pulse: 135

Respiratory Rate: 25 on ventilation

Blood Pressure: 85/40

Oxygen Saturation: 100% on 100% O_2

Progression

This patient is sedated, paralyzed, and intubated, with improved color and capillary refill and strong peripheral pulses. Abdominal distention decreased with nasogastric/orogastric tube in place.

ASK YOURSELF

■ What is the most likely diagnosis for this patient?

Abdominal injury secondary to physical abuse is the most likely diagnosis in this patient. The chin, ear, and particularly the sternum are unusual sites of bruising for an 8-month-old child who is incapable of independent bipedal ambulation. In addition, the mother's history of the patient developing abdominal symptoms after "falling over the edge of a box" is inconsistent with the severity of the symptoms. The severity of symptoms may be attributed to a delay in seeking medical care, a common element in many cases of child abuse. Before CT scan results are available, it is difficult to determine whether a solid organ or hollow viscous organ has been injured.

The most commonly injured organs associated with blunt abdominal trauma are the liver, spleen, and kidneys. In this patient with vomiting, abdominal distention, heme-negative rectal examination, and hypotension easily corrected by isotonic fluid, a forceful injury to the duodenum also must be considered. Duodenal injuries are found in up to 14% of patients with blunt abdominal injury.[2] Blunt duodenal injuries are a diagnostic and therapeutic challenge because of nonspecific signs and symptoms, associated injuries, unreliable history, and the difficulty in imaging the retroperitoneum.[3]

Differentiation between types of duodenal injuries, namely duodenal perforation and hematoma, is essential because different treatment courses are required. Persistent abdominal pain or vomiting in a child with signs of upper abdominal trauma and an abdominal CT scan with findings of free fluid, air, or intestinal mural wall thickening without evidence of solid organ injury indicates a need for surgical exploration of the abdomen. Free air also can be seen on the initial chest radiograph or on a cross-table lateral abdominal film in duodenal perforation. Duodenal perforations are thought to develop from shearing forces in the abdomen or from simultaneous closure of the pylorus and fourth portion of the duodenum, resulting in increased intraluminal pressure and rupture of the bowel.[3] Perforations of the bowel are treated with closure of the perforation and drainage or, in severe cases, with blind pouch creation and ostomy. Duodenal hematomas result from compression of the epigastrium and duodenum against the vertebral column, and mural thickening on CT is diagnostic in this clinical picture. Duodenal hematomas are generally treated nonoperatively with nasogastric/orogastric tube decompression and parenteral nutrition.

■ What additional studies should be done in a patient with suspected nonaccidental trauma?

The key to the diagnosis of nonaccidental injury is obtaining a history that is inconsistent with the results of a careful physical examination. The force needed to cause the symptoms in this patient could not be explained by falling over the edge of a box. Any infant or child who is acutely ill with a history that is not believable or consistent, who has had a previous history of abuse in the household, or who was not in the care of the primary caretaker at the onset of symptoms should be considered as a victim of abuse. Often, physical evidence can be found to show multiple injuries in various stages of healing.

If physical abuse is suspected, the following studies should be performed in a timely fashion to rule out occult injury: head CT, skeletal survey, CBC, coagulation studies, liver function tests, amylase, lipase, urinalysis, abdominal CT with contrast, and retinal examination by an ophthalmologist.[4]

Objectives of This Scenario

1. Recognize and manage an acutely ill patient with poor perfusion and altered mental status.

This patient presented with waning mental status, hypotension, and poor perfusion. Immediate recognition of the need for resuscitation is important. Equally crucial is an understanding of the importance of providing an adequate airway and fluid resuscitation.

2. Recognize and manage trauma as a possible etiology for a patient presenting with altered mental status and shock.

Recognizing that a patient with altered mental status and shock with evidence of bruising could be a victim of trauma is important in the early management of the patient in the emergency department. First, when opening the airway, one must maintain in-line stabilization of the cervical spine to prevent a spinal cord injury secondary to cervical vertebral manipulation. Second, intravenous access is of paramount importance in maintaining a blood pressure to perfuse all vital organs. Third, a possible traumatic etiology must be recognized and a search for occult injury must be made with a careful physical examination and appropriate laboratory and radiologic studies.

3. Recognize and manage abdominal trauma.

The patient's presentation with bilious emesis, hypotension, absent bowel sounds, and bruising to the sternum should point the physician in the direction of the upper abdomen as the primary point of injury. Obtaining an early surgical consultation and appropriate laboratory studies as well as an abdominal CT (in the hemodynamically stable patient) is important to determine the presence and magnitude of abdominal injuries. Early diagnosis of blunt abdominal and particularly duodenal injuries is critical to minimize the morbidity and mortality associated with late presentation or late diagnosis of these injuries.

4. Recognize and manage possible nonaccidental trauma.

A recent National Pediatric Trauma Registry review of cases of blunt abdominal trauma in children found that child abuse accounted for approximately 24% of pediatric ICU admissions for blunt trauma.[5] In addition, abuse may be responsible for about 1% of cases of abdominal trauma seen in urban hospitals and for 4% of children seen in a pediatric emergency department for trauma.[6] Children with abuse-related abdominal trauma are younger than most trauma patients, usually younger than 5 years. Accurate histories are difficult to obtain in these often nonverbal patients because the caretaker responsible for the injury is often the only source of information. Because of the unreliable history, the difficulty in diagnosing severe occult injuries, and the frequently prolonged delay in seeking medical care, mortality rates are as high as 40% in these patients.[2]

Since the advent of abdominal CT as a diagnostic tool, the abdominal organs found to be most commonly injured traumatically have been the liver (27%), spleen (27%), kidneys (25%), gastrointestinal tract (21%), and genitourinary tract (5%). The most common presentations of nonaccidental abdominal trauma include shock secondary to significant abdominal bleeding, peritonitis secondary to hollow viscous rupture, and bilious vomiting.[2] Associated injuries that are seen in patients with nonaccidental abdominal trauma are soft tissue injuries (95%), head trauma (45%), long bone fractures (27%), and skull fractures (18%).[7]

Physicians must consider abuse in all patients presenting with symptoms and physical findings inconsistent with the caretaker's history or with evidence of possible nonaccidental trauma on physical examination.

References

1. Bell LM. Shock. In: Fleisher GR, Ludwig S, eds. *Textbook of Pediatric Emergency Medicine*. 4th ed. Philadelphia, Pa: Lippincott Williams and Wilkins; 2000:47-59.
2. Rothrock SG, Green SM, Morgan R. Abdominal trauma in infants and children: prompt identification and early management of serious and life-threatening injuries. Part 1: injury patterns and initial assessment. *Pediatr Emerg Care*. 2000;16:106-115.
3. Desai KM, Dorward IG, Minkes RK, et al. Blunt duodenal injuries in children. *J Trauma*. 2003;54:640-646.
4. Zenel J, Goldstein B. Child abuse in the pediatric intensive care unit. *Crit Care Med*. 2002;30:S515-S523.
5. Discala C, Sege R, Li G, et al. Child abuse: a 10-year retrospective. *Arch Pediatr Adolesc Med*. 2000;154:16-22.
6. Sivit CJ, Taylor GA, Eichelberger MR. Visceral injury in battered children: a changing perspective. *Radiology*. 1989;173:659-661.
7. Cooper A, Floyd T, Barlow B, et al. Major blunt abdominal trauma due to child abuse. *J Trauma*. 1988;28:1483-1487.
8. Rothrock SG, Green SM, Morgan R. Abdominal trauma in infants and children: prompt identification and early management of serious and life-threatening injuries. Part II: specific injuries and ED management. *Pediatr Emerg Care*. 2000;16:189-195.

SCENARIO #20

Shock

Debra Weiner, MD, PhD

Brief Presenting History

A 17-year-old girl presents to the emergency department with a 12-hour history of worsening abdominal pain and vaginal bleeding.

Pediatric Assessment Triangle

Appearance: Alert, anxious, obese, diaphoretic, in moderate discomfort

Work of Breathing: Rapid, deep inspirations with prolonged expirations

Circulation to the Skin: Well-perfused

Initial Vital Signs

Pulse: 120

Respiratory Rate: 24

Blood Pressure: 110/70

Temperature: 37°C (98.6°F) oral

ASK YOURSELF

- **What is the range of normal vital signs for a 17-year-old girl?**

  Pulse of 60 to 120, respiratory rate of 10 to 16, and minimum systolic blood pressure of 100 (see Appendix A).

Physical Examination on Arrival to the Emergency Department

Airway: Patent with no evidence of obstruction

Breathing: Rapid, labored respirations; breath sounds symmetric, clear to auscultation, good aeration

Circulation: Capillary refill less than 2 seconds in hands and feet with bounding peripheral pulses

Disability: Alert, responsive but distracted by pain in the lower abdomen

ASK YOURSELF

- **What is the initial assessment? What is the patient's physiologic status?**

  The patient is alert, tachycardic, tachypneic, and in moderate pain and has normal mental status. The tachycardia could be a manifestation of pain; however, with vaginal bleeding one must consider early, compensated hemorrhagic shock.

- **What is the most likely differential diagnosis of the vaginal bleeding in this patient?**

  Gynecologic etiologies include menses with menstrual cramps and vaginal trauma. Obstetric etiologies include ectopic pregnancy, abortion, threatened abortion, placenta previa, placental abruption, and active labor with bloody show.

Additional History and Physical Examination Findings

The patient describes pain that is constant but also crampy. It is moderate in severity but alternating with severe episodes that are worsening. It began slowly after a motor vehicle crash the previous night. She was the front seat passenger (wearing a lap belt and shoulder harness) in a car that was struck in the rear, causing moderate rear bumper damage. She felt no obvious initial injuries but this morning awoke with much more severe abdominal pain and vaginal bleeding.

Her last menstrual period was approximately 8 months ago. She is sexually active and using no contraception.

Past Medical History: The patient denies major medical problems. She reports no prior pregnancies or history of sexually transmitted diseases. She reports use of one pack per day of cigarettes and occasional alcohol consumption but denies use of illegal drugs.

Medications: None

Allergies: Shellfish

Physical Examination: Abdomen is obese with a large, firm mass with its upper edge palpable up to the midepigastrium. She is tender throughout her lower abdominal quadrants. She has palpable contractions and moderate to severe vaginal bleeding composed of dark blood with clots.

ASK YOURSELF

■ What is the most likely diagnosis?

By history and physical examination, this young woman has a hemorrhagic complication of pregnancy. The most likely is placental abruption, which is separation of the placenta from the uterus. This generally occurs after 20 weeks' gestation and involves vaginal bleeding from the cervical os (80% of cases) or concealed hemorrhage with blood trapped behind the placenta (20% of cases).

■ If the patient had presented with only abdominal pain, what other diagnoses would have been in the differential?

Abdominal trauma to a solid organ or hollow viscus; appendicitis/perforation; ovarian torsion; ruptured ovarian cyst; pelvic inflammatory disease; duodenal ulcer/perforation; and spontaneous peritonitis.

■ What are this patient's risk factors for placental abruption?

Her risk factors include trauma and cigarette smoking.

■ What are other risk factors for placental abruption?

Other risk factors include maternal age of 35 years or older; maternal hypertension, preeclampsia; maternal coagulopathy, congenital or acquired; increasing parity; cocaine use; male fetus; multiple gestations; prolonged rupture of membranes; chorioamnionitis; and previous abruption.

■ How is the diagnosis made?

The initial diagnosis of placental abruption is made clinically. The classic findings are vaginal bleeding, abdominal pain, uterine tenderness with increased uterine tone, and uterine contractions. Even without vaginal bleeding, this constellation of findings should suggest abruption with concealed hemorrhage. Ultrasonography may support the diagnosis, but it detects abruption in only 50% of cases.[1] The diagnostic sonographic finding is retroplacental clot. Ultrasonography also is helpful to confirm pregnancy and to rule out other etiologies of bleeding.

■ What interventions should be made at this time? What complications might be expected?

Interventions:

- Consult obstetric and neonatology services as available; consult surgery if obstetrics not available.
- Position mother on left side or in Trendelenburg position.
- Place mother on cardiac monitor.
- Provide supplemental oxygen.
- Insert two large-bore intravenous lines and begin fluid resuscitation with **normal saline or lactated Ringer 20 mL/kg** infused over 10 to 20 minutes.
- Place Foley catheter to monitor urine output, which should be at a rate of more than 30 mL/hr.

- Laboratory studies include CBC, BUN and creatinine, prothrombin time (PT), partial thromboplastin time (PTT), and fibrinogen.
- Type and cross 4 units of packed RBCs.
- Begin fetal monitoring if available.

Potential Complications (maternal):

- Hypovolemia
- Shock
- Disseminated intravascular coagulation (DIC)
- Amniotic fluid embolism
- Death

Potential Complications (fetal):

- Fetal distress; fetal bradycardia, late decelerations
- Prematurity
- Fetal death

Progression

Over the next 30 minutes, the young woman's pain intensifies, and her bleeding increases. Peripheral capillary refill is now 3 seconds in her extremities.

Repeat Vital Signs

Pulse: 140

Respiratory Rate: 30

Blood Pressure: 82/42

ASK YOURSELF

■ What is the patient's physiologic status now?

She has developed hypovolemic, decompensated shock manifested by increasing tachycardia and tachypnea, decreased perfusion, and new hypotension. Although pregnancy is accompanied by some increase in heart rate and decrease in blood pressure, these changes are extreme.

Initial Laboratory Results

WBC count of 22,000 with 88% neutrophils; hematocrit 26%; platelets 98,000. BUN 12, creatinine 1.2, PT 14, PTT 33, fibrinogen 160, blood type O negative.

ASK YOURSELF

■ What do these laboratory results indicate?

Anemia due to blood loss; hypofibrinogenemia with possible impending DIC.

■ What interventions should be made at this time? What complications might be expected?

Interventions:

- Blood transfusion of cross-matched packed RBCs, starting with 2 units over 30 minutes, titrated to response of heart rate and blood pressure. Alternatively, if cross-matched blood is not immediately available, type O negative uncrossed blood could be used.
- Consider fresh frozen plasma, cryoprecipitate, and/or platelets.
- Prepare immediately for a newborn delivery. If possible, delivery should take place in the operating room (emergent cesarean section) or a delivery room (if labor has progressed and delivery is imminent)

Potential Complications (maternal):

- Hemorrhage, if uncontrollable, could necessitate hysterectomy.[2]
- Transfusion reaction, especially with uncrossed blood

Potential Complications (fetal)

- Fetal distress
- Death from acute placental deficiency

■ What would you have done differently if bleeding were mild and the patient were hemodynamically stable?

If a patient is not in labor, monitor the mother and fetus in the hospital until bleeding stops. If a patient is in labor and near term, allow delivery. If the patient is in labor and the fetus is preterm, consider tocolysis to delay delivery at least long enough to assess fetal lung maturity or until corticosteroids can be given to promote lung maturity.[2]

Objectives of This Scenario

1. Recognize that two patients are involved.

Early recognition that the patient is pregnant and that delivery may be imminent or necessary is critical. A separate team should attend to each patient. Each team should ideally consist of at least two health care professionals and at least one physician. Appropriate equipment must be available for both adult and infant resuscitation.

2. Know the impact of pregnancy on vital signs and laboratory values.

- Pulse increases 10 to 15 beats/min.
- Respiratory rate does not change although minute ventilation increases.
- Blood pressure: 5 to 10 mm Hg decrease in systolic and 10 to 15 mm Hg decrease in diastolic. The nadir is reached in the 2nd trimester; pressures are near normal at term.
- WBC count: 10,000 to 15,000, can increase to 25,000 at delivery
- Hematocrit decreases to 30% to 35%.
- Platelets can decrease during pregnancy.
- BUN/creatinine decrease by 25% to 50%, especially in first and second trimesters.
- PT/PTT can be shortened in pregnancy.
- Fibrinogen increases by fourth month, increases one third by term.

3. Know the differential diagnosis and manage pregnancy with vaginal bleeding.[3]

The history and physical examination should be directed at identifying the type and degree of bleeding. Attempt to determine the gestational age of the fetus; solicit history of any maternal conditions that predispose to obstetric bleeding; and identify the character, quantity, and site of bleeding and pain, maternal hemodynamic status, fetal position, and presence or absence of uterine contractions.

Do not perform a vaginal or rectal examination when there is vaginal bleeding near term that could be due to placental abruption, placenta previa, or rupture of the uterus, as this can induce severe hemorrhage. Emergency delivery is indicated when delivery is imminent or when the amount of bleeding is a threat to maternal or fetal well-being.

Obstetric causes of vaginal bleeding:

Placental abruption, defined as the premature separation of the placenta from the uterus, occurs in 1% of pregnancies and results in stillbirth in approximately 0.1% of deliveries. Bleeding can be external or concealed behind the placenta; therefore, the amount of bleeding is not necessarily indicative of clinical status.[4] The severity of abruption determines management. There are three categories:

- **Mild abruption (Grade I).** Vaginal bleeding is scant to moderate and dark with mild lower abdominal discomfort and no uterine contractions. Mother is hemodynamically stable and blood loss is minimal with no fetal distress and no coagulopathy. The mother is not in labor. Mother and fetus can be monitored, preferably in an obstetric unit or ICU until bleeding stops.
- **Moderate abruption (Grade II).** There is moderate vaginal bleeding unless hemorrhage is concealed. There is moderate, continuous uterine pain. Pain may be more severe if there is concealed hemorrhage. There is minimal maternal risk despite significant risk of fetal distress, and fetal death is possible. If the fetus is term or near term, a cesarean delivery is indicated. If the fetus is preterm and the mother and fetus are stable, tocolysis and corticosteroids should be used to promote lung maturity before delivery. Without fetal delivery, grade II usually progresses to grade III.
- **Severe abruption (Grade III).** Vaginal bleeding is severe unless there is concealed hemorrhage. There is continuous, severe, stabbing uterine pain, usually with maternal shock, and often with DIC, renal failure, and severe fetal distress or death. Emergent delivery is indicated. If the fetus is viable, cesarean section is preferred, after correction of maternal hypovolemia and coagulopathy. Packed RBCs are administered to correct hematocrit to 25% to 30% or higher; platelets, to restore count to 60,000 to 100,000/mm^3 or higher; and fresh frozen plasma or cryoprecipitate, to increase fibrinogen to 150 to 200 mg/dL or higher. Vaginal delivery is preferred if fetal death has occurred.

Placenta previa is defined as implantation of the lower pole of the uterus near or over the os. It can present with painless bright red bleeding secondary to separation of the placenta from the uterus. Usually presenting after 20 weeks' gestation, it can be complete (the entire cervix is covered) or marginal (the edge of the placenta covers the cervix). Its incidence is 1:200 pregnancies; 80% of the cases occur in multiparous women. Other risk factors include maternal age of greater than 35 years, previous cesarean section, multiple gestation, and abnormal fetal position.[5]

Abortion or threatened abortions are most common in the first trimester. Spontaneous abortion is more likely if bleeding is minimal to moderate and accompanied by cramping.

Bloody show can be one of the first signs of imminent labor. Usually occurring near term, it involves the painless discharge of blood and mucus before delivery.

Ectopic pregnancy is defined as a pregnancy implanted outside of the uterus, usually in a fallopian tube.[6] It most commonly presents at 8 to 12 weeks of pregnancy and involves a classic triad of vaginal bleeding, abdominal pain, and amenorrhea. Vaginal bleeding is usually light; 90% have pain. If the conceptus is unruptured, pain is usually unilateral in the pelvis. If the conceptus is ruptured, the pain may be diffuse throughout the pelvis and abdomen with peritonitis. Its incidence is 1:50 pregnancies; the incidence is higher in women with previous ectopic pregnancy, previous pelvic inflammatory disease, previous tubal surgery, and an intrauterine device.

Ruptured uterus presents with lower abdominal pain and vaginal or concealed bleeding. Its incidence is 1:100 women previously delivered by cesarean section.[7]

Gynecologic causes of vaginal bleeding:

These causes include menses, endometriosis, dysfunctional uterine bleeding, lower genital tract trauma, pelvic infection, bleeding diathesis, mass, cyst, abscess, and neoplasm.

4. Recognize maternal conditions associated with and resulting from obstetric bleeding.

Maternal conditions *predisposing* to obstetric bleeding and precipitous preterm delivery include hypertension, infection, inherited thrombophilia, injury secondary to trauma, cigarette use, cocaine use, multiple gestation, advanced maternal age, multiparity, and previous abruption.

Maternal conditions *resulting* from obstetric bleeding and precipitous preterm delivery include hypovolemic shock, DIC, respiratory failure, cardiac arrest, renal failure, and death.

References

1. Moore C, Promes SB. Ultrasound in pregnancy. *Emerg Med Clin North Am.* 2004;22:697-722.
2. Shevell T, Malone FD. Management of obstetric hemorrhage. *Semin Perinatol.* 2003;27:86-104.
3. Papp Z. Massive obstetric hemorrhage. *J Perinat Med.* 2003;31:408-414.
4. Korby J. Abruptio placentae. *Nursing.* 2004;34:96.
5. Faiz AS, Ananth CV. Etiology and risk factors for placenta previa: an overview and meta-analysis of observational studies. *J Matern Fetal Neonatal Med.* 2003:13:175-190.
6. Sowter MC, Farquhar CM. Ectopic pregnancy: an update. *Curr Opin Obstet Gynecol.* 2004;16:289-293.
7. Guise JM, McDonagh MS, Osterweil P, et al. Systematic review of the incidence and consequences of uterine rupture in women with previous caesarean section. *BMJ.* 2004;329:19-25.

SCENARIO #21

Cardiac – Cyanotic Spell

Brent J. Barber, MD, and Grant Burch, MD

Brief Presenting History

A 3-month-old boy is brought in by his mother. He has had increasing upper respiratory infection symptoms during the past several days, and while he was waiting to be seen in the emergency department, he began coughing and then crying, and then he turned blue.

Pediatric Assessment Triangle

Appearance: Minimally responsive

Work of Breathing: Tachypneic, hyperpneic

Circulation to the Skin: Profoundly cyanotic

Initial Vital Signs

Pulse: 180

Blood Pressure: 76/44

Respiratory Rate: 65

Temperature: 37.6°C (99.7°F) axillary

Oxygen Saturation: 52% in room air

ASK YOURSELF

- **What is the normal respiratory rate of a 2-month-old child? What is hyperpnea?**

  The normal rate for a neonate is 40 to 50; a 0- to 1-year-old, 24 to 38; and a 1- to 3-year-old, 22 to 30.[1] Hyperpnea is energetic (deep and rapid) respiration that occurs normally after exercise or abnormally with fever or various disorders.

Physical Examination

Airway: Patent, moving air freely, no secretions in the mouth

Breathing: Deep, gasping respirations; lungs clear bilaterally without wheeze

Circulation: Skin slightly cool, deeply cyanotic both centrally and peripherally; capillary refill time 2 seconds

ASK YOURSELF

- **How would you differentiate peripheral from central cyanosis?**

  Peripheral cyanosis is best noted in the nail beds—a comparison of the patient's nailbeds with those of the examiner can reveal cyanosis. Central cyanosis is noted in the tongue and mucosal membranes. In central cyanosis, the oxygen saturation of the arterial blood is reduced. Note that perioral cyanosis is common in infants secondary to the proximity of the blood vessels to the skin and is *not* a sign of peripheral or central cyanosis.[2]

Disability: Eyes closed, pupils equal and reactive to light 4 mm to 2 mm bilaterally

ASK YOURSELF

- **What is the initial assessment? What is the patient's physiologic status?**

  Patient presents with respiratory distress, cyanosis, and altered mental status.

- **What determines the degree of cyanosis?**

  For cyanosis to be apparent, 3 to 5 g/dL of hemoglobin must be desaturated. Therefore, it is easier to appreciate cyanosis in a patient with polycythemia than it is in one with anemia. For example, an oxygen saturation of 85% in a patient with a hemoglobin of 20 g/dL can result in cyanosis (3 g/dL desaturated hemoglobin), whereas in a patient with a hemoglobin of 9 g/dL, the oxygen saturation must drop below 67% before cyanosis is observed. Thus, in neonates during their period of postnatal physiologic anemia, cyanosis will be more difficult to observe than in an older child or an adult.

- **What is postnatal physiologic anemia?**

  Postnatal physiologic anemia is a normal decrease in hemoglobin from 14 to 20 g/dL at birth to 9 to 11 g/dL at 8 to 12 weeks of age. This is caused by the decrease in renal erythropoietin production in response to the increase in Pa_{O_2} postnatally.[3]

- **What interventions are needed at this time?**
  - Administer 100% O_2 by face mask for respiratory distress and hypoxia.
  - Place the patient on a cardiorespiratory monitor with pulse oximetry.
  - Attempt intravenous access and begin fluid resuscitation with **normal saline 20 mL/kg.**

Additional History and Physical Examination Findings

The patient's mother says he has gastroesophageal reflux disease (GERD) and was told that he had a heart murmur. They have an appointment next week with a pediatric cardiologist. He has been growing and feeding well until today, although he occasionally turns blue when crying. Today he has been more irritable, is not nursing well, and has had decreased urine output.

Past Medical History: The patient was delivered via a normal-term vaginal delivery. He stayed in the nursery for 2 weeks after a possible seizure was observed and was noted to have a low calcium level, which required calcium supplementation for a few weeks. He was diagnosed with GERD at 3 weeks because he is a very "spitty" baby.

Medications: Ranitidine for GERD.

Physical Examination: Generalized cyanosis with a percutaneous oxygen saturation of 60% while on 10 L O_2 via face mask. The child exhibits a bizarre deep and rapid respiratory pattern with good bilateral air entry. There is tachycardia with *no murmur*. The abdominal examination is normal.

ASK YOURSELF

- **What is in the differential diagnosis for this patient?**

  The most likely etiology in this age group is a respiratory problem, but this is less likely for this patient, because he has good air movement and no wheezing, stridor, or rales. Also, the lack of a response to oxygen suggests an etiology other than a primary alveolar problem.

  A patient with a positive history for GERD and infants with reflux can present with apparent life-threatening events, usually manifested by apnea, cyanosis, and limpness. However, this patient has not experienced apnea with his cyanotic spell. Aspiration is a consideration but, again, it is unlikely for the reasons already mentioned.

  A cardiac etiology is an important consideration in this case, with respiratory causes being less likely; however, the patient does not have a murmur.

  Seizures are in the differential for a blue and minimally responsive infant, but no history and no evidence of seizure activity make this diagnosis less likely.

  Methemoglobinemia is possible, associated with exposure to nitrates/nitrites and other toxins; also, the condition does not respond to oxygen. Suspicion would be aroused with history of exposure or if ABGs showed normal Pa_{O_2} with decreased oxygen saturation.

Additional Studies

Chest Radiograph: Showing clear lung fields with decreased pulmonary vascular markings and a "boot-shaped" heart. Image courtesy of Laura Fenton, MD.

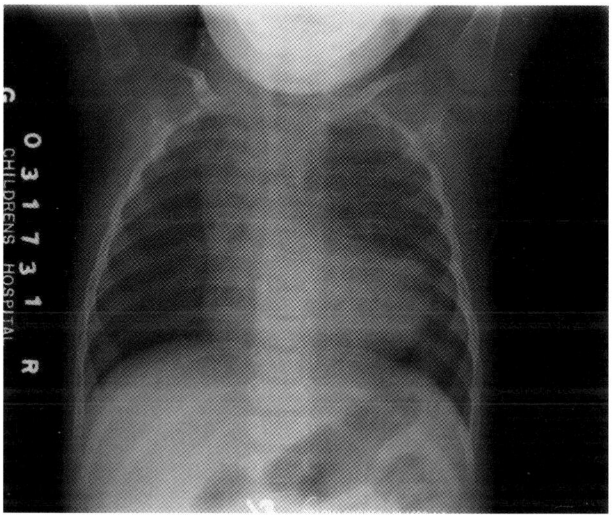

ABG: pH 7.36, Pco_2 32, Po_2 35 (on 100% Fio_2), HCO_3^- 17

ASK YOURSELF

■ What is your interpretation of the ABGs?

The ABGs show a metabolic acidosis with respiratory compensation and hypoxemia. This patient has clear lungs on examination and chest radiography, and his response to a hyperoxia test suggests right-to-left shunting. The hyperoxia test is performed by placing the patient in 100% oxygen for 5 to 10 minutes and obtaining a right radial arterial blood gas. A Pao_2 of less than 150 mm Hg is strongly suggestive of cyanotic congenital heart disease.[2]

■ What is the most likely diagnosis?

Hypercyanotic spell secondary to congenital heart disease.

■ What is the most likely underlying heart defect?

Tetralogy of Fallot (the tetrad comprises infundibular and pulmonary valve stenosis, ventricular septal defect [VSD], overriding aorta, and right ventricular hypertrophy). Other lesions associated with hypercyanotic or "tet" spells include tricuspid atresia, single ventricle with pulmonary stenosis, and transposition of the great arteries if also associated with VSD and pulmonary stenosis. The boot-shaped heart on chest radiography is classic for tetralogy of Fallot and is caused by the diminutive pulmonary artery segment and right ventricular hypertrophy.[4]

■ What causes a hypercyanotic spell?

Although the trigger for a hypercyantoic spell is still debated, the spell is manifested by an acute increase in right-to-left shunting and dynamic changes in the degree of subpulmonic (infundibular) obstruction. Some believe that the infundibular spasm is the primary event. Others argue that the initial event is a drop in systemic vascular resistance that leads to increased right-to-left ventricular septal defect shunting.[5]

■ What interventions are needed at this time?

- Oxygen is administered to maximize oxygen delivery.
- Knees to chest: this maneuver increases systemic vascular resistance by "kinking" the femoral arteries. Older children with unrepaired tetralogy of Fallot are known to squat, especially after exercise-induced vasodilation. Squatting or placing an infant's knees to the chest results in increased systemic vascular resistance and decreased right-to-left shunting through the ventricular septal defect and increases pulmonary blood flow.
- Intravenous fluid bolus (**10 to 20 mL/kg**) with **normal saline** or **lactated Ringer** is given to promote right ventricular filling, which is hoped to improve pulmonary blood flow.
- **Morphine sulfate 0.1 mg/kg IV/IM.** The mechanism is not completely known, but this therapy is thought to break the cycle of agitation and hyperpnea and may have direct effects on the infundibulum. It also reduces oxygen consumption by providing some degree of sedation.[4-6]
- **Phenylephrine 0.5 to 5 mcg/kg/min continuous IV infusion.** Phenylephrine is an α-agonist that decreases right-to-left shunting by raising systemic vascular resistance. Some experts advocate phenylephrine as first-line therapy.[4-6]

- **Propranolol 0.15 to 0.25 mg/kg/dose slow IV push.** This may be repeated once in 15 minutes. β-Blockade decreases heart rate, promotes right ventricular filling, and decreases contractility, which may promote infundibular relaxation. Oral propranolol is also used to prevent recurrent spells.[4-6]

If all of these interventions fail to halt the spell, emergent surgery to increase pulmonary blood flow must be considered. This is usually accomplished through a systemic-to-pulmonary (Blalock-Taussig) shunt. There have been reports of the spells breaking while under general anesthesia before surgery. Care must be taken during sedation/anesthesia with these patients because agents that acutely decrease systemic vascular resistance can precipitate or worsen a spell. Some recommend using ketamine, which increases systemic vascular resistance, or having phenylephrine available at the time of induction.[4,5]

Objectives of This Resuscitation

1. Recognize a hypercyanotic or "tet" spell.

The patient in this scenario presents with an acute episode of severe cyanosis characteristic of a hypercyanotic spell. The cardinal symptoms are cyanosis, hyperpnea, agitation, and mental status changes that can eventually progress to coma. The usual duration is 15 to 30 minutes, but severe spells can continue and require urgent intervention. Spells occur more commonly in the mornings and during intercurrent illness. They can be precipitated by crying or occur spontaneously. This patient had a history of a murmur, but no murmur was appreciated during this event, which is classic for hypercyanotic spells. In patients with tetralogy of Fallot, the systolic murmur is secondary to right ventricular outflow tract obstruction. The ventricular septal defect in these patients is typically large with nonturbulent flow, so no ventricular septal defect murmur is produced from right ventricular blood being ejected through the ventricular septal defect into the overriding aorta. During a spell, the pulmonary-to-systemic vascular resistance ratio increases, and it is thought that the infundiblum undergoes dynamic obstruction. This yields a severe decreased flow out of the right ventricular outflow tract; therefore, the murmur decreases in intensity or disappears altogether. The deoxygenated blood in the right ventricle is then forced through the ventricular septal defect and out of the aorta, resulting in deep cyanosis.

With the trend toward early surgical repair of tetralogy and other congenital heart lesions, hypercyanotic spells are becoming less common. In fact, the occurrence of a spell is now an indication for surgery. Spells should not be seen in the postoperative tetralogy patient after ventricular septal defect closure and right ventricular outflow tract augmentation. Infants with congenital heart disease requiring a Blalock-Taussig shunt can present with acute cyanosis and no murmur if the shunt becomes obstructed. This requires prompt recognition and usually surgical or transcatheter intervention.

2. Manage a hypercyanotic spell.

The goals of management are to maximize oxygen delivery, to minimize oxygen consumption, and to favorably influence the systemic and pulmonary vascular resistances to improve pulmonary blood flow.

3. Consider additional diagnoses.

This infant also had a past history of hypocalcemia and difficulty with feedings. These findings, in addition to suspected congenital heart disease (especially tetralogy and other conotruncal malformations), should raise suspicion for DiGeorge syndrome caused by chromosome 22q11 deletion.

References

1. Greenfield MM. Pulmonology. In: Gunn VL, Nechyba C, Barone MA, eds. *The Harriet Lane Handbook: A Manual for Pediatric House Officers*. 16th ed. St Louis, Mo: CV Mosby; 2002:513-527.
2. Momma K. Approach to the cyanotic infant. In: Moller JH, Hoffman JIE, eds. *Pediatric Cardiovascular Medicine*. New York: Churchill Livingstone; 2000:249-254.
3. Glader B. Physiologic anemia of infancy. In: Berman RE, Kliegman RM, Jenson HB, eds. *Nelson Textbook of Pediatrics*. 17th ed. Philadelphia, Pa: WB Saunders; 2003:1610-1611.
4. Siwik ES, Patel CR, Zahka KG, et al. *Tetralogy of Fallot*. In: Allen HD, Gutgesell HP, Clark EB, et al, eds. *Moss and Adams' Heart Disease in Infants, Children, and Adolescents*. 6th ed. Philadelphia, Pa: Lippincott Williams & Wilkins; 2001:880-902.
5. Doyle TP, Kavanaugh-McHugh A, Graham TP. Tetralogy of Fallot and pulmonary atresia with ventricular septal defect. In: Moller JH, Hoffman JIE, eds. *Pediatric Cardiovascular Medicine*. New York: Churchill Livingstone; 2000:391-408.
6. Siegfried BH, Henderson TO. Cardiology. In: Gunn VL, Nechyba C, Barone MA, eds. *The Harriet Lane Handbook: A Manual for Pediatric House Officers*. 16th ed. St Louis, Mo: CV Mosby; 2002:156.

SCENARIO #22

Cardiac – Irritability

Brian H. Shear, MD, and Katherine Bakes, MD

Brief Presenting History

An 8-month-old boy presents to the emergency department with fever, irritability, and poor feeding for the past 2 days. His mother reports he has some nasal congestion and a cough.

Pediatric Assessment Triangle

Appearance: Pale, crying

Work of Breathing: Slightly tachypneic, no retractions or nasal flaring

Circulation to the Skin: Mottled skin, hands and feet slightly cyanotic and cool

Initial Vital Signs

Pulse: Too fast to accurately assess (>200)

Blood Pressure: Unable to register

Respiratory Rate: 50

Temperature: 38.9°C (102°F) rectal

Pulse Oximetry: 93% on room air

Weight: 8 kg

ASK YOURSELF

- **Where is the best place to feel for the pulse in an infant?**

  The brachial pulse is the recommended site, although the femoral pulse may be used as an alternative. The carotid is not recommended because it can be difficult to palpate in babies with chubby necks and can cause excessive vagal stimulation.

- **What is the normal pulse range for an 8-month-old?**

  The normal awake pulse range for an infant aged 3 months to 2 years is 100 to 190, with a mean of 130.[1]

- **What is the differential diagnosis for a pulse rate this high?**

  The differential diagnosis includes sinus tachycardia, supraventricular reentrant arrhythmia, or ventricular tachycardia. A heart rate above 220 in an infant makes it unlikely that fever, anxiety, pain, or dehydration is the cause. Toxic ingestion is a possibility. A reentrant tachyarrhythmia is likely in this infant.

Physical Examination on Arrival to the Emergency Department

Airway: Patent, moving air freely, no secretions in mouth

Breathing: Increased respiratory rate with mild increased work of breathing, clear breath sounds without retractions

Circulation: Skin pale, slightly mottled and cool to the touch; capillary refill time of 3 seconds

Disability: The patient is crying and difficult to console. He is moving all extremities equally.

ASK YOURSELF

- **What is the initial assessment? What is the patient's physiologic status?**

  The patient presents with mild respiratory distress and compensated shock.

- **What interventions are needed at this time?**
  - Administer 100% O_2 by face mask
  - Place the patient on a cardiorespiratory monitor with pulse oximetry.
  - Obtain intravenous access.
  - Antipyretic therapy: **acetaminophen 15 mg/kg PO/PR** or **ibuprofen 10 mg/kg PO**

ECG Monitor:

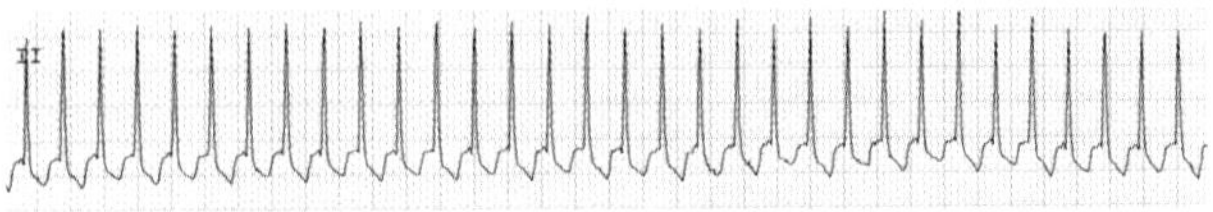

Progression

ECG monitor shows a narrow complex tachycardia with a rate of 270.

ASK YOURSELF

- **What is the cause of the patient's respiratory distress and shock?**

  The patient is febrile, with mild increased work of breathing. This could be an early septic shock; however, the high heart rate is concerning for an arrhythmia.

- **What further studies could help establish his diagnosis?**

  A 12-lead ECG would be the most helpful in this case. A chest radiograph would help evaluate for cardiomegaly. If intravenous fluids are given to a patient with cardiogenic shock, his condition may deteriorate rather than improve.

Additional History and Physical Examination Findings

Past Medical History: The patient had a normal birth by vaginal delivery without complications. He has been healthy up until this episode. He is up to date on his immunizations (including three documented Prevnar vaccinations). He is in day care 3 days a week. His family history is negative.

Medications: The mother has been giving the patient over-the-counter infant cold medication at the recommended doses. He has no known drug allergies.

Physical Examination: The anterior fontanel is soft and flat, nares with nonpurulent discharge, and oropharynx with dry mucous membranes. The patient has a rapid heartbeat and no murmurs, and the brachial pulse is weak but easily palpable. The abdomen is soft, with the liver edge just below right costal margin. Extremities are cool without edema.

ECG:

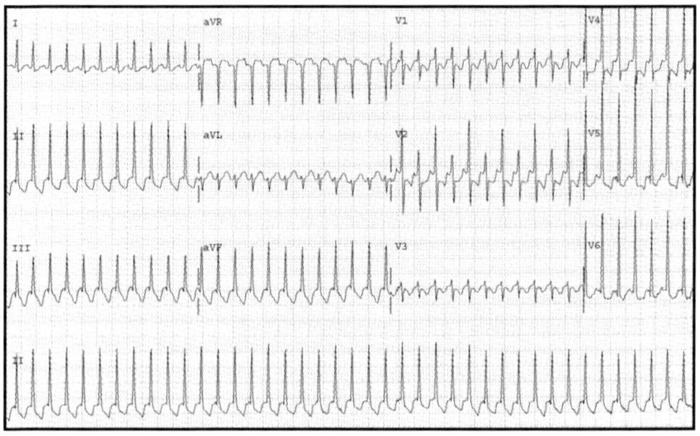

ASK YOURSELF

- **What does this ECG reveal?**

  The ECG shows a narrow tachycardia at 270 with absent P waves, a very high rate, and no RR variability or abrupt changes in rhythm. These characteristics indicate supraventricular tachycardia.

- **What interventions are needed at this time?**
  - First line: Vagal maneuvers. These are safe to perform without an intravenous line if necessary.
    - Bag of ice over face ("diving reflex": do not put pressure on the eyes or occlude the mouth/airway)
    - Nasal suction or rectal stimulation for infants (for children able to cooperate, have them blow through an obstructed straw or hold their breath)

- Monitor rhythm continuously during all maneuvers.
- Contact pediatric cardiology.

■ What are the possible complications of vagal maneuvers?

Complications, predominantly bradycardia and rarely asystole, can result from carotid sinus massage and the diving reflex but are virtually absent when the Valsalva maneuver is used. This emphasizes the need for continuous electrocardiographic monitoring during all vagal maneuvers. Rare complications include cervicomediastinal hematoma after carotid massage and fat necrosis after application of ice to the face. Ocular pressure is an unacceptable vagal maneuver as it may cause retinal trauma.[2]

Progression

The patient continues to be irritable, and the heart rate remains at 270 after vagal maneuvers. At this time, the brachial pulse is weak but palpable.

ASK YOURSELF

■ What should be done next?

With continuous electrocardiographic monitoring, administer **adenosine 0.1 mg/kg** IV. If unsuccessful, repeat at **0.2 mg/kg** (maximum first dose 6 mg, maximum second dose 12 mg).[3]

■ No effect is seen with adenosine. What is the most likely explanation?

Adenosine has a very short half-life. It can fail to convert the tachycardia if the drug is given through a small vein distal to the heart, which does not facilitate rapid administration, or is not followed immediately by a saline flush.[3]

Progression

The patient has received two doses of adenosine without effect.

ASK YOURSELF

■ What should be done now?

Reassess the patient. If the patient is hemodynamically stable, there is time to consult with cardiology to discuss alternative methods of converting the rhythm to sinus.

Progression

The patient acutely becomes more tachypneic and diaphoretic. Brachial pulse is thready, and the patient now is responsive only to pain.

ASK YOURSELF

■ What should be done next?

Perform emergent **synchronized cardioversion** at 0.5 to 1 J/kg. Joules may be increased to a maximum of 2 J/kg if the initial dose is ineffective. If the patient is awake, provide sedation and analgesia. Short-acting agents with minimal physiologic effects should be used. Midazolam and fentanyl are commonly used; however, both can compromise cardiac output. Importantly, if the patient is unstable, sedation should not delay cardioversion.[3]

■ What paddle size should be used?

Infant or small paddles (4.5 cm) should be used in infants up to 1 year of age or 10 kg (approximately 30 inches on a length-based resuscitation tape). Adult or large paddles (8 to 13 cm) should be used for children over these parameters. If the larger paddle fits entirely on the chest wall, it is preferred because the larger the paddle, the lower the intrathoracic impedance and the more effective the current flow.[1]

■ What are the alternatives if the patient is stable and adenosine fails to convert the rhythm?

It should be emphasized that adenosine and synchronized cardioversion provide the safest and most likely mechanisms for success in converting SVT in the hands of ALS providers who are not experts (cardiologists).[1] Patients may be in and out of this rhythm for hours to days without acutely decompensating. Alternative methods of conversion are typically used with expert consultation. Digoxin, short-acting β-blockers, overdrive pacing, amiodarone, or procainamide may be used to treat SVTs in infants and children. Amiodarone and procainamide must not be used together because both can cause prolongation of the QT interval.[4] Verapamil, a calcium channel blocker, has been reported to result in hypotension and cardiac arrest when administered to infants and should not be used in this setting.[1]

■ What disposition is appropriate for this patient?

Admission of children converted from SVT is generally not useful unless there is underlying cardiac disease that must be evaluated and treated or significant intervention was required in conversion. A cardiology consultation and outpatient followup are definitely needed. If a patient has symptoms or signs of congestive heart failure, admission is recommended, as these patients are more likely to have immediate recurrences of the arrthymia.[3] It is important to always check an ECG after conversion to identify the presence of accessory pathways, as in Wolff-Parkinson-White syndrome, which has also been shown to increase the risk of recurrent SVT.[5] Some patients with recurrent SVT will require chronic medical therapy, whereas others may require radiofrequency ablation of an accessory pathway. Because this arrhythmia can spontaneously resolve in infants, ablation therapy is usually delayed until the patient is 4 to 5 years of age unless the tachycardia is life threatening or medically refractory.[3]

Objectives of This Scenario

1. Distinguish supraventricular tachycardia from sinus tachycardia.

Sinus tachycardia usually occurs in patients with fever, dehydration, an injury, or pain. Anxiety also will result in pediatric sinus tachycardia. In sinus tachycardia, the P waves are present and normal, the heart rate often varies with activity, and the RR interval may be variable with a constant PR.

Below is a rhythm strip showing SVT at a rate of 230 converting to normal sinus rhythm, rate 160, with administration of adenosine.

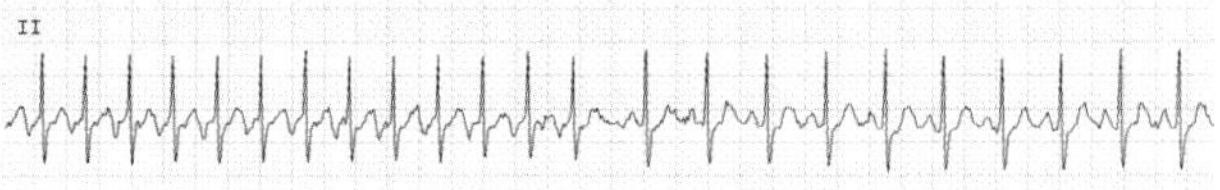

SVT is a reentrant type of tachycardia in which the presenting history is often nonspecific, P waves are absent or abnormal, and the heart rate does not vary with activity. In SVT, the onset and cessation are abrupt, the QRS complex is narrow, and the rate is very regular. As in the patient of this scenario, the tachycardia is not responsive to control of fever or volume resuscitation, both of which are typical of sinus tachycardia. An ECG reveals a regular, narrow complex tachycardia, usually 220 to 320 beats per minute in infants and between 180 and 250 beats per minute in a child.[6]

2. Manage SVT without hemodynamic compromise.

Many reentrant tachycardias can be managed with vagal maneuvers. In some children, the Valsalva maneuver can be used at home as a chronic treatment if the episodes occur infrequently. A bag of ice placed on the face will convert some children (90% to 100% in young infants).[3]

Adenosine is the drug of choice for pharmacologic conversion. It has an extremely short half-life (15 seconds) and is given as a rapid bolus followed immediately by a normal saline bolus. Because of the short half-life, it has rare serious side effects. The initial dose is 0.1 mg/kg (maximum 6 mg), and if unsuccessful, a second dose of 0.2 mg/kg (maximum 12 mg) can be given. Rare arrhythmias may be induced by adenosine, and an ECG should be monitored and recorded during administration. Patients often complain of chest discomfort, shortness of breath, and flushing, but these symptoms subside within 1 to 2 minutes.[3]

If adenosine fails to convert the rhythm, consultation with cardiology is recommended. Other measures for converting the hemodynamically stable patient are discussed earlier. If at any time the patient is deemed unstable, synchronized cardioversion is indicated.

3. Recognize when aggressive management of SVT is indicated.

Synchronized cardioversion is always an acceptable technique to terminate SVT and is the recommended treatment if a patient becomes unstable with hypotension or altered mental status from compromised blood flow to the brain. The energy dose is 0.5 to 2 J/kg. Unless the patient is in critical condition, infants should receive sedation and analgesia before cardioversion. The electrode position can be either anterior-anterior or, in the case of a small infant, anterior-posterior. Remember, if vagal maneuvers are unsuccessful in a patient whose stability is in question and vascular access is difficult to obtain, move directly to cardioversion.[3]

References

1. Zaritsky AL, Nadkarni VM, Hickey RW, et al, eds. *PALS Provider Manual.* Dallas, Tex: American Academy of Pediatrics and American Heart Association; 2002:200-203.
2. Atkins D, Chameides L, Fallat M, et al. Resuscitation science of pediatrics. *Ann Emerg Med.* 2001;37:41-48.
3. Atkins D. Advances in pediatric resuscitation: diagnosis and management of supraventricular tachycardia in children. *Clin Pediatr Emerg Med.* 2001;2:107-113.
4. Atkins D, Dorian P, Gonzalez E, et al. Treatment of tachyarrhythmias. *Ann Emerg Med.* 2001;37:91-109.
5. Tortoriello T, Snyder C, Smith E, et al. Frequency of recurrence among infants with supraventricular tachycardia and comparison of recurrence rates among those with and without preexcitation and among those with and without response to digoxin and/or propanolol therapy. *Am J Cardiol.* 2003;92:1045-1049.
6. Gewitz M. Cardiac emergencies. In: Fleisher GR, Ludwig S, eds. *Textbook of Pediatric Emergency Medicine.* 4th ed. Philadelphia, Pa: Lippincott Williams & Williams; 2000:676-681.

SCENARIO #23

Cardiac – Unresponsive

Leticia Manning Ryan, MD

Brief Presenting History

An 8-year-old boy is brought to the emergency department from an adjacent playground by his parents after he collapsed while playing basketball.

Pediatric Assessment Triangle

Appearance: Limp, pale, cyanotic, unresponsive

Work of Breathing: No respiratory effort

Circulation to the Skin: Extremities cool and mottled

Initial Vital Signs

Pulse and Blood Pressure: Unable to palpate pulse or auscultate heart sounds

Respiratory Rate: 0

Temperature: 36°C (96.8°F) tympanic

ASK YOURSELF

- **How much should this 8-year-old weigh?**

  An estimated weight for an 8-year-old is 25 kg. One can use the length-based Broselow Pediatric Emergency Tape or a pediatric table to determine weight based on age. See Appendix A.

- **What is the initial assessment? What is the patient's physiologic status?**

  This child presents in cardiopulmonary arrest.

- **What could be causing this arrest?**

  In pediatrics, the most common primary cause of cardiopulmonary arrest is a respiratory problem.[1] However, the brief history provided of sudden collapse in a previously well child is suspicious for a cardiac etiology. In the presence of certain structural and conductive cardiovascular diseases, physical exertion can trigger ventricular tachyarrhythmias and result in sudden collapse and cardiopulmonary arrest.[2] Such arrhythmias also can occur in children without cardiovascular disease who have sustained blunt nonpenetrating trauma to the chest (commotio cordis). Survival is uncommon and dependent on prompt initiation of CPR and defibrillation.[2,3]

  Additional noncardiac etiologies of a sudden cardiopulmonary arrest among child athletes include heat stroke, head trauma, severe asthma exacerbation, pulmonary embolism, and a ruptured cerebral artery aneurysm.[2]

- **What interventions are needed at this time? What complications might be expected?**

  Interventions:

  - Initiate algorithm for pediatric pulseless arrest. See "Evaluation and Management: Circulation," Figure 1.
  - Position airway and initiate BMV with cricoid pressure at a rate of 20 with 100% O_2. Suction airway as needed.

- Place board under child and begin chest compressions at a rate of 100 per minute in synchrony with BMV at a ratio of 5:1. Check for pulses with compressions.
- Attach cardiorespiratory monitor and turn on defibrillator.
- Attempt to establish intravenous access.

Potential Complications:

- Ineffective BMV due to poor positioning or failure to suction.
- Ineffective chest compressions because of poor compression method or failure to check pulse with compressions.
- Inability to obtain venous access, necessitating intraosseous or central venous line placement.

Additional History and Physical Examination Findings

This child was previously well with no known history of cardiac disease. He had an episode of syncope that occurred during basketball practice last month. There was no history of trauma during today's game, but the patient complained of pain in his chest before collapse.

There is a family history of an uncle with a "heart problem" who suddenly collapsed and died during a football game more than 10 years ago.

No defibrillator was available at the playground. Parents and bystanders initiated CPR and drove the child to the hospital, which took 8 to 10 minutes.

Past Medical History: No known illnesses or operations.

Medications: None

Allergies: None known

Physical Examination: Symmetric adequate chest rise with BMV, femoral pulse present with chest compressions, pupils 4 mm, symmetric, unreactive.

ECG Monitor:

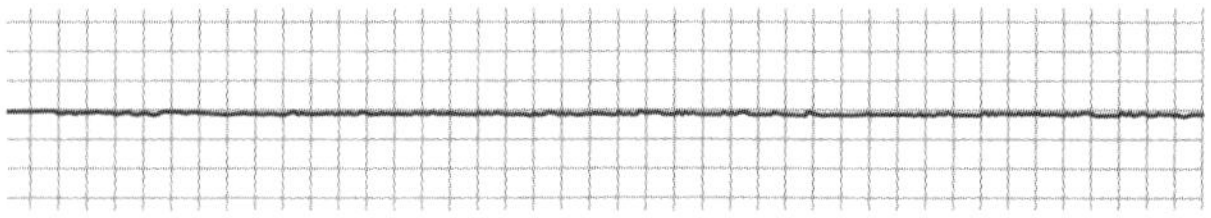

ASK YOURSELF

■ What is the most likely diagnosis?

The association of symptoms with exercise and reported complaint of chest pain before collapse strongly suggests a cardiac etiology. The family history is suggestive of a genetic cardiac disease. Possible cardiovascular conditions include congenital and genetic disorders such as hypertrophic cardiomyopathy, congenital coronary artery anomalies, valvular heart disease, and conduction disorders such as the long QT syndrome, as well as acquired conditions such as myocarditis.[2] Given the lack of access to immediate defibrillation and the elapsed time, the presumed initial ventricular dysrhythmia has deteriorated into asystole.

■ What interventions are needed at this time? What complications might be expected?

Interventions:

- Continue CPR (check electrode position and contact; confirm rhythm in two different leads).
- Perform endotracheal intubation with #2 or #3 Miller (straight) or MacIntosh (curved) blade and 6.0 cuffed ET tube using suction as needed and cricoid pressure. Medications for RSI are not indicated.
- Continue chest compressions at a rate of 100. Check for pulse or rhythm change every 5 minutes.
- If intravenous access has not been obtained by this point, place an intraosseous line.
- **Epinephrine 0.01 mg/kg (1:10,000; 0.1 mL/kg) IV/IO** with saline flush or **0.1 mg/kg (1:1,000; 0.1 mL/kg)** via ET tube if other access not obtained.
- When access is obtained, check glucose, blood gas, CBC, electrolytes. Administer **normal saline 20 mL/kg IV/IO.**

Potential Complications:

- Inability to visualize airway if not properly suctioned or positioned
- Either intubation of esophagus with auscultation of breath sounds over stomach or intubation of right mainstem bronchus if tube position not verified

- Extravasation of fluid into surrounding tissues if intraosseous line improperly placed

Reassessment

No spontaneous respiratory effort; bilateral symmetric breath sounds and chest rise with ventilation through ET tube; no breath sounds auscultated over epigastrium; femoral pulses present with chest compressions; femoral pulses absent without compressions; end-tidal CO_2 detector fails to register expired CO_2.

ECG Monitor:

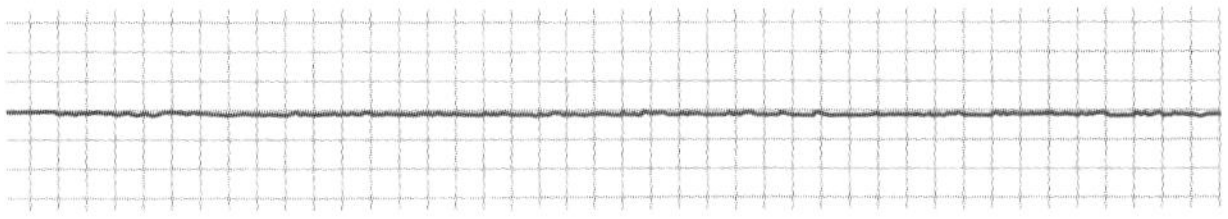

ASK YOURSELF

Does failure to detect expired CO_2 indicate that the ET tube has been erroneously placed in the esophagus?

A colorimetric end-tidal CO_2 detector uses a filter paper that changes color on contact with CO_2. The filter paper begins as purple and should change to yellow with the exhalation phase as CO_2 makes contact with the paper.[4] Both esophageal ET tube placement and a lack of a perfusing rhythm in the patient can result in the absence of a color change from purple to yellow. This patient has been in asystole with no spontaneous pulse throughout the resuscitation. Given the presence of other confirmatory signs of proper ET tube placement (bilateral symmetric breath sounds, chest rise, lack of breath sounds over epigastrium), the persistent purple color is most likely due to lack of a perfusing rhythm.

What interventions are needed at this time? What complications might be expected?

Interventions:

- Continue manual ventilation through ET tube at a rate of 20.
- Continue chest compressions at a rate of 100.
- Repeat **epinephrine** every 3 to 5 minutes at **0.01 mg/kg (1:10,000; 0.1 mL/kg) IV/IO** with saline flush or **0.1 mg/kg (1:1,000; 0.1 mL/kg) via ET tube.**
- Continue to check for pulse or rhythm change every 5 minutes. If rhythm changes, continue along the appropriate specific algorithm.
- Repeat fluid bolus of **normal saline 20 mL/kg** over 5 to 10 minutes.
- Consider **sodium bicarbonate 1 mEq/kg IV/IO.**
- Identify and treat the four Hs (hypoxemia, hypovolemia, hypothermia, hyperkalemia/hypokalemia and other metabolic disorders) and the four Ts (tamponade, tension pneumothorax, toxins, thromboembolism) if clinically indicated.
- Place NG tube to decompress air from stomach and possibly improve ventilation.

Potential Complications:

- Pneumothorax requiring percutaneous anterior needle aspiration or chest tube placement if barotrauma induced by excessive tidal volume
- Impaired ventilation of patient due to abdominal distention if NG tube not placed
- ET tube dislodged if not secured with tape

Progression

The resuscitation has continued for 30 minutes. The patient has received three doses of epinephrine. There has been no return of spontaneous circulation or respiratory effort. The pupils are fixed and dilated.

ASK YOURSELF

What is this patient's prognosis?

The prognosis is very poor. Survival after prolonged asystolic arrest is uncommon and is most likely when CPR and defibrillation are prompt.[2,3] In addition, return of spontaneous circulation is unlikely if the child fails to respond to effective advanced resuscitation efforts and two or more doses of epinephrine.[5]

■ When should resuscitation efforts be discontinued?

This is a difficult decision, particularly in pediatric cases. The Guidelines 2000 for Cardiopulmonary Resuscitation and Emergency Cardiovascular Care (ECC)[5] state that "if a child fails to respond to two doses of epinephrine with a return of spontaneous circulation the child is unlikely to survive." The guidelines also suggest that resuscitative efforts may be ceased in pediatric cardiopulmonary arrest victims after 30 minutes in the absence of ventricular fibrillation, ventricular tachycardia, toxic drug exposure, and primary prearrest hypothermia.[5]

Given the likely etiology of the arrest as well as the duration of CPR, it is unlikely that this child will respond to further resuscitation and it is reasonable to terminate resuscitation efforts.

Note: If this scenario is to be used as a mock code, please refer to Guidelines for Conducting the Mock Code for the discussion on the pitfalls of mock codes ending in the death of the mannequin. Instructors must approach this issue with great sensitivity.

Objectives of This Scenario

1. Recognize the presentation of a primary cardiac arrest.

In contrast to cardiac arrest in adults, cardiopulmonary arrest in children is rarely sudden and is more frequently caused by progression of respiratory distress or shock than by primary cardiac arrhythmias.[6] If a previously well child experiences a sudden collapse, however, primary cardiac arrest may be the cause. Risk for arrhythmia and sudden death is associated with myocarditis, a sudden sharp blow to the chest, underlying cardiac disease including cardiomyopathy, prolonged QT syndrome, severe electrolyte abnormality, profound hypothermia, drug intoxication, and a family history of sudden death.[7,8]

2. Initiate management for asystole.

Asystole is the most common rhythm in pediatric cardiopulmonary arrest and is usually the result of a prolonged arrest. Remember to treat the patient and not the monitor. If the monitor rhythm is asystole, be sure to do the following:

- Check for pulses. If the patient does not have pulses, do not delay the initiation of CPR while confirming rhythm. Proceed directly to pediatric pulseless arrest algorithm.
- Check placement of leads.
- Confirm in two different leads to be sure that the rhythm is not fine ventricular fibrillation.
- Verify that chest compressions are producing palpable pulses.
- Continue to check for pulses or rhythm changes every 5 minutes.

3. Recognize when termination of resuscitation efforts is appropriate.

Prolonged resuscitation for children with pulseless arrest is not likely to be successful.[9] In general, resuscitation efforts may be discontinued if a child has not responded with spontaneous circulation after 20 to 30 minutes.[6,10] It has been noted that failure to respond to two doses of epinephrine greatly decreases the chance of survival for a child. After such attempts, and in the absence of ventricular fibrillation, ventricular tachycardia, toxic drug exposure, and primary prearrest hypothermia, resuscitation can be discontinued if there is no return of spontaneous circulation.[5] It should be noted that nonreactive pupils have little predictive value in the outcome of a case and should not be the sole criterion for the termination of resuscitation efforts. In one study of pediatric resuscitation, 33% of children with nonreactive pupils survived.[11]

References

1. Fitzmaurice L, Gerardi MJ. Cardiovascular system. In: Gausche-Hill M, Fuchs S, Yamamoto L, eds. *APLS: The Pediatric Emergency Medicine Resource.* 4th ed. Sudbury, Mass: American Academy of Pediatrics, American College of Emergency Physicians, Jones and Bartlett Publishing Co; 2004:133.
2. Maron BJ. Medical progress: sudden death in young athletes. *N Engl J Med.* 2003;349:1064-1075.
3. Maron BJ, Gohman TE, Kyle SE, et al. Clinical profile and spectrum of commotio cordis. *JAMA.* 2002;287:1142-1146.
4. Ward KR, Yealy DM. End-tidal CO_2 monitoring in emergency medicine. Part 1. Basic principles. *Acad Emerg Med.* 1998;5:628-636.
5. American Heart Association in collaboration with International Liaison Committee on Resuscitation. Guidelines 2000 for Cardiopulmonary Resuscitation and Emergency Cardiovascular Care: International Consensus on Science. *Circulation.* 2000;102(suppl 1).
6. Young KD, Seidel JS. Pediatric cardiopulmonary resuscitation: a collective review. *Ann Emerg Med.* 1999;33:195-205.
7. Liberthson RR. Sudden death from cardiac causes in children and young adults. *N Engl J Med.* 1996;334:1039-1044.

8. Zaritsky A, Nadkarni V, Getson P, et al. CPR in children. *Ann Emerg Med.* 1987;16:1107-1111.

9. American Academy of Pediatrics, Committee on School Health and Committee on Bioethics. Do not resuscitate orders in schools. *Pediatrics.* 2000;105:878-879.

10. Rosenberg N, Klein E, Nozicka CA. When to start and when to stop. *Pediatr Emerg Care.* 2001;17:126-129.

11. Nichols DG, Kettrick RG, Swedlow DB, et al. Factors influencing outcome of cardiopulmonary resuscitation in children. *Pediatr Emerg Care.* 1986;2:1-5.

SCENARIO #24

Cardiac – Unresponsive

Michael Quinn, MD

Brief Presenting History

A 10-year-old boy presents to the emergency department via ambulance; CPR is being administered by paramedics. He collapsed after being struck in the chest by a pitched baseball at Little League practice. Bystanders trained in basic life support began CPR at the scene, and 911 personnel were called immediately via cell phone.

Pediatric Assessment Triangle

Appearance: Unresponsive; no spontaneous movement

Work of Breathing: No spontaneous respiratory effort

Circulation to the Skin: Cool, pale, clammy

Initial Vital Signs

Pulse: 0

Respiratory Rate: 0

Blood Pressure: Not obtainable

Temperature: 37°C (98.6°F) oral

Physical Examination on Arrival to the Emergency Department

Airway: Maintained by chin lift during BMV

Breathing: No spontaneous effort; good air movement with rescue breaths

Circulation: Pulse palpable only with compressions

Disability: Unresponsive

ASK YOURSELF

- **What is the initial assessment? What is the patient's physiologic status?**

  The patient presents with sudden onset of cardiopulmonary arrest after a blunt injury to the chest.

- **What could have caused his collapse?**

  The clinical entity of commotio cordis (sudden death after a blunt chest blow) comes immediately to mind. Other causes of cardiopulmonary arrest after chest trauma include pericardial tamponade, coronary artery or large central vessel laceration, heart wall contusion or laceration, pneumothorax, airway crush injury, and airway or pulmonary hemorrhage. Nontraumatic causes are low in incidence but myriad in number and include dysrhythmias provoked by myocarditis, ischemic heart disease, or previously unrecognized or unknown structural heart disease. Noncardiac causes include CNS events such as seizures or intracranial hemorrhage, metabolic causes such as an adverse medication reaction or hypoglycemia, and respiratory problems such as acute laryngospasm or bronchospasm.[1,2]

- **What additional history is necessary at this point?**

  A rapid primary survey and a focused history are essential. Rapid review with witnesses of the events preceding the collapse is important. Any reliable past medical history related to underlying illnesses, particularly involving the cardiac, pulmonary, and nervous systems, should be sought. Time should not be spent seeking extensive history of obscure, occult disease.

Additional History and Physical Examination Findings

The child had been at practice after school. The coach was pitching, "not fast," and he reports that he is sure the ball hit the boy's chest anteriorly.

Past Medical History: Healthy 10-year-old boy with no history of heart, lung, or neurologic illness

Medications: None

Allergies: Rash in past with penicillins

Physical Examination: No evidence of trauma on primary survey, particularly of the head, neck, and chest

ASK YOURSELF

■ What interventions are needed at this time? What complications might be expected?

Interventions:

- **Airway:** Suction and maintain the airway to facilitate BMV while preparations for intubation begin. Intubate the trachea at the first available opportunity. A #3 Miller or Macintosh blade is acceptable; a 6.0 or 6.5 cuffed ET tube is appropriate for a 10-year-old.
- **Breathing:** Continue BMV with 100% oxygen; when an ET tube is secured, continue hand ventilation through it.
- **Circulation:** Continue chest compressions at a rate of 100/min. Check frequently for pulses. Establish intravenous access. Apply a cardiac monitor and determine the underlying electrical rhythm. If the rhythm is determined to be ventricular fibrillation (VF) or pulseless ventricular tachycardia (VT), asynchronous defibrillation should be delivered immediately, even if intubation or attempts at intravenous access must be briefly delayed as a result.

Note: In this pulseless patient in whom cardiac arrhythmia is strongly suspected, the single most important intervention (after initiation of CPR) is to place monitors to confirm the rhythm and then defibrillate if indicated.

Potential Complications:

- Failure to immediately establish rhythm type, delaying the definitive, life-saving intervention (defibrillation)
- Failure to intubate properly (esophageal intubation, right mainstem bronchus intubation)
- Emesis during intubation with suction not available
- Failure to obtain intravenous access, which necessitates intraosseous placement

Progression

There are no pulses without compressions.

ECG Monitor:

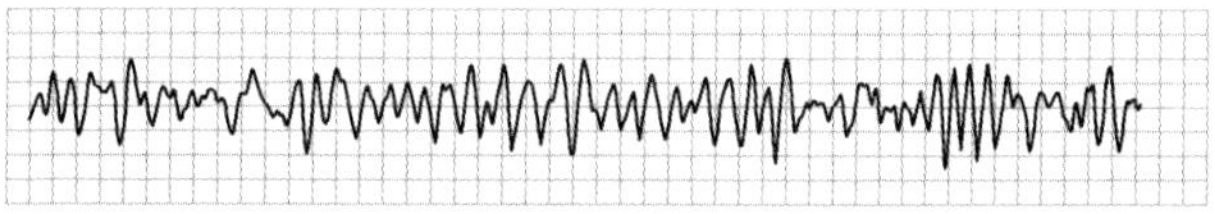

ASK YOURSELF

■ What is this rhythm? What does it mean?

The rhythm is VF. It is a nonperfusing rhythm. If it is not addressed immediately, death will result.

■ What should be done immediately?

The rhythm is VF. It is treated with CPR and defibrillation. The dose of energy is calculated using a weight-based method. The initial dose should be 2 J/kg (asynchronous mode). The second dose should be 2 to 4 J/kg, and the third and any subsequent doses should be 4 J/kg.[3,4] See "Evaluation and Management: Circulation," Figure 1 for pulseless arrest algorithm. Two practical considerations come into play: the patient's weight may not be known, and the defibrillator in use may provide only a limited menu of dose options below 50 J. A patient's weight may be estimated based on standardized norms or length-based methods (see Appendix A). If the defibrillator has limited dose options, it should be set to the closest available dose. Many clinicians suggest "rounding up" to the next highest available dose.

Progression

The patient's weight is estimated to be 35 kg. The defibrillator is powered, set to defibrillation mode, and charged to 70 J.

ASK YOURSELF

■ **How do you defibrillate this patient?**

1. The defibrillator operator will apply standard-sized paddles, each to its appropriate location on the chest (apex and base, usually indicated on the paddles), using a low-impedance interface material (electrode cream, paste, or pads) between the paddles and the skin. Some defibrillators have self-adherent pads instead of hand-held paddles; these are acceptable if they are available.
2. A shock of 70 J is delivered after the operator provides sufficient warning to the other staff to clear themselves from physical contact with the patient.[4]

■ **What complications might be expected?**

- The defibrillator fails to deliver the shock because of mechanical or operator failure; for example, the appropriate cables are not connected or the defibrillator is not powered or charged.
- The paddles or pads are not physically separated, or electrode paste from the two sites is touching.
- Oxygen is allowed to flow freely over the patient's chest, leading to ignition and risk of fire and burns.
- Staff member fails to clear from the patient, risking injury to that individual.

Progression

A first shock is delivered at 70 J, after the operator provides a warning cadence to the staff. VF persists. A second shock is delivered, this time at 150 J (4 J/kg), leading to brief asystole followed by sinus bradycardia at a rate of 30/min.

ASK YOURSELF

■ **What interventions are needed at this time?**

- Rapid assessment of circulatory status, beginning with assessment of pulses and perfusion
- Resumption of previous resuscitative efforts, including monitoring, supported respirations, chest compressions, and intravenous or intraosseous access attempts

Progression

A weak carotid pulse is palpable with the monitored complexes. Blood pressure cannot be detected, and skin perfusion is poor. Attempts at peripheral intravenous access remain unsuccessful.

ASK YOURSELF

■ **What interventions are needed at this time?**

- Continue CPR.
- Intubate if ET tube is not already in place.
- Place an intraosseous line.
- Initiate algorithm for bradycardia with poor perfusion (see "Evaluation and Management: Circulation," Figure 2). Continue compressions.
- Administer epinephrine. There are two alternatives at this point:
  1. **Epinephrine 0.1 mg/kg ET (0.1 mL/kg of 1:1,000 solution)**, followed by 2 to 3 mL of saline and positive pressure ventilations. Although a vascular route is preferable, this method can be immediately accomplished in this patient.
  2. **Epinephrine 0.01 mg/kg IV/IO (0.1 mL/kg of 1:10,000 solution)** can also be administered. Although not instantly available, intraosseous needle insertion can provide reliable access within 30 to 60 seconds.

Progression

Epinephrine is administered endotracheally, and the patient now has a sinus rhythm with a rate of 80 to 100 with palpable central pulses and a blood pressure of 90/40. There are no spontaneous respirations. Hand ventilation through the ET tube continues. Central venous access is obtained, and a continuous epinephrine infusion at 0.1 mcg/kg/min is started. This child is transferred to the ICU.

ASK YOURSELF

- **What additional complications might be expected for this patient?**

  This patient remains in a state of decompensated shock, and he has sustained an unknown degree of ischemic insult to vital organs, including the heart. He is at risk for recurrent dysrhythmia and heart pump failure. He will need critical care monitoring, continued mechanical ventilation, and vasoactive medications such as antiarrhythmics and pressor agents. He may have experienced complications related to his intubation and supported ventilation (barotrauma). He also may have sustained injuries such as rib fracture during the period of CPR.

- **If an automated external defibrillator (AED) had been available at the scene, how would the sequence be affected?**

  This patient arrived at the emergency department in VF. However, the availability of AEDs in public places is increasing. Had an AED been available at the scene, its application and use would have been acceptable and indicated. AEDs are now recommended for use in patients aged 1 year and older.[5] Newer generations of AEDs capable of delivering doses of electricity appropriate for smaller individuals are becoming more widely available.[4,6]

Objectives of This Scenario

1. Recognize VF.

This patient presented with sudden cardiorespiratory arrest and was found to be in VF. Although it is the most common collapse rhythm in adults, VF is less common than asystole as the terminal rhythm in children. Several recent studies have reported that VF may be more common in children than previously recognized.[7,8] It is essential, therefore, to keep the possibility of VF in mind, particularly in cases of sudden collapse like the one illustrated here, despite the vast differential diagnosis involved. CPR must be provided to the pulseless patient, and the rhythm must be sought and recognized. When found, the pediatric resuscitation paradigm (which heavily emphasizes respiratory resuscitation) must be modified to allow for early defibrillation. Survival from VF is most likely when defibrillation occurs as soon as possible after the collapse. Effective CPR should be provided until defibrillation can be performed but should not delay defibrillation.[4,6]

2. Be able to use a defibrillator.

Defibrillation is not a common event in the care of children, even in busy pediatric emergency departments and ICUs. Staff may be unfamiliar and uncomfortable with use of the device, and mechanical and operator error may therefore be encountered. Several common pitfalls are pointed out in the scenario. It is incumbent on individuals and emergency departments to ensure familiarity with the use of these devices through ongoing education and practice.[4]

3. Recognize a rare but devastating sport-related injury.

Commotio cordis, sometimes called cardiac concussion, is sudden death caused by nonpenetrating trauma to the chest in the absence of structural damage to the chest wall and intrathoracic structures. Once thought to be a rare, sports-related injury, it is reported with increasing frequency and is found to occur in nonsporting situations. Many reports include instances of seemingly very low impact injury leading to commotio cordis. Blows to the chest with baseballs, softballs, hockey pucks, and other projectiles remain the most frequent cause, and male athletes aged 5 to 18 make up the majority of victims. Death is usually immediate, and resuscitation is rarely successful.[1] Child safety advocates encourage the use of chest protective devices and "safety" balls, particularly for young athletes. These have not won universal acceptance, and there are insufficient data to make definitive recommendations for their use.[9,10]

References

1. Link MS, Wang PJ, Maron BJ, et al. What is commotio cordis? *Cardiol Rev.* 1999;7:265-269.
2. Ludwig S. Resuscitation. In: Fleisher GR, Ludwig S, eds. *Textbook of Pediatric Emergency Medicine.* 4th ed. Philadelphia, Pa: Lippincott Williams and Wilkins; 2000:3-23.
3. Chameides L, Brown GE, Raye JR, et al. Guidelines for defibrillation in infants and children: report of the American Heart Association target activity group: cardiopulmonary resuscitation in the young. *Circulation.* 1977;56:502A-503A.
4. Rhythm disturbances. In: Hazinski MF, Zaritsky AL, Nadkarni VM, et al, eds. *PALS Provider Manual.* Dallas, Tex: American Academy of Pediatrics and American Heart Association; 2000:185-228.
5. Samson RA, Berg RA, Bingham R, et al. Use of automated external defibrillators for children: an update: an advisory statement from the Pediatric Advanced Life Support Task Force, International Liaison Committee on Resuscitation. *Circulation.* 2003;107:3250-3255.
6. VF treated with CPR and automated external defibrillation. In: Cummins RO, ed. *ACLS Provider Manual.* Dallas, Tex: American Heart Association; 2000:63-73.
7. Young KD, Seidel JS. Pediatric cardiopulmonary resuscitation: a collective review. *Ann Emerg Med.* 1999;33:195-205.
8. Mogayzel C, Quan L, Graves JR, et al. Out-of-hospital ventricular fibrillation in children and adolescents: causes and outcomes. *Ann Emerg Med.* 1995;25:484-491.
9. Luckstead EF, Patel DR. Catastrophic pediatric sports injuries. *Pediatr Clin North Am.* 2002;49:581-591.
10. Maron BJ, Gohlman TE, Kyle SB, et al. Clinical profile and spectrum of commotio cordis. *JAMA.* 2002;287:1142-1146.

SCENARIO #25

Altered Mental Status

Richard A. Greenberg, MD

Brief Presenting History

A 2-month-old boy is brought to the emergency department by his mother after she found him in his crib "limp and blue," with gagging respirations.

Pediatric Assessment Triangle

Appearance: Pale, limp, difficult to arouse

Work of Breathing: Labored respirations with subcostal and suprasternal retractions

Circulation to the Skin: Mottled

Initial Vital Signs

Pulse: 180

Respiratory Rate: 44

Blood Pressure: 95/70

Temperature: 38°C (100.4°F) rectal

ASK YOURSELF

- **How much should this 2-month-old child weigh?**

  This child should weigh about 4 kg. One can use the length-based Broselow Pediatric Emergency Tape or a pediatric table to determine weight based on age. See Appendix A.

Physical Examination

Airway: Patent with a weak cry; moderate secretions in the mouth

Breathing: Labored respirations, no wheezes or crackles

Circulation: Mottled, cool extremities; capillary refill time 4 seconds centrally

ASK YOURSELF

- **Where would you best feel the central pulse in this 2-month-old patient?**

  Femoral or brachial pulses are easiest to palpate in infants and young children. Carotid pulses can be difficult to palpate due to the relatively short necks of children.[1] This patient has 1+ femoral and brachial pulses.

Disability: Eyes closed and do not open with painful stimulation; pupils equal, round, reactive to light, 5 to 3 mm bilaterally

Exposure: Patient's clothes removed and warming lights turned on; no obvious bruising or deformity of extremities

ASK YOURSELF

- **What is the initial assessment? What is the patient's physiologic status?**

The child presents with altered mental status and compensated shock.

- **What is the differential diagnosis of altered mental status in this 2-month-old infant?**

Infection is common in this age group and should be considered high on the differential diagnosis. Infectious causes include meningitis, sepsis, and encephalitis. Metabolic causes include hypoglycemia, hyponatremia, and inborn errors of metabolism. Pulmonary causes include hypoxia and/or hypercapnia with pulmonary disease (eg, pneumonia, bronchiolitis). Nonaccidental trauma (including shaken baby syndrome) is a possibility. Neurologic etiologies are seizures and hydrocephalus. Congenital heart disease, gastrointestinal conditions of volvulus and intussusception, and CNS tumor[2,3] also should be included in the differential. Toxic ingestion is a common cause of altered mental status but would have to be intentional (Munchausen syndrome by proxy) or related to an exposure like carbon monoxide poisoning in a patient of this age (infant). Shock of any etiology, with associated decreased cerebral perfusion, also can cause alterations in mental status.

- **What additional history and physical examination findings would help you to establish the diagnosis?**

The presence of fever suggests an infectious cause of the patient's symptoms, although the lack of fever in a 2-month-old does not rule out an infectious cause. Septic infants can present with hypothermia and altered mental status. Cough, congestion, tachypnea, and increased work of breathing would likely be present with pulmonary disease. Nonaccidental trauma may be suggested by a history that is inconsistent with the physical examination findings and/or the developmental ability of the child.[4] Shaken baby syndrome often presents with a variety of nonspecific symptoms, such as poor feeding, lethargy, irritability, and vomiting. Nonaccidental trauma cases are more common with premature infants, patients with chronic medical problems, and "colicky" infants and in homes with a high level of stress.[5] A bulging fontanel implies increased intracranial pressure (ICP) (hemorrhage, infection, or hydrocephalus). A thorough evaluation of the skin for signs of bruising or trauma should be performed. An ophthalmoscopic examination that reveals retinal hemorrhages confirms the diagnosis of shaken baby syndrome.

Additional History and Physical Examination Findings

The patient has had cough and congestion for 3 days. He has been afebrile. The patient had been home alone with the mother's boyfriend for 4 hours when his mother came home and found him "limp and blue" in his crib.

Past Medical History: Premature birth at 32 weeks, gastroesophageal reflux disease, colic

Medications: Ranitidine, simethicone

Physical Examination: Anterior fontanel bulging and retinal hemorrhages present bilaterally. Heart is tachycardic with regular rhythm without murmur. The abdomen is soft and nondistended.

ASK YOURSELF

- **What interventions should be made at this time? What complications might be expected?**

Interventions:

- Administer 100% O_2 via face mask.
- Suction oropharynx.
- Place in cervical spine collar, because shaken baby syndrome can be associated with cervical spine injuries.[6]
- Place patient on a cardiorespiratory monitor with pulse oximetry.
- Place rectal temperature probe.
- Attempt intravenous access, and start fluid resuscitation with **20 mL/kg of normal saline.** Order laboratory tests if blood is available (rapid glucose, arterial or venous blood gas, CBC, blood culture, chemistry panel, urinalysis with culture).

- Consider giving empiric intravenous antibiotics for a possible infectious etiology of altered mental status.

Potential Complications:

- Vomiting, requiring suction, while log rolling and maintaining in-line cervical spine immobilization
- Inability to secure intravenous access, requiring intraosseous line placement.

Initial Laboratory Test Results: Hematocrit 34, glucose 129

Repeat Vital Signs

Pulse: 95

Respiratory Rate: 12

Blood Pressure: 100/70

Oxygen Saturation: 82% with 100% O_2 via face mask

ASK YOURSELF

■ What is the physiologic status now?

Impending respiratory failure with agonal respirations and bradypnea

■ What interventions should be made at this time? What complications might be expected?

Interventions:

- BMV with 100% O_2. Prepare for RSI. Apply cricoid pressure.
- RSI
  1. #1 Miller laryngoscope blade, 3.5 ET tube
  2. Continue to preoxygenate and apply cricoid pressure.
  3. Ensure suction with a stiff tonsillar-tip suction device is set up.
  4. **Atropine 0.01 to 0.02 mg/kg** IV (minimum dose 0.1 mg)
  5. **Lidocaine 1 mg/kg** IV (use to blunt increased ICP response to intubation)[7]
  6. **Etomidate 0.3 mg/kg** IV (has the benefit of lowering ICP without significantly decreasing blood pressure)[7]
  7. **Rocuronium 0.6 to 1 mg/kg IV** (succinylcholine has the potential to raise ICP but is not contraindicated and may be used in head-injured patients)[7]
- In-line cervical spine immobilization while placing ET tube
- End-tidal CO_2 monitor
- Chest radiograph to confirm ET tube placement
- Secure ET tube, and place NG or orogastric tube.

Potential Complications:

- Abdominal distention leading to impaired ventilation or vomiting if an NG or orogastric tube is not placed.
- Right mainstem intubation if ET tube is inserted too far. Use Broselow Pediatric Emergency Tape to approximate correct depth for ET tube placement. To confirm correct placement, observe for symmetric chest rise, auscultate breath sounds over both lungs, confirm that the patient is well saturated, and obtain a chest radiograph.

Progression

The patient becomes unresponsive to painful stimuli, and agonal respirations develop. Right pupil is 7 mm and fixed; left pupil is 5 mm and reactive to light. Decerebrate posturing (rigid extension of upper and lower extremities) is noted on the left.

Repeat Vital Signs

Pulse: 60

Respiratory Rate: Ventilated at 40

Blood Pressure: 125/85

ASK YOURSELF

■ What is the physiologic status now?

Bradycardia, hypertension, and irregular respirations (Cushing triad) are late findings of increased ICP and signify impending herniation. This patient exhibits tentorial herniation, which is accompanied by ipsilateral pupillary dilation and contralateral hemiparesis/decerebrate posturing relative to the mass lesion.[8]

■ **What interventions should be made at this time?**

- Hyperventilation. The use of hyperventilation should be reserved for acute neurologic deterioration. Without acute deterioration, use controlled ventilation with a goal of $Paco_2$ of 35 to 40 mm Hg.[9]
- **Mannitol 0.25 to 1 g/kg** IV[9,10]

Progression

Decerebrate posturing resolves, and pupils become equal and reactive to light.

Repeat Vital Signs

Pulse: 160

Respiratory Rate: Ventilated at 60

Blood Pressure: 100/75

ASK YOURSELF

■ **What interventions should be made at this time?**

- Stop acute hyperventilation.
- When the patient is stable enough to go to radiology, obtain a CT scan of the brain to evaluate the extent of intracranial injury and a CT of the abdomen to rule out blunt abdominal trauma.
- Consult neurosurgery and trauma surgery, and contact child protective services.

Progression

CT scan of the brain reveals diffuse cerebral edema and a large right-sided subdural hematoma with midline shift.

ASK YOURSELF

■ **What disposition and additional management would be expected for this patient?**

After it has been determined that no other injuries require immediate operative intervention (intra-abdominal bleeding, etc.), the patient should be taken to the operating room for emergent evacuation of the subdural hematoma. After decompression, the patient will be admitted to the pediatric ICU for ongoing treatment. A further work-up for other injuries, including a cervical spine series, skeletal survey, and a formal ophthalmologic examination, should be performed when the patient's condition has stabilized.

Objectives of This Scenario

1. Recognize the presentation of shaken baby syndrome.

Child abuse should be high on the differential diagnosis list in any child younger than 1 year who presents with altered consciousness.[11] Physical abuse often is difficult to recognize in an infant because the patient frequently has no outward signs of trauma and may present with various nonspecific symptoms. These presenting complaints can include respiratory complaints, irritability, lethargy, altered mental status, vomiting, poor feeding, and seizures.[4] The caregivers often provide a history that is not consistent with the injuries sustained by the infant.

The shaking of an infant is often accompanied by an impact as the child is thrown against a wall, crib, or other hard surface. This mechanism provides acceleration and deceleration forces that lead to tearing of cortical bridging veins, causing a subdural hematoma.[12,13] As the subdural bleeding increases, the child becomes symptomatic as a result of increased ICP. The presentation of the infant can be several days after the shaking event, as a subdural collection can increase slowly. The violent nature of the abuse also can lead to injuries of the neck, chest, abdomen, and extremities, as well as retinal hemorrhages.

2. Recognize evolving respiratory failure.

Respiratory failure is the inability to meet the body's

need for oxygen or to adequately clear carbon dioxide. Clinical signs of respiratory failure can include altered mental status, skin changes (cyanosis, pallor), and respiratory abnormalities, including tachypnea, bradypnea, agonal respirations/apnea, retractions, stridor, and wheezing. Cardiac changes (tachycardia, bradycardia, cardiac arrest) also can be present in respiratory failure. Cardiorespiratory monitoring, pulse oximetry, and blood gas values can be used to aid in the diagnosis of respiratory failure. To properly manage and prevent respiratory failure, it is important to recognize the early warning signs of respiratory distress.[14]

3. Recognize and initiate management of increased ICP.

Early signs and symptoms of increased ICP include headache, vomiting, and altered mental status. It is important to recognize the early warning signs before later manifestations such as irregular respirations, abnormal posturing, hypertension, bradycardia, and pupillary dilation occur. These later signs can indicate impending herniation.[8] The treatment for increased ICP includes RSI, hyperventilation, and mannitol. For more details, see the section on increased ICP in "Evaluation and Management: Neurologic Emergencies."

References

1. Dieckman RA. Pediatric assessment. In: Gausche-Hill M, Fuchs S, Yamamoto L, eds. *APLS: The Pediatric Emergency Medicine Resource.* 4th ed. Sudbury, Mass: American Academy of Pediatrics, American College of Emergency Physicians, Jones and Bartlett Publishing Co; 2004:40.

2. Issacman DJ, Trainor JL, Rothrock SG. Central nervous system. In: Gausche-Hill M, Fuchs S, Yamamoto L, eds. *APLS: The Pediatric Emergency Medicine Resource.* 4th ed. Sudbury, Mass: American Academy of Pediatrics, American College of Emergency Physicians, Jones and Bartlett Publishing Co; 2004:150-152.

3. Nelson DS. Coma and altered level of consciousness. In: Fleisher GR, Ludwig S, eds. *Textbook of Pediatric Emergency Medicine.* 4th ed. Philadelphia, Pa: Lippincott Williams and Wilkins; 2000:166-170.

4. Berkowitz CD, Carroll ML. Child maltreatment. In: Gausche-Hill M, Fuchs S, Yamamoto L, eds. *APLS: The Pediatric Emergency Medicine Resource.* 4th ed. Sudbury, Mass: American Academy of Pediatrics, American College of Emergency Physicians, Jones and Bartlett Publishing Co; 2004:326-327.

5. Castiglia PT. Shaken baby syndrome. *J Pediatr Health Care.* 2001;15:78-80.

6. Conway EE. Nonaccidental head injury in infants: "the shaken baby syndrome revisited." *Pediatr Ann.* 1998;27:677-690.

7. King BR, King C, Coates WC. Critical procedures In: Gausche-Hill M, Fuchs S, Yamamoto L, eds. *APLS: The Pediatric Emergency Medicine Resource.* 4th ed. Sudbury, Mass: American Academy of Pediatrics, American College of Emergency Physicians, Jones and Bartlett Publishing Co; 2004:702-707.

8. Greenes DS, Madsen JR. Neurotrauma. In: Fleisher GR, Ludwig S, eds. *Textbook of Pediatric Emergency Medicine.* 4th ed. Philadelphia, Pa: Lippincott Williams and Wilkins; 2000:1273-1277.

9. Tepas JJ, Fallat ME, Moriarty TM. Trauma. In: Gausche-Hill M, Fuchs S, Yamamoto L, eds. *APLS: The Pediatric Emergency Medicine Resource.* 4th ed. Sudbury, Mass: American Academy of Pediatrics, American College of Emergency Physicians, Jones and Bartlett Publishing Co; 2004:294-298.

10. Adelson PD, Bratton SL, Carney NA, et al. Guidelines for the acute medical management of severe traumatic brain injury in infants, children, and adolescents. Chapter 11. Use of hyperosmolar therapy in the management of severe pediatric traumatic brain injury. *Pediatr Crit Care Med.* 2003;4(3 suppl):S40-S44.

11. Bruce DA, Zimmerman RA. Shaken impact syndrome. *Pediatr Ann.* 1989;18:482-494.

12. American Academy of Pediatrics. Shaken baby syndrome: inflicted cerebral trauma. *Pediatrics.* 1993;92:872-875.

13. Duhaime AC, Christian CW, Rorke LB, et al. Nonaccidental head injury in infants: the "shaken-baby syndrome." *N Engl J Med.* 1998;338:1822-1829.

14. Stenklyft PH, Cataletto ME, Lee BS. The pediatric airway in health and disease. In: Gausche-Hill M, Fuchs S, Yamamoto L, eds. *APLS: The Pediatric Emergency Medicine Resource.* 4th ed. Sudbury, Mass: American Academy of Pediatrics, American College of Emergency Physicians, Jones and Bartlett Publishing Co; 2004:94-96.

SCENARIO #26

Altered Mental Status

Elizabeth A. Edgerton, MD, MPH

Brief Presenting History

A 4-year-old girl is brought to the emergency department by ambulance. Her parents report that she has been vomiting intermittently during the past 2 weeks and is losing weight and has new onset of enuresis. Emergency medical services personnel describe her as being irritable and complaining that her head hurts.

Pediatric Assessment Triangle

Appearance: Awake but very irritable and intermittently somnolent

Work of Breathing: Rapid, deep

Circulation to the Skin: Mottled with delayed capillary refill

Initial Vital Signs

Pulse: 130

Respiratory Rate: 30

Blood Pressure: 90/50

Temperature: 36.2°C (97.1°F) axillary

ASK YOURSELF

- **What is the differential diagnosis for altered mental status in this patient?**

  Primary CNS disorders include closed head injury, atypical seizure disorder, atypical migraine, infection (eg, meningitis or encephalitis), neoplasm with inflammation and raised intracranial pressure (ICP), and ischemic or hemorrhagic vascular event (eg, stroke).

  Secondary CNS problems include hypoxia, accidental ingestion of psychoactive substance, metabolic derangement, and a mental health issue.

Physical Examination on Arrival to the Emergency Department

Airway: Moving air freely

Breathing: Rapid deep breathing, lung fields clear

Circulation: Mucous membranes dry; peripheral pulses rapid and weak; capillary refill time 3 to 4 seconds in the feet

Disability: Responds to voice; pupils equally round, reactive to light; normal reflexes

Additional History and Physical Examination Findings

Past Medical History: Previously well child; despite weight loss seems to be eating and drinking well

Medications: None

Allergies: None known

Physical Examination: Skin mottled, dry, and cool; neck supple, abdomen soft and nontender

ASK YOURSELF

- **What is the most likely diagnosis for this patient? How do the vital signs and physical examination support this diagnosis?**

Given the history of weight loss despite good oral intake and new-onset enuresis in a patient who presents dehydrated and with Kussmaul breathing, diabetic ketoacidosis (DKA) must be strongly considered. In this afebrile patient, tachycardia and diminished peripheral perfusion are consistent with dehydration. Kussmaul breathing pattern (rapid and deep) is seen in patients with a metabolic acidosis and represents a compensatory respiratory alkalosis.

- **What degree of dehydration is expected in patients with DKA?**

Estimation of dehydration is inexact. Comparing a child's current weight with her most recent recorded weight can be useful, but this does not account for loss of lean body mass. It is best to estimate the degree of dehydration in moderate to severe DKA to be at least 10% and to replace the fluid loss over the next 24 to 48 hours.

- **What initial bedside testing could be performed to assess the severity of DKA?**

Simple bedside tests include capillary blood glucose determination, "dipstick" urinalysis, and venous blood gases (VBGs). Capillary blood glucose will help determine the level of hyperglycemia. It is important to confirm this value with serum assessment. The urinalysis can provide confirmation of DKA if glucose and ketones are present. Finally, a VBG analysis assesses the level of acidosis.

- **What are the usual biochemical criteria for classifying DKA as mild, moderate, or severe?**

DKA is usually classified based on the severity of acidosis: *mild*—venous pH 7.21 to 7.30, bicarbonate concentration 10 to 15 mmol/L; *moderate*—pH 7.11 to 7.2, bicarbonate 5 to 10 mmol/L; and *severe*—pH <7.1, bicarbonate <5 mmol/L.

- **Why is it important to determine the severity of DKA?**

Assessing the severity of DKA will assist in predicting which patients may require ICU management (moderate and severe) and which can be expected to clear the acidosis in the emergency department (mild).[1] Disposition will vary greatly depending on institutional variations in management and available resources.

Initial Bedside Laboratory Tests

Rapid glucose: >500 mmol/L

Urine dipstick: 4+ glucose and 4+ ketones

VBGs: pH 7.0, P_{CO_2} 25, bicarbonate 4 mmol/L, calculated base deficit –21

ASK YOURSELF

- **What is the recommended initial fluid resuscitation for this patient?**

Patients with moderate to severe DKA are generally estimated to be at least 10% dehydrated. Initial fluid resuscitation should include isotonic fluids at a volume of 10 to 20 mL/kg infused over 1 to 2 hours. It is vital to not overhydrate patients with DKA or hydrate too quickly; the concern is that rapid changes in osmolarity result in changes in intracellular and extracellular volumes that can contribute to cerebral edema.

- **What is the role of bicarbonate in the resuscitation of patients with severe DKA?**

Similar to rapid and overzealous fluid resuscitation, the use of bicarbonate has been associated with rapid changes in intracellular and extracellular volumes in the brain. Rapid shifts in these volumes in the brain are thought to lead to cerebral edema, because the cerebral autoregulatory mechanism appears to be impaired in patients with DKA. Although severe acidosis is of concern, bicarbonate therapy is not recommended unless hyperkalemia is so significant as to impair cardiac function. Hyperkalemia is uncommon in association with DKA. Most patients with DKA are total-body potassium depleted.

- **What is the recommended dosage and route of administration for insulin therapy?**

DKA is a result of an absolute or a relative deficit of insulin that results in glycogenolysis and ultimately the breakdown of fats, resulting in ketone formation. Supplemental insulin is needed to stop this catabolic pathway and to halt the production of serum ketones. The recommended starting dose is **regular insulin 0.1 unit/kg/hr** as a continuous infusion. The use of insulin boluses is no longer recommended because of the potential for rapid changes in osmolarity and secondary intracellular and extracellular fluid shifts within the brain. Intramuscular or subcutaneous injections of insulin are not recommended because if there is poor perfusion to the tissues in a state of dehydration, inconsistent insulin absorption will result.

- **What is the recommended maintenance fluid for a patient with DKA?**

Initially, 0.45% normal saline is recommended as the maintenance fluid for the management of DKA. As the serum glucose approaches 200 to 300 mmol/L, dextrose (D_5) can be added to the intravenous fluid. If the serum glucose continues to drop, the amount of insulin can be decreased or the amount of dextrose can be increased (D_{10}). Insulin is necessary to correct the metabolic acidosis, and halting the infusion of insulin in response to decreasing serum glucose levels should be avoided.

- **What is the role of potassium and phosphate replacement?**

A patient with DKA has a total body deficit of potassium and phosphate. As a result of the acidosis, intracellular potassium moves into the extracellular space, which explains why the initial serum potassium may be normal or elevated. As the acidosis clears, the serum potassium will drop as potassium returns to the cells. **Potassium 40 mEq/L** should be added to the maintenance fluid of a patient with DKA.

Phosphate is primarily lost through the significant diuresis caused by hyperglycemia. Controversy exists over whether to add phosphate in the maintenance fluids to or to allow levels to correct on their own. If phosphate is added with maintenance fluids, it is recommended to replace electrolytes as **20 mEq KCl/L** and **20 mEq KPO_4/L**.

- **Once initial therapy is started for a patient with DKA, what should be closely monitored in the emergency department?**

All patients should receive continuous cardiorespiratory monitoring. Vital signs, including pulse, respiratory rate, and blood pressure, should be recorded frequently, and fluid input and output closely followed. Bedside glucose determinations are typically made every hour, whereas electrolytes, BUN, and VBGs are usually followed every 2 to 4 hours.

Frequent physical examination is essential. Close attention must be paid to complaints of headache, recurrence of vomiting, and changes in mental status, which can manifest as restlessness, irritability, or increased drowsiness. The signs and symptoms of developing cerebral edema must be watched for actively. The Cushing triad of bradycardia, hypertension, and abnormal breathing is a late finding of increased ICP.

Progression

One hour later, when the patient is reassessed, she is found to be unresponsive.

Repeat Vital Signs

Pulse: 70

Respiratory Rate: 8

Blood Pressure: 130/80

ASK YOURSELF

- **What is the most likely cause of the patient's deterioration?**

The patient has the clinical signs of increased ICP described as Cushing triad. She has decreased pulse and respiratory rates, with elevated blood pressure. The most likely cause of her deterioration is cerebral edema associated with DKA.

■ Is there a role for CT scanning in diagnosing cerebral edema?

Cerebral edema associated with DKA is primarily a clinical diagnosis. Although the use of CT can confirm the diagnosis, obtaining imaging can delay appropriate therapy. Furthermore, radiographic evidence of cerebral edema may lag the clinical presentation.[2]

■ What interventions are needed at this time? What complications might be expected?

Interventions:

- Stop fluid bolus and other fluid administration.
- **Mannitol 1 g/kg IV** is currently recommended for the treatment of cerebral edema.[3,4] Mannitol may be given every 15 to 20 minutes.
- In this case, intubation and hyperventilation are indicated as well to protect the airway and to ventilate to a P_{CO_2} of 35 to 40. Recommended drugs for RSI include the following:
  1. **Lidocaine 1 mg/kg IV** (may blunt rise in ICP associated with intubation)
  2. **Atropine 0.02 mg/kg IV** (if succinylcholine is used)
  3. **Etomidate 0.3 mg/kg IV** (Although thiopental decreases ICP as well, it may not be a good choice in this patient with intravascular depletion because it will exacerbate hypotension.)
  4. **Rocuronium 0.6-1 mg/kg IV** (Succinylcholine also may be used, but it is associated with an increase in ICP.)

Potential Complications:

- Progression of cerebral swelling with herniation and cardiorespiratory arrest
- Emesis during attempts at intubation if cricoid pressure not maintained
- Failure to adequately secure or assess airway: esophageal intubation, right mainstem intubation

Progression

With intubation and mannitol, the patient's condition stabilizes, and she is transferred to the pediatric ICU for continued management of increased ICP, ketoacidosis, and dehydration.

Objectives of This Scenario

1. Recognize the signs and symptoms of cerebral edema among patients with DKA.

Cerebral edema accounts for 30% to 60% of the fatalities and 20% of the morbidity associated with DKA.[2,5] Although 60% of patients diagnosed with cerebral edema associated with DKA survive without impairment, an estimated 21% to 24% die, and 7% to 35% are left in a permanent vegetative state or with severe neurologic impairment.[2,6,7] The incidence of DKA has been decreasing with increasing patient education, but the incidence of cerebral edema among those patients presenting with DKA has remained constant at 0.7% to 1%.[2,5]

The clinical course of cerebral edema among patients with DKA is rapid, usually between 1 and 24 hours. It is crucial that patients with DKA be frequently assessed. Marcin et al[6] found no correlation of clinical outcome with time of diagnosis of cerebral edema. As might be expected, patients receiving intervention with less severe neurologic compromise at presentation have better long-term outcomes. Predictors of cerebral edema vary among studies but include the degree of neurologic depression at time of diagnosis, the degree of dehydration (as assessed by serum urea nitrogen concentration), the degree of acidosis, and younger age.[6-8] In addition, one study found that newly diagnosed diabetes was associated with three times the likelihood of cerebral edema compared with the incidence in known diabetics.[2]

2. Understand the components of the initial management of DKA.

The goal of managing DKA is to replace the water and salt deficits while reversing acidosis with the use of insulin. Fluid management guidelines are primarily based on expert consensus panels.[9] Current recommendations support the use of isotonic crystalloid and not colloid. Fluid resuscitation begins with isotonic fluids (normal saline or lactated Ringer). Subsequent fluid management involves the use of fluid solutions of at least 0.45% saline. Fluid deficits should be replaced over 24 to 48 hours. Daily fluid replacement should rarely exceed 1.5 to 2 times the usual maintenance requirements of the patient.

Data to support the replacement of potassium in patients with DKA exist, but little evidence is available to recommend the amount and method of replacement.[9] Replacement of phosphate does not appear to have any clinical benefit and can be associated with hypocalcemia. In addition, the use of bicarbonate therapy has been found to be associated with the development of cerebral edema.[7]

Clear evidence supports the guidelines on managing insulin deficiency.[9] These guidelines include the use of low doses of insulin at 0.1 unit/kg/hr continuous IV infusion. Intravenous insulin should be continued until the acidosis corrects to at least pH 7.3 with closure of the anion gap. When a patient's serum glucose is below 250 mmol/L, supplemental dextrose should be added to fluids so that the insulin infusion can continue until the metabolic acidosis resolves. Insulin delivered as either an intravenous bolus or an intramuscular or a subcutaneous injection is not recommended in patients with compromised perfusion.

3. Understand the management of cerebral edema and the prevention of its complications.

Prevention of cerebral edema is related to the overall prevention of DKA. Although cerebral edema is a known and highly fatal complication of DKA, it is often unpredictable. In one study, only 50% of patients had neurologic symptoms before progressing to respiratory arrest.[2] Once severe neurologic signs or respiratory arrest is present, the effectiveness of medical management such as mannitol administration or hyperventilation is diminished. Furthermore, all patients who presented with respiratory arrest either died or sustained significant neurologic impairment.

Identifying the severity of DKA on presentation can guide appropriate clinical management. Patients with moderate and severe DKA need repeated neurologic assessments and staff who are prepared to identify and managed cerebral edema.

References

1. Linares MYR, Schunk JE, Lindsay R. Laboratory presentation in diabetic ketoacidosis and duration of therapy. *Pediatr Emerg Care.* 1996;12:347-351.
2. Edge JA, Hawkins MM, Winter DL, et al. The risk and outcome of cerebral oedema developing during diabetic ketoacidosis. *Arch Dis Child.* 2000;85:16-20.
3. Roberts M, Slover R, Chase H. Diabetic ketoacidosis with intracerebral complications. *Pediatr Diabetes.* 2001;2:103-114.
4. Carlotti AP, Bohn D, Halperin ML. Importance of timing of risk factors for cerebral oedema during therapy for diabetic ketoacidosis. *Arch Dis Child.* 2003;88:170-173.
5. Kaufman FR. Diabetes in children and adolescents. Areas of controversy. *Med Clin North Am.* 1998;82:721-738.
6. Marcin JP, Glaser N, Barnett P, et al. Factors associated with adverse outcomes in children with diabetic ketoacidosis-related cerebral edema. *J Pediatr.* 2002;141:793-797.
7. Glaser N, Barnett P, McCaslin I, et al. Risk factors for cerebral edema in children with diabetic ketoacidosis. *N Engl J Med.* 2001;344:264-269.
8. Edge JA. Cerebral oedema during treatment of diabetic ketoacidosis: are we any nearer to finding a cause? *Diabetes Metab Res Rev.* 2000;16:316-324.
9. Dunger DB, Sperling MA, Acerini CL, et al. ESPE/LWPES consensus statement on diabetic ketoacidosis in children and adolescents. *Arch Dis Child.* 2004;89:188-194.

SCENARIO #27

Altered Mental Status

Michael C. Bachman, MD, MBA

Brief Presenting History

A mother brings her 36-month-old son to the emergency department because he has a fever, is irritable, and has been vomiting. She has been treating the child with an over-the-counter cough and cold syrup for the past 4 days.

Pediatric Assessment Triangle

Appearance: Awake and crying

Work of Breathing: Breathing comfortably

Circulation to the Skin: Skin very dry, cheeks flushed

Initial Vital Signs

Pulse: 160

Respiratory Rate: 42

Blood Pressure: 105/62

Temperature: 40°C (104°F) rectal

Physical Examination on Arrival to the Emergency Department

Airway: Patent, moving air freely, no secretions in the mouth

Breathing: Good air entry bilaterally without rales, ronchi, or wheezes; no use of accessory muscles

Circulation: Capillary refill less than 2 seconds with strong central and peripheral pulses; skin markedly warm and dry

Disability: Alert, eyes open, extremely combative; inconsolable with mother; moving all extremities

ASK YOURSELF

- **What is the initial assessment? What is the patient's physiologic status?**

  This child presents with altered mental status (agitation and inconsolability), fever, tachycardia, and flushed skin. The differential diagnosis includes early sepsis, meningoencephalitis, a toxic ingestion, and simple fussiness caused by high fever (sometimes called "fever delirium").

- **What additional history would help you establish the diagnosis?**

  Further information about the length of the fever and any ill contacts would help elucidate an infectious etiology. Other essential information would be the content and amount of the over-the-counter cold remedy given to the child.

Additional History and Physical Examination Findings

This child has had cough and rhinorrhea for 4 days. His mother had been giving him an over-the-counter cold medicine containing acetaminophen and diphenhydramine. Because the symptoms were not improving, the mother has given him twice the recommended dose for the past 2 days.

Past Medical History: Healthy child with history of one febrile seizure; no chronic medical conditions

Medications: Cold medicine

Allergies: None known

Physical Examination: Agitation persisting, mucous membranes dry and tacky, skin red and hot, pupils markedly dilated

ASK YOURSELF

■ What is the most likely diagnosis?

The history of cold medicine ingestion and the presenting signs indicate anticholinergic toxicity. The child has the classic symptoms of "dry as a bone, red as a beet, hot as a hare, mad as a hatter, and blind as a bat."

■ What interventions should be made at this time?

- Place the patient on a cardiorespiratory monitor with pulse oximetry.
- Obtain IV access and administer a **20-mL/kg bolus of normal saline** over the first hour. The child can be expected to have had increased fluid losses from hyperthermia.
- Administer **activated charcoal** at a dose of **0.5 to 1 kg**. Most children can be induced to take charcoal by mouth, however an NG tube may be needed in some cases.

■ What diagnostic tests should be performed?

- Laboratory tests: Serum electrolytes can guide supportive fluid therapy. Although toxicology screening is rarely useful in the diagnosis of patients with anticholinergic poisoning, it should be considered because of the high incidence of combined ingestions. Acetaminophen and salicylate levels should be checked if their ingestion cannot be ruled out by a careful history.
- ECG: Patients with diphenhydramine toxicity can have a wandering pacemaker, prolonged QRS and QT intervals, nonspecific ST-T wave changes, and a left bundle-branch block that resolve with recovery.

Progression

As the patient's mother is attempting to console her child, he arches his back, his eyes roll back, and generalized tonic-clonic seizure activity begins.

Repeat Vital Signs

Pulse: 160

Respiratory Rate: 36

Blood Pressure: 122/70

Temperature: 40°C (104°F) rectal

Oxygen Saturation: 92% on room air

ASK YOURSELF

■ What has happened?

Although rare, seizures can occur during an anticholinergic crisis. This child also has a history of febrile seizures and is currently hyperthermic.

■ What interventions are needed at this time? What complications might be expected?

Interventions:

- Administer 100% O_2 via nonrebreather mask. Assess airway integrity.
- Administer a benzodiazepine: **lorazepam 0.05 to 0.1 mg/kg** IV.
- If seizure activity persists, repeat the dose.
- Administer rectal **ibuprofen 10 mg/kg** for the persistent fever.

Potential Complications:

- Airway cannot be maintained during or after seizure, requiring RSI.
- Use of repetitive doses of benzodiazepines induces hypoventilation, necessitating ventilatory support and possibly intubation.
- Emesis occurs, requiring suctioning and airway management.

■ What specific antidotes are available?

Most patients with anticholinergic syndrome can be managed supportively, but **physostigmine 0.02 mg/kg** IV, a reversible inhibitor of acetylcholinesterase, can be given to patients with evidence of severe toxicity (hyperthermia, severe delirium, and tachycardia). It is generally indicated only for a pure anticholinergic ingestion. Severe side effects can occur, including atrioventricular block, asystole, and seizures. It should not be used in tricyclic antidepressant ingestions.

Progression

The seizure activity ceases after the second dose of lorazepam, and the child becomes postictal. The child remains somnolent for 1 hour and then becomes more alert and starts to interact with his mother. The child is admitted to an observation unit for monitoring overnight and is discharged in the morning when he is asymptomatic and tolerating fluids well.

Objectives of This Scenario

1. Recognize the importance of a thorough history of medication use, including over-the-counter preparations.

The average child has 6 to 10 colds per year, and each cold can last 10 to 14 days, providing several days and nights of discomfort for the child and the caregivers.[1] Parents often turn to one of dozens of over-the-counter and other home cough and cold preparations for relief. Although no studies in children have proved the efficacy of cough and cold preparations in facilitating recovery from these illnesses,[2,3] a small number of children experience significant adverse effects from the administration of these over-the-counter preparations.

2. Recognize the anticholinergic toxidrome.

The patient in this scenario presents with progressive signs and symptoms of anticholinergic toxicity with dry mucous membranes, flushed red skin, fever, and agitation. Anticholinergic poisoning can be caused by jimson weed, deadly nightshade, potato leaves, and a number of medications, including antihistamines, benztropine, atropine, phenothiazines, and tricyclic antidepressants.[4]

Dry mucous membranes and hot, dry, flushed skin result from inhibition of secretions from salivary glands, bronchioles, and sweat glands ("dry as a bone"). A flushed appearance results from vasodilation of peripheral blood vessels ("red as a beet"). The inability to sweat and altered CNS thermoregulation result in hyperthermia ("hot as a hare"). Central anticholinergic syndrome can cause disorientation, agitation, short-term memory impairment, incoherent speech, and visual hallucinations ("mad as a hatter"). Pupils become markedly dilated and vision can be blurred with the loss of accommodation ("blind as a bat").[5]

3. Prevent absorption.

Activated charcoal is sufficient decontamination for most patients. Although this is most effective within 1 hour of ingestion, it may be of benefit even several hours after ingestion because of the anticholinergic effect of decreased gastrointestinal motility.[6]

4. Detect rhabdomyolysis.

Rhabdomyolysis and myoglobinuric renal failure are serious complications of prolonged seizures in a febrile patient. As muscle cells break down, they release their intracellular contents, including myoglobin, creatine phosphokinase (CPK), potassium, and phosphate in the plasma. The circulating myoglobin is then excreted in the urine and can cause acute renal failure as the myoglobin casts obstruct the renal tubules. Laboratory findings in rhabdomyolysis include a CPK at least five times the upper normal limit. The release of CPK occurs rapidly after muscle injury, peaking at 24 to 36 hours and persisting for several days. Urine from patients with rhabdomyolysis appears dark and tests are positive for blood with a dipstick urinalysis, but no red blood cells are detected on microscopy.[7]

References

1. Pappas DE, Hayden GF, Hendley JO. Treating colds: keep it simple. *Contemp Pediatr.* 1999;16:109-119.
2. Smith MB, Feldman W. Over-the-counter cold medications: a critical review of clinical trials between 1950 and 1991. *JAMA.* 1993;369:2258-2263.
3. Clemens CJ, Taylor JA, Almquist JR, et al. Is an antihistamine-decongestant combination effective in temporarily relieving symptoms of the common cold in preschool children? *J Pediatr.* 1997:99:918-920.
4. Dieckmann RA. Pediatric assessment. In: Gausche-Hill M, Fuchs S, Yamamoto L, eds. *APLS: The Pediatric Emergency Medicine Resource.* 4th ed. Sudbury, Mass: American Academy of Pediatrics, American College of Emergency Physicians, Jones and Bartlett Publishing Co; 2004:243-244.
5. Delaney KA. Anticholinergics and antihistamines. In: Ford MD, Delaney KA, Ling LJ, et al (eds). *Clinical Toxicology.* Philadelphia, Pa: WB Saunders; 2001:473-474.
6. Chyka PA, Seger D. Position statement: single-dose activated charcoal. American Academy of Clinical Toxicology, European Association of Poison Centres and Clinical Toxicologists. *Clin Toxicol.* 1997;35:721-736.
7. Cronan K, Norman ME. Renal and electrolyte emergencies. In: Fleisher GR, Ludwig S, eds. *Textbook of Pediatric Emergency Medicine.* 4th ed. Philadelphia, Pa: Lippincott Williams and Wilkins; 2000:856-857.

SCENARIO #28

Altered Mental Status

Jason A. Levy, MD, and Richard G. Bachur, MD

Brief Presenting History

A 4-year-old boy is brought to the emergency department by his father. He tells the triage nurses that his son has been especially cranky and tired with an increasingly "white" appearance over the past 1 to 2 days.

Pediatric Assessment Triangle

Appearance: Awake and alert, intermittently crying, moderately pale

Work of Breathing: No increased respiratory effort

Circulation to the Skin: Pale but without cyanosis

Initial Vital Signs

Pulse: 115

Respiratory Rate: 28

Blood Pressure: 129/88

Temperature: 37.8°C (100°F) oral

Oxygen Saturation: 99% on room air

ASK YOURSELF

■ Which of this child's vital signs are abnormal for a 4-year-old?

This child has mild tachycardia and an elevated blood pressure. Categories of potential causes of acute hypertension in a child are renal (poststreptococcal glomerulonephritis or acute renal failure of any cause), vascular (renal artery thrombosis), medication induced (steroids, decongestants, sympathomimetics, illicit drugs, albuterol, caffeine), trauma (burns, increased intracranial pressure), and miscellaneous (inappropriate cuff size, volume overload, anxiety or pain, seizures).[1]

■ How much should this 4-year-old weigh?

An estimated weight for a 4-year-old child is 15 kg. One can use the length-based Broselow Pediatric Emergency Tape or a pediatric table to determine weight based on age. See Appendix A.

Physical Examination on Arrival to the Emergency Department

Airway: Patent, moving air freely without obstruction as evidenced by crying

Breathing: No tachypnea, retractions, tracheal tugging, or flaring

Circulation: Skin slightly cool and very pale, capillary refill time 2 seconds, peripheral pulses strong; a few petechiae noted on the trunk and upper extremities

Disability: Eyes open; responds to verbal commands but difficult to engage

ASK YOURSELF

- **What is the initial assessment? What is the patient's physiologic status?**

  This patient presents with irritability, pallor, and hypertension but with stable respiratory and cardiovascular status.

- **What additional history would help you establish the diagnosis?**

  A history of trauma can point to internal injury and hemorrhage as a reason for pallor, although this child is hypertensive. A history of fever can suggest infection and sepsis. A history of hematuria or dark urine can raise suspicion for a urologic or renal etiology or hemolysis. In addition, a history of anuria or oliguria would further suggest acute renal failure and would account for this child's hypertension. Finally, a history of preceding bloody diarrhea would suggest bacterial enteritis and subsequent hemolytic uremic syndrome (HUS).

Additional History and Physical Examination Findings

The father says that the child was well until 6 days ago, when he developed abdominal pain and bloody diarrhea. The patient then developed the acute onset of pallor and irritability seen on presentation. On questioning, the father also says that the child has not produced any urine today as far as he knows.

Past Medical History: Otherwise healthy with no chronic illnesses

Medications: None

Allergies: None known

Physical Examination: Vital signs unchanged; additional petechiae noted over trunk and upper extremities; mild abdominal tenderness noted diffusely without guarding or rebound; no hepatosplenomegaly appreciated; stools positive for blood

ASK YOURSELF

- **What are some possible etiologies of this child's presentation?**

  This child initially presented with acute onset of pallor and hypertension. Acute pallor suggests an acute hemolytic process, blood loss, shock, or metabolic disorder such as hypoglycemia. In a normotensive patient without a history of trauma, blood loss is unlikely without an underlying bleeding disorder. Acute hemolysis can be drug induced or caused by autoimmune disease, HUS, disseminated intravascular coagulation (DIC), or cavernous hemangioma. Less commonly, sickle cell anemia or erythrocyte membrane or enzyme defects may have gone unrecognized and can present as an aplastic crisis, splenic crisis, or hemolytic process, respectively. As noted above, the acute onset of hypertension can have numerous etiologies, including renal, vascular, and medication-induced disease as well as trauma, pain, or anxiety. In the young child, however, true acute hypertension is most commonly the result of renal disease.[1] The additional history of oliguria without signs of significant dehydration suggests acute renal failure. A history of bloody diarrhea, fatigue, and decreased urine output in a fussy child with acute onset of pallor and hypertension strongly suggests HUS with acute renal failure. His irritability and fatigue could be explained by hypertension, severe anemia, or uremia.

- **What interventions are needed at this time? What complications might be expected?**

  Interventions:

  - Administer supplemental oxygen (anyone who is profoundly anemic can benefit from oxygen even if the oxygen saturation level is normal).
  - Place the patient on a cardiorespiratory monitor with pulse oximetry.
  - Obtain intravenous access.

  Potential Complications:

  - Inability to obtain intravenous access.
  - Administration of an intravenous bolus of fluid in a patient with acute renal failure, hypertension, and oliguria can lead to volume overload and subsequent pulmonary edema.

■ **Which laboratory and radiologic studies are warranted for this patient?**

A CBC with differential, Coombs test, reticulocyte count, PT/PTT, blood culture, electrolytes with BUN and creatinine, blood bank sample, and an ECG should be obtained. Chest radiography could also be considered.

Repeat Vital Signs

Pulse: 200

Respiratory Rate: 32

Blood Pressure: 132/90

Oxygen Saturation: 99%

ECG Monitor:

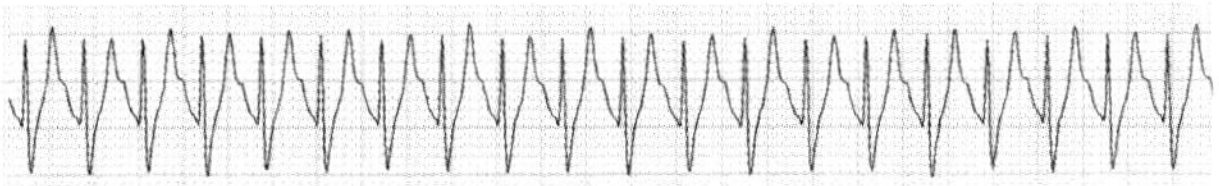

ASK YOURSELF

■ **What is the etiology of the electrocardiographic findings?**

The patient has developed tachycardia. The ECG shows a sinus tachycardia at a rate of 200 with markedly peaked T waves. In a patient with acute renal failure, hyperkalemia should be suspected.

■ **What interventions are needed at this time? What complications might be expected?**

Interventions:

- In any patient with acute renal failure and electrocardiographic findings consistent with hyperkalemia, treatment should be initiated.
  1. Intravenous calcium administration: **10% calcium gluconate 100 mg/kg (1 mL/kg)** or **10% calcium chloride 20 mg/kg (0.2 mL/kg)** diluted in saline
  2. **Sodium bicarbonate IV** 7.5% (1 mEq = 1 mL) **1 to 2 mL/kg** over 30 to 60 minutes
  3. Consider insulin and glucose IV: D_{10} **5 mL/kg** (or equivalent) with **1 unit of regular insulin for every 5 g of dextrose given (~0.1 unit/kg)**. Insulin can be given subcutaneously as well. Potential for hypoglycemia necessitates use with caution.
  4. **Sodium polystyrene (Kayexalate) 1 g/kg** in either 10% glucose solution (1 g in 4 mL) or 20% sorbitol solution PO or PR
  5. Nebulized albuterol could also be considered.

Potential Complications:

- Giving calcium with solution containing $NaHCO_3$ can lead to precipitation of $CaCO_3$.
- Calcium can cause infiltrative burns, especially if not diluted with saline.

Progression

The patient suddenly becomes unresponsive and loses his pulse.

ECG Monitor:

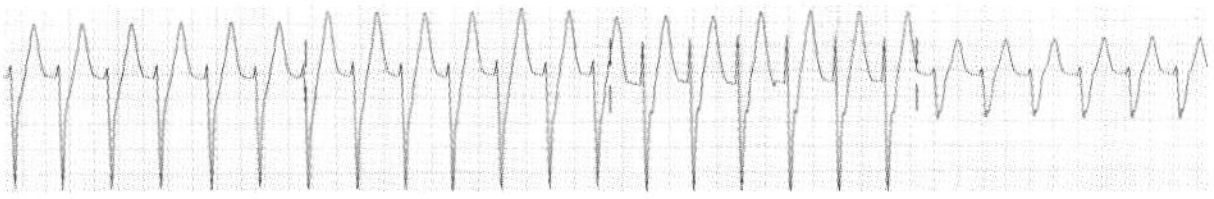

ASK YOURSELF

■ **What is this rhythm, and what has happened?**

The patient's rhythm is ventricular tachycardia at a rate of 150, secondary to hyperkalemia.

■ **What interventions are needed at this time? What complications might be expected?**

Interventions:

- Confirm lack of pulse.
- Initiate algorithm for pulseless arrest ("Evaluation and Management: Circulation," Figure 1).
  1. Initiate BMV (with cricoid pressure) and chest compressions.
  2. Defibrillate up to 3 times with 2 J/kg, 4 J/kg, and 4 J/kg with pulse checks between attempts.
  3. If no response, **1:10,000 epinephrine 0.1 mL/kg** followed by defibrillation at 4 J/kg
- After control of airway with BMV initially, perform endotracheal intubation
  1. #2 Miller blade, 5.0 ET tube
  2. Cricoid pressure

- Treat the patient for hyperkalemia as noted above.

Potential Complications:

- Delay in therapy for hyperkalemia: If not initiated, defibrillation is less likely to convert rhythm. Waiting for laboratory values would be detrimental to this patient.
- Problems with defibrillation: Paddles of an incorrect size, no gel used, improper placement of paddles, synchronized mode
- Problems with intubation: Vomiting, failure to confirm placement of ET tube

Progression

With the combination of treatment for hyperkalemia and appropriate defibrillation, the ECG displays a sinus rhythm with a narrow QRS complex and normal T waves.

Repeat vital signs

Pulse: 120

Respiratory Rate: 30

Blood Pressure: 124/78

Oxygen Saturation: 100%

ASK YOURSELF

- **What other therapies may be used?**

  For patients with renal failure, hemodialysis should be considered for severe metabolic derangements or respiratory failure from volume overload.

Objectives of This Scenario

1. Recognize HUS with acute renal failure.[2-5]

HUS is characterized by the combination of hemolytic anemia, thrombocytopenia, and acute renal failure. Commonly, the clinical picture is one of a previously healthy child who develops bloody diarrhea followed 5 to 7 days later by pallor and oliguria. The diarrhea is usually due to a toxin produced by *Escherichia coli* 0157:H7. The toxin binds to endothelial cells, especially in the kidney, causing endothelial cell injury and release of inflammatory mediators. The injured endothelium leads to a microangiopathic hemolytic anemia with consumption of platelets. Schistocytes and helmet cells are seen on the peripheral smear.

Severe renal involvement is characterized by anuria, renal cortical necrosis, and acute renal failure with subsequent hypertension. The combination of acute renal failure and hemolysis can result in a variety of fluid and electrolyte imbalances, including hyponatremia, hyperkalemia (from reduced glomerular filtration rate and hemolysis), acidosis, and volume overload. The latter can lead to edema and congestive heart failure. HUS also can have CNS involvement with lethargy and seizures. As seen in this case, electrolyte abnormalities can lead to cardiac dysrhythmias.

The treatment of HUS is supportive and aimed at correcting severe anemia and managing the fluid balance in the face of acute renal failure. Fluid management, especially with the need for RBC transfusion, is delicate. Intravenous fluids or blood products can precipitate pulmonary edema and congestive heart failure. Hemodialysis may be necessary to correct electrolyte abnormalities or fluid overload.

2. Recognize and manage hyperkalemia.

One should maintain a high index of suspicion for hyperkalemia in any patient who presents with anuria. It is a potentially lethal condition, primarily because of its effect on the myocardium and cardiac conduction. It is very rare for hyperkalemia to occur in the absence of renal disease, as the healthy kidney can excrete hundreds of milliequivalents of potassium per day, 4 to 6 times the usual daily intake. Several factors and conditions can contribute to an elevation of potassium in the setting of impaired renal function: excessive potassium intake, drugs (potassium-sparing diuretics, ACE inhibitors, nonsteroidal anti-inflammatory drugs, trimethoprim-sulfamethoxazole), acute hemolysis, rhabdomyolysis or tumor lysis syndrome, and metabolic acidosis.[6]

Although the ECG is not always a reliable test for the presence of mild to moderate hyperkalemia, once hyperkalemia is suspected, the severity and risk of cardiotoxicity should be assessed with an ECG. The classic finding consists of tall, peaked T waves, the earliest electrocardiographic change of hyperkalemia. Other electrocardiographic findings also can be present, including widened QRS complexes, PR prolongation, low-amplitude or absent P waves, and ST-segment elevation.[7-9] Electrocardiographic evidence of hyperkalemia is a true electrolyte emergency, and prompt therapy is warranted. **One should not wait for laboratory confirmation before treatment is initiated.**

Therapies for hyperkalemia can be divided into three groups: 1) those that minimize the cardiac effects, 2) those that induce potassium uptake by cells, and 3) those that remove potassium from the body.

Intravenous calcium specifically protects the myocardium from the abnormal ionic balance created by hyperkalemia. It has rapid onset of effect and should be the initial treatment for patients with hyperkalemia and ECG-related abnormalities. Calcium can be administered as calcium gluconate or calcium chloride. Although it was once thought that calcium chloride is preferred for resuscitation because of better bioavailability, recent evidence indicates that either drug is acceptable. Calcium chloride has a higher incidence of extravasation and local tissue damage and should always be diluted before administration.[6]

Cellular uptake of potassium is promoted by administering insulin, which stimulates potassium uptake primarily in hepatocytes and myocytes. Glucose should be administered concomitantly to avoid hypoglycemia. The amount of dextrose should be **0.5 g/kg** as D_{50}-, D_{25}-, or D_{10}-containing solution. The insulin dose is **1 unit/4 to 5 g of dextrose** administered. Sodium bicarbonate at a dose of **1 mEq/kg** should also be given in the presence of electrocardiographic changes associated with hyperkalemia and acidosis and can enhance cellular uptake.[10,11] A β_2-agonist such as albuterol may also be administered via nebulized treatment. The dose has not been established in children, but in adults it is 10 to 20 mg.[11]

Finally, potassium removal from the body should be undertaken. **Sodium polystyrene** (Kayexalate) at a dose of **1 g/kg** can be administered either orally or rectally (adult dose: 15 g orally, 30 g rectally) every 6 hours. Each gram of Kayexalate reduces serum potassium by 0.5 to 1 mEq/L.[6] If hyperkalemia is persistent and severe, dialysis should be considered.

References

1. Norwood VF. Hypertension. *Pediatr Rev.* 2002;23:197-209.
2. Eddy AA. Hemolytic uremic syndrome. In: Rudolph AM, Rudolph CD, eds. *Rudolph's Pediatrics.* 21st ed. New York, NY: McGraw-Hill Medical Publishing; 2003:1696-1698.
3. Corrigan JJ, Boineau FG. Hemolytic uremic syndrome. *Pediatr Rev.* 2001;22:365-369.
4. Kaplan BS, Meyers KE, Schulman SL. Disease of the month: the pathogenesis and treatment of hemolytic uremic syndrome. *J Am Soc Nephrol.* 1998;9:1126-1132.
5. Cronan K, Norman ME. Renal and electrolyte emergencies. In: Fleisher GR, Ludwig S, eds. *Textbook of Pediatric Emergency Medicine.* 4th ed. Philadelphia, Pa: Lippincott Williams and Wilkins; 2000:847-848.
6. Hyperkalemia. In: *Brenner & Rector's The Kidney.* 6th ed. Philadelphia, Pa: WB Saunders; 2000:1020-1026.
7. Webster A, Brady W, Morris F. Recognizing signs of danger: ECG changes resulting from an abnormal serum potassium concentration. *Emerg Med J.* 2002;19:74-77.
8. Mattu A, Brady WJ, Robinson DA. Electrocardiographic manifestations of hyperkalemia. *Am J Emerg Med.* 2002;18:721-729.
9. Wrenn KD, Slovis CM, Slovis BS. The ability of physicians to predict hyperkalemia from the ECG. *Ann Emerg Med.* 1991;20:1229-1232.
10. Ahee P, Crowe AV. The management of hyperkalemia in the emergency department. *J Accid Emerg Med.* 2000;17:188-191.
11. Greenberg A. Hyperkalemia: treatment options. *Semin Nephrol.* 1998;18:46-57.

SCENARIO #29

Altered Mental Status

Molly B. Hasty, MD, and Erica L. Liebelt, MD

Brief Presenting History

An 18-month-old girl was found sleeping on the living room floor by her mother, who was unable to arouse her. The mother states that her daughter was fine earlier in the day and has not been sick recently.

Pediatric Assessment Triangle

Appearance: Comatose, moaning with stimulation

Work of Breathing: Spontaneous respirations, no tachypnea or distress

Circulation to the Skin: Tachycardic; well perfused, flushed, dry skin

Initial Vital Signs

Pulse: 150

Respiratory Rate: 22

Blood Pressure: 120/58

Temperature: 37.3°C (99.1°F) rectal

ASK YOURSELF

- **How much should this 18-month-old weigh?**

  An estimated weight for a 18-month-old is 12 kg. One can use the length-based Broselow Pediatric Emergency Tape or a pediatric table to determine weight based on age. See Appendix A.

Physical Examination on Arrival to the Emergency Department

Airway: Patent without evidence of obstruction

Breathing: Spontaneous respirations with clear lung fields bilaterally

Circulation: Tachycardic, capillary refill less than 2 seconds, dry skin, flushed face

Disability: Localizing and moaning with painful stimulation, no eye opening on command, pupils 4 to 5 mm and reactive

Exposure: No obvious signs of external injury

ASK YOURSELF

- **What is the initial assessment? What is the patient's physiologic status?**

  This patient is hemodynamically stable with altered mental status of unknown etiology and responds only to pain (the **P** of the mnemonic AVPU [**A** = Alert, **V** = responds to Voice, **P** = responds to Pain, **U** = Unresponsive]).

- **What is the differential diagnosis of altered mental status?**

  Broad categories include infectious, metabolic, traumatic (especially child abuse), hypoxia, hypercarbia, neurologic due to CNS lesions, and toxicologic due to ingestions.

■ **What additional history would be helpful to establish the diagnosis?**

Because injuries due to child abuse are in the differential diagnosis, a detailed social history including information about recent caretakers of the child is warranted. In addition, any history of recent fever, changes in diet, gastrointestinal complaints, weight loss, and change from neurologic or behavioral baseline are important to elicit. Because toxic ingestion is in the differential diagnosis, the presence of any medications in the house should be determined.

Additional History and Physical Examination Findings

Earlier that day, the child had been cared for by the grandmother, who has a history of depression and is known to take an antidepressant medication.

Past Medical History: Significant only for recurrent otitis media, which resolved after placement of tympanostomy tubes at age 12 months

Medications: None

Allergies: Rash following penicillins

Physical Examination: There are no obvious external signs of injury or any focal neurologic abnormalities. The patient remains comatose but localizes painful stimuli.

Laboratory Findings: Glucose 120; ABG: pH 7.32, Pco_2 47, Po_2 126, HCO_3^- 18

Progression

The patient abruptly develops a generalized and symmetric tonic-clonic seizure.

ASK YOURSELF

■ **What interventions are needed at this time? What complications might be expected?**

Interventions:

- Place the patient on a cardiorespiratory monitor with pulse oximetry.
- Administer **lorazepam 0.1 mg/kg IV**
- RSI
  1. #1 Miller (straight) blade, 4.5 uncuffed ET tube
  2. Consider **atropine 0.02 mg/kg IV** (the patient is older than 1 year)
  3. **Etomidate 0.3 mg/kg IV**
  4. **Vecuronium 0.1 mg/kg IV** (*Note:* Rocuronium or succinylcholine [with atropine] may also be used.)
- Cricoid pressure
- Place NG tube and end-tidal CO_2 monitor.
- Confirm ET tube position with chest radiography.
- **Activated charcoal 1 g/kg NG** after protection of airway and lavage with normal saline (15 mL/kg)
- Perform ECG and continue cardiac monitoring.

Potential Complications:

- Vomiting with NG tube placement if airway not controlled
- Difficulty with intravenous access necessitating intraosseous line placement

Repeat Vital Signs

Pulse: 150

Respiratory Rate: 30 with bag ventilations

Blood Pressure: 70/40

ECG Monitor:

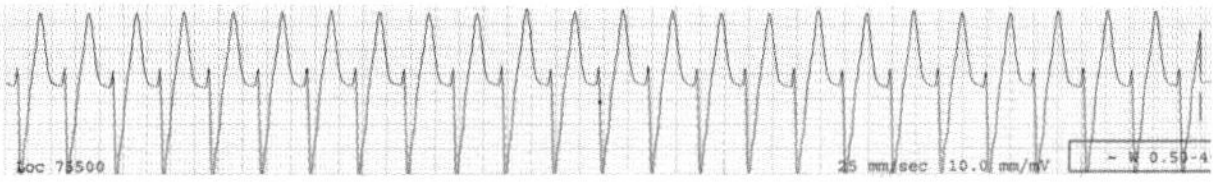

ASK YOURSELF

■ **What does this ECG show?**

Wide-complex tachycardia at 150

■ **What interventions are needed at this time?**

- If the patient becomes unstable, the wide-complex tachycardia seen on ECG prompts the need for cardioversion to prevent deterioration into asystole, which would require chest compressions and resuscitation drugs.

- The patient's blood pressure has now dropped and requires aggressive management with isotonic crystalloid. Two or three initial boluses of **20 mL/kg of normal saline** are appropriate with careful monitoring of response. If the hypotension is refractory to crystalloids, vasopressors and ionotropes should be started.
- Seizures should be treated acutely with a benzodiazepine. **Phenobarbital** should be administered if seizures are long lasting or recurrent.
- Toxic etiologies of QRS prolongation and hypotension should be considered. Repetitive boluses of **sodium bicarbonate (1 to 2 mEq/kg) IV** over 2 to 3 minutes should be administered while monitoring the QRS duration, blood pressure, and pH.

Progression

After giving multiple boluses of sodium bicarbonate and putting the child on a continuous sodium bicarbonate drip, the QRS complex narrowed to normal.

Disposition

To pediatric ICU for continued cardiorespiratory monitoring.

Objectives of This Scenario

1. Appropriately evaluate and manage altered mental status.[1,2]

There are numerous etiologies of altered mental status in children. Starting with the basic principles of ABCs is prudent. Potential causes include head trauma (accidental and nonaccidental), increased intracranial pressure from a space-occupying CNS lesion, infectious causes, hypercarbia, hypoxemia, metabolic derangements (hypoglycemia), and toxic effects of ingested drugs. This patient had no obvious external signs of trauma and no focal neurologic deficits. This patient's age and history of being watched earlier by a caretaker with depression prompt investigation of and treatment for potential ingestants like antidepressants or other medications that can cause this clinical picture.

Naloxone is indicated for altered mental status due to opioid toxicity. Instead of pinpoint pupils, bradycardia, and bradypnea that is associated with opioid toxicity, this child had tachycardia and large pupils. Thus, naloxone is not indicated. Flumazenil should not be used routinely in any potential overdose patient with altered mental status because it can precipitate or worsen seizure activity. It is contraindicated, for example, in patients who receive benzodiazepines for a seizure disorder or acute seizure activity.

In a patient with altered mental status and a suspected tricyclic antidepressant ingestion, securing the airway is a priority.

2. Understand the role for gastrointestinal decontamination.[3,4]

Although gastric lavage is no longer routinely recommended after potentially toxic ingestions, there are certain instances when it should still be considered: ingestion of a potentially life-threatening agent like tricyclic antidepressants and some cardiovascular agents, ingestion of an agent not absorbed by charcoal (eg, iron), ingestants known to have a propensity to form bezoars (eg, iron, large amounts of aspirin tablets), and when gastric lavage can be undertaken within 60 minutes of ingestion.

Tricyclic antidepressants are considered life threatening, especially when the patient presents with serious symptoms. Activated charcoal is of greatest benefit when given within 1 hour of ingestion and should be administered after the lavage effluent is clear. For this particular clinical scenario, given the depressed mental status, gastric lavage with 15 mL/kg of normal saline per cycle (maximum of 200 mL) was performed and activated charcoal via nasogastric tube (1 g/kg) was administered once the airway was secured with an endotracheal tube.

3. Recognize the signs and symptoms of tricyclic antidepressant ingestion.[1]

Recognizing the signs and symptoms of tricyclic antidepressant ingestions is critical given the significant morbidity and mortality these drugs continue to cause. Signs and symptoms of toxicity usually occur within the first 2 to 4 hours. Patients can present with peripheral anticholinergic symptoms, CNS dysfunction, or cardiovascular effects. Typica anticholinergic effects include tachycardia, mydriasis, and flushed, dry skin, as were exhibited by the patient in this scenario. Central nervous system dysfunction ranges from agitation, delirium, and psychosis to seizures, unresponsiveness, and coma. Seizures are usually brief and most often occur within 1 to 2 hours of ingestion.

Potential toxic cardiovascular effects include conduction delays, dysrhythmias, and hypotension. On ECG, cardiac toxicity manifests as a sinus tachycardia with prolonged QRS duration or wide-complex tachycardia that resembles ventricular tachycardia. Both a QRS duration of 120 milliseconds or longer and an R wave measured in lead aVR of greater than 3 mm have a high sensitivity in predicting further complications. Persistent hypotension refractory to standard treatments is the most common cause of death.

4. Manage complications of tricyclic antidepressant toxicity.[1,5,6]

Adequate airway protection with intubation should be initiated in any comatose patient or any patient with significantly depressed mental status. Recurrent seizures, prolonged seizures, and status epilepticus require prompt treatment with benzodiazepines as first-line therapy. If this therapy fails, barbiturates should be administered.

Continuous cardiac monitoring and serial ECGs are necessary to monitor for potential cardiac complications. Alkalinization and sodium loading with **sodium bicarbonate** (1 to 2 mEq/kg IV bolus) should be initiated for prolonged QRS duration and wide-complex tachycardia until the QRS complex narrows. The management of hypotension should include volume expansion with isotonic saline and alkalinization/sodium loading with hypertonic sodium bicarbonate and/or hypertonic saline. Continuous alkalinization may be carried out with 150 mEq of sodium bicarbonate in 1 L of D_5W at 1.5 to 2 times maintenance fluid rate. Hypotension unresponsive to these therapeutic interventions necessitates the use of vasopressors and ionotropes (norepinephrine with low-dose dopamine is recommended). Other therapies include correcting hypoxia and acidosis.

5. Discuss the etiology and differential diagnosis for wide-complex tachycardia.[7]

Wide-complex tachycardia is the characteristic potentially life-threatening dysrhythmia observed in patients with severe tricyclic antidepressant toxicity and is probably multifactorial in etiology. These medications block the rapid inward movement of sodium ions into the fast sodium channels, slowing phase 0 depolarization of the action potential in the distal His-Purkinje system, as well as the ventricular myocardium. Impaired depolarization is manifested as prolongation of the QRS interval on the ECG. It is likely that most cases of wide-complex tachycardia are actually sinus tachycardia with rate-dependent aberrancy. However, ventricular tachycardia also can occur in the setting of hypoxia and metabolic acidosis. Congenital or acquired heart disease, electrolyte imbalance, untreated hypoxemia and acidosis, and drugs are the primary causes of wide-complex tachycardia in the pediatric population. Other drugs that can cause wide-complex tachycardia include cocaine, diphenhydramine, thioridazine, propoxyphene, and quinidine.

6. Discuss the usefulness of determining tricyclic antidepressant levels in the management of this toxicity.[1]

Quantitative determination of tricyclic antidepressant plasma concentration has limited use in the immediate evaluation and management of patients with acute overdoses. Because of the large volumes of distribution, long distribution half-lives, wide interpatient variability of terminal elimination half-lives, and development of tolerance among people chronically on these medications, the value of plasma concentrations in predicting acute toxicity is very limited. Thus, evaluation and management should be guided by a combination of clinical signs and symptoms and the ECG.

References

1. Liebelt E. Toxicology reviews: targeted management strategies for cardiovascular toxicity from tricyclic antidepressant overdose: the pivotal role for alkalinization and sodium loading. *Pediatr Emerg Care.* 1998;14:293-298.
2. Osterhoudt KC, Shannon M, Henretig FM. Toxicologic emergencies. In: Fleischer GR, Ludwig S, eds. *Textbook of Pediatric Emergency Medicine.* 4th ed. Philadelphia, Pa: Lippincott Williams & Wilkins; 2000:925-926.
3. Krenzelok E, Vale A. Position statements: gut decontamination. American Academy of Clinical Toxicology; European Association of Poisons Centres and Clinical Toxicologists. *J Toxicol Clin Toxicol.* 1997;35:695-786.
4. Erickson TB. Toxicology: ingestions and smoke inhalation. In: Gausche-Hill M, Fuchs S, Yamamoto L, eds. *APLS: The Pediatric Emergency Medicine Resource.* 4th ed. Sudbury, Mass: American Academy of Pediatrics, American College of Emergency Physicians, Jones and Bartlett Publishing Co; 2004:238-239.

5. Liebelt EL, Ulrich A, Francis PD, et al. Serial electrocardiogram changes in acute tricyclic antidepressant overdoses. *Crit Care Med.* 1997;25:1721-1726.

6. Liebelt EL, Francis PD, Woolf AD. ECG lead aVR versus QRS interval in predicting seizures and arrhythmias in acute tricyclic antidepressant toxicity. *Ann Emerg Med.* 1995;26:195-201.

7. Gewitz MH, Vetter VL. Cardiac emergencies. In: Fleischer GR, Ludwig S, eds. *Textbook of Pediatric Emergency Medicine.* 4th ed. Philadelphia, Pa: Lippincott Williams & Wilkins; 2000:682-686.

SCENARIO #30

Altered Mental Status

Amir Kimia, MD, and Richard G. Bachur, MD

Brief Presenting History

A 12-year-old girl presents to the emergency department via ambulance because of a staring gaze and confusion that were noted at school 45 minutes before her arrival.

Pediatric Assessment Triangle

Appearance: Awake, thin girl, no apparent distress, staring into space

Work of Breathing: Tachypneic without any stridor or labored breathing

Circulation to the Skin: Good perfusion, normal peripheral pulses, capillary refill less than 2 seconds

Initial Vital Signs

Pulse: 140

Respiratory Rate: 36

Blood Pressure: 105/41

Temperature: 35.7°C (96.3°F) oral

Physical Examination on Arrival to the Emergency Department

Airway: Airway patent, no stridor or drooling, normal voice although mumbled speech

Breathing: Tachypnea without hyperpnea or retractions; clear breath sounds; excellent aeration

Circulation: Distal extremities cold, normal peripheral pulses, no cyanosis, capillary refill 2 seconds

Disability: Speech slurred and incomprehensible, able to follow simple commands, eyes open to speech and pain

ASK YOURSELF

- **What is the initial assessment? What is the patient's physiologic status?**

  The patient is presenting with an acutely altered mental status. In addition, she has tachycardia and tachypnea without other signs of respiratory distress or shock.

- **What is this patient's Glasgow Coma Scale (GCS) score?**

  Her GCS is 11: 3 for eye opening, 6 for motor response, and 2 for verbal response. See Appendix C.

- **What are possible causes of the patient's altered mental status?**

  Primary CNS disorders include trauma, postictal state, infection (eg, meningitis or encephalitis), neoplasm, and vascular problems (eg, stroke). Secondary CNS problems include hypoxia, ingestion, metabolic derangement, and psychiatric disease (conversion reaction).

- **What additional history would help you at this point?**

  History of trauma, seizure activity, medication or illicit drug use, fever, infectious contacts, psychiatric illness, and recent illness and past medical history would all be helpful.

Additional History and Physical Examination Findings

The patient is a good student, and there are no previous medical or social concerns. Recently, she joined a gym. She was in her usual state of good health this morning, but one of her classmates noted that she excused herself several times during the day to go the school's bathroom. There was no history of trauma at school.

Past Medical History: Eating disorder, in counseling

Medications: Vitamin supplements

Allergies: Sulfa drugs have caused rashes.

Physical Examination: Pupils 3 mm bilaterally and briskly reactive, confused but not combative or somnolent, no scalp contusions or hematomas, normal tone to extremities, normal and symmetric deep tendon reflexes, cranial nerves including gag intact, skin dry

ASK YOURSELF

■ **What interventions are needed at this time? What complications might be expected?**

Interventions:

- Administer 100% O_2 by face mask. A staff member should be assigned and ready to manage the patient's airway and to monitor breathing.
- Intravenous access should be obtained. If circulation becomes compromised, a bolus of **normal saline 20 mL/kg** should be considered.
- Place the patient on a cardiorespiratory monitor with pulse oximetry.
- Perform appropriate laboratory tests for a patient with altered mental status: Bedside glucose test, venous blood gas, CBC, electrolytes, BUN, creatinine, serum glucose, calcium, magnesium, serum aspirin and acetaminophen levels, urine toxicology screen, urine pregnancy test
- Twelve-lead ECG

Potential Complications:

- Further mental status deterioration
- Development of seizure, posturing
- Patient becomes combative with interventions
- Circulatory compromise

■ **Why should a 12-lead ECG be obtained?**

Arrhythmias or other findings (widened QRS) associated with specific ingestions could be causing the patient's altered mental status.

Repeat Vital Signs

Pulse: 122

Respiratory Rate: 40

Blood Pressure: 108/68

Oxygen Saturation: 98% on room air

Progression

The patient suddenly develops generalized tonic-clonic activity with urinary incontinence and eye deviation, stertorous breathing, and copious oral secretions.

ASK YOURSELF

■ **What interventions are needed at this time?**

- Maintain airway with midline positioning and suctioning; use head tilt and jaw thrust as needed.
- Consider BMV if respiratory effort falters.
- Administer anticonvulsants: **Lorazepam 0.1 mg/kg IV**, repeat if no response in 3 minutes; for persistent seizure activity load with **fosphenytoin 15 to 20 mg PE/kg IV.**

Progression

Seizure activity ceases and spontaneous respirations continue, but the patient requires gentle jaw thrust for sonorous breathing.

Repeat Vital Signs

Pulse: 152

Respiratory Rate: 18

Blood Pressure: 102/60

Oxygen Saturation: 98% on blow-by oxygen

Laboratory Results

Hematocrit 44%, WBC count 11.2, platelets 325

Other initial laboratory results: glucose 67, Na^+ 115, K^+ 3.3, CO_2 31, BUN 20, creatinine 1.1, Cl^- 92, Ca^{2+} 8.7, Mg^{2+} 1.7

Urine toxicology screen, negative for substances of abuse

Progression

The patient has another seizure, a generalized motor seizure lasting for 45 seconds. It resolves spontaneously, and the girl remains postictal with spontaneous respirations.

ASK YOURSELF

■ **What is your differential diagnosis for hyponatremia?**

- Increased water accumulation relative to sodium. Causes include congestive heart failure, cirrhosis, acute renal failure, the syndrome of inappropriate secretion of antidiuretic hormone, and water intoxication.
- Decreased sodium stores relative to water. Causes include gastrointestinal and renal losses of sodium, adrenal (aldosterone) insufficiency, and third spacing of fluids.
- "Pseudohyponatremia" or measured low sodium level secondary to presence of serum hyperglycemia, hyperlipidemia, or hyperproteinemia.

■ **What interventions are needed at this time? What complications might be expected?**

Interventions:

- Because of the persistent seizures likely caused by hyponatremia, rapid correction of the serum sodium to 125 mEq/L should be attempted using **3% NaCl solution 10 to 12 mL/kg IV** over 60 minutes.

Potential Complications:

- The risks of administration of hypertonic saline include the osmotic demyelination syndrome (central pontine myelinolysis). Rapid correction should therefore be reserved only for symptomatic patients such as the one presented here.

■ **What is the etiology of hyponatremia resulting in altered mental status and seizures in this patient?**

This teenage girl with an eating disorder abused diuretics (furosemide) and as a result presented with altered mental status and seizures due to hyponatremia. The etiology of the hyponatremia is suggested by the medical history and confirmed by the laboratory findings of hyponatremia, hypocalcemia, hypochloremia, and metabolic alkalosis consistent with diuretic abuse.

Objectives of This Scenario

1. Have a knowledgeable approach to altered mental status.

This patient presented with a progressive alteration in mental status, eventually leading to seizures. The differential diagnosis is extensive in this case. It is best reviewed as two subgroups: primary CNS disorders such as trauma, intracranial hemorrhage, intracranial mass, CNS infections, and infarct; and secondary CNS involvement such as hypoxia, hypercarbia, shock, intoxication/ingestion (carbon monoxide), metabolic derangement (hypoglycemia, hyponatremia, uremia, hyperammonemia), and psychiatric disorders.

Many of the conditions described in the differential diagnosis have similar clinical characteristics, so detailed history taking is very important. In this scenario, the patient has no history of trauma, fever, or antecedent infection. She visited the bathroom several times that morning, and one should consider diarrhea or emesis (due to gastroenteritis or a toxic ingestion) or frequent urination (due to diabetes mellitus/DKA or diuretic abuse). Her physical examination and directed laboratory work-up further narrow the differential diagnosis.

2. Manage the patient with seizures.

The patient in our scenario had an intractable seizure that did not respond to conventional sequence of anticonvulsants: **lorazepam 0.1 mg/kg IV** followed by **fosphenytoin 15 to 20 mg PE/kg IV**. During the seizure, the clinical team should focus on ensuring adequate oxygenation and ventilation. Faced with intractable seizures, aggressive pursuit of possible etiologies for the seizure including underlying metabolic derangements must be undertaken. For this patient, hyponatremia was the cause of the seizures. The other electrolyte abnormalities presented here, such as the mild hypocalcemia, would not cause seizures.[1] See the section on seizures in "Evaluation and Management: Neurologic Emergencies."

3. Manage acute hyponatremia with neurologic manifestations.

Severe hyponatremia with neurologic manifestations represents a medical emergency. This condition should to be treated with intravenous hypertonic saline (3% NaCl); if this is not available, normal saline in combination with a loop diuretic also can rapidly raise the serum sodium concentration. The exact amount of hypertonic saline required to raise the serum sodium can be calculated as described next, although in practice, hypertonic saline is often given slowly up to 10 mL/kg until seizures resolve. Once the seizures resolve, the sodium can be further normalized based on the etiology of the hyponatremia.[1,2]

- Rapid elevation of serum sodium by 10 mEq/L up to levels of around 125 mEq/L may bring immediate relief.
- NaCl 3% contains sodium of 0.5 mEq/mL.
- Because sodium is primarily distributed in the extracellular space, the volume of distribution will be 0.6 L/kg times body weight (kg).
- In this case, the amount of 3% NaCl required to elevate the serum sodium by 10 mEq/L is [10 mEq/L × body weight (kg) × 0.6 L/kg]/0.5 mEq/mL or 10 to 12 mL/kg of 3% NaCl. The dose should be given over 60 minutes.

Rapid intervention with hypertonic saline carries the risk of osmotic demyelination syndrome. Osmotic demyelination syndrome is a neurologic disorder that can occur after rapid correction of hyponatremia. Initially named central pontine myelinolysis, this disease is now known to also affect extrapontine brain areas. Manifestations of myelinolysis usually evolve several days after correction of hyponatremia. Typical features are disorders of upper motor neurons, spastic quadriparesis and pseudobulbar palsy, and mental disorders ranging from mild confusion to coma. Death can occur.

The exact pathogenesis of myelinolysis has not been determined. Optimal management of hyponatremic patients involves weighing the risk for illness and death from untreated hyponatremia against the risk for myelinolysis from correction of the hyponatremia. Experiments in animals and clinical experience suggest that correction of chronic hyponatremia should be kept at a rate of less than 10 mmol/L in any 24-hour period.[3]

References

1. Moritz ML, Ayus JC. Disorders of water metabolism in children: hyponatremia and hypernatremia. *Pediatr Rev.* 2002;23:371-380.
2. Cheng JC, Zikos D, Peterson DR, et al. Symptomatic hyponatremia: pathophysiology and management. *Acute Care.* 1989;15:270-292.
3. Laureno R, Karp BI. Myelinolysis after correction of hyponatremia. *Ann Intern Med.* 1997;126:57-62.

SCENARIO #31

Seizure

Tom Langston, MD, and Joe E. Wathen, MD

Brief Presenting History

An 8-year-old girl with cerebral palsy and developmental delay is brought to the emergency department by EMS personnel with a report of seizures. The child experienced generalized tonic-clonic seizure activity for 20 minutes before EMS responders arrived at the child's day care facility. En route to the hospital, she received 2 mg of rectal diazepam after several attempts at intravenous access were unsuccessful. The patient arrives on blow-by oxygen with continued tonic-clonic activity. The total seizure time is now approximately 30 minutes.

Pediatric Assessment Triangle

Appearance: Tonic-clonic seizure activity, eyes deviated to the right

Work of Breathing: Substernal retraction

Circulation to the Skin: Distal extremities are mottled; perioral area has slight cyanosis

Initial Vital Signs

Pulse: 140

Respiratory Rate: 25

Blood Pressure: 100/70

Temperature: 37.9°C (100°F) rectal

Oxygen Saturation: 91% on blow-by O_2

ASK YOURSELF

- **What is the definition of status epilepticus?**

It has been estimated that more than 60,000 pediatric patients experience status epilepticus annually in the United States.[1] Despite this large number, there is no consensus definition for this condition. The World Health Organization defines status epilepticus as "a condition characterized by an epileptic seizure that is sufficiently prolonged or repeated at sufficiently brief intervals so as to produce an unvarying or enduring epileptic condition."[2] The Working Group on Status Epilepticus of the Epilepsy Foundation of America recommends that any seizure lasting longer than 10 minutes be treated with anticonvulsant therapy. For most research studies, status epilepticus is defined as seizures or repetitive seizures lasting at least 30 minutes.

Practically speaking, any child who arrives to the emergency department displaying active seizure activity should be assumed to be in status epilepticus and managed accordingly.[1,2]

Physical Examination on Arrival to the Emergency Department

Airway: Patent, copious secretions

Breathing: Moderate increase in work of breathing; coarse breath sounds throughout all lung fields

Circulation: Mottled skin; capillary refill time 2

seconds centrally and 3 seconds distally

Disability: Eyes open and deviated to the right; moaning, actively seizing

ASK YOURSELF

- **What is the initial assessment? What is the patient's physiologic status?**

  The patient presents with altered mental status due to status epilepticus. There is also a degree of respiratory distress due to seizure activity and to copious oral secretions.

- **How much should this 8-year-old weigh?**

  An estimated weight for a normal 8-year-old child is 25 kg. When estimating weight based on age for a child with special needs such as cerebral palsy, remember that the length-based Broselow Pediatric Emergency Tape or a pediatric table (Appendix A) gives average weights for healthy children; the patient's weight may be overestimated.

- **After the patient's ABCs are addressed, what bedside test would be appropriate to order for this patient?**

  A rapid assay for blood glucose should be performed in the field or quickly at the bedside for any patient who is considered to be in status epilepticus. Hypoglycemia is a known cause of seizures. In addition, hypoglycemia can occur in a seizing patient because of the increased metabolic demands from this hyperkinetic, hypermetabolic state.

Additional History and Physical Examination Findings

The child was sitting in her wheelchair at the daycare center and began repetitive lip smacking movements; next, she began to shake all over. The child's aunt, who is now in the emergency department, says that she has been taking care of the child for the past 10 days while the mother is out of town. When questioned about the past medical history, the aunt says that the child has had seizures before and is "on some medicine" to prevent them. However, the child's prescription ran out about 1 week ago, and the aunt does not know how to get this medicine refilled.

Past Medical History: Premature birth at 27 weeks, ventriculoperitoneal shunt (VPS) secondary to hydrocephalus

Medications: Unknown medicine for seizures

Physical Examination: G-tube in place, chronic contractures, no visible signs of trauma

ASK YOURSELF

- **Knowing this history, what is the most likely cause of this patient's current seizure activity?**

  The patient has a known disorder for which she takes an anticonvulsant. Given the aunt's history of running out of this unknown medicine "about a week ago," the child's anticonvulsant medication level may now be subtherapeutic, precipitating the seizures. However, other important etiologies of seizures must be considered. Increased intracranial pressure must be considered in any patient with a VPS, which could malfunction. Central nervous system infection is less likely in this afebrile patient but certainly is a consideration, especially in a patient with a VPS. Ingestion, hypoxia, and metabolic abnormalities also must be considered. In addition, this child's chronic underlying conditions (cerebral palsy, seizure disorder) place her at a higher risk for nonaccidental trauma.[3] Closed head injury, whether nonaccidental or accidental, commonly causes altered mental status and seizures.

Repeat Vital Signs

Pulse: 190

Respiratory Rate: 24

Blood Pressure: 95/70

Temperature: 37.8°C (100°F)

Oxygen Saturation: 95% via face mask

Rapid Glucose: 98

Progression

The child continues to have tonic-clonic seizure activity. The total seizure time is now approximately 40 minutes.

ASK YOURSELF

■ **What interventions are needed at this time?**

- Continue 100% O_2 via face mask for respiratory distress despite adequate pulse oximeter reading.
- Suction child's airway to control secretions.
- Place the patient on a cardiorespiratory monitor with pulse oximetry.
- Attempt intravenous access and begin fluid resuscitation with **normal saline 20 mL/kg.**
- Administer medications to control seizure activity.

■ **What medications should be considered as first-line therapy for a child in status epilepticus?**

Benzodiazepines should be considered as the first-line drugs for treatment of a child in status epilepticus. These drugs act rapidly and cause most seizure activity to end with one or two doses, usually 2 to 3 minutes after the dose is given. It is important to remember that all drugs within this class cause some level of respiratory depression.[1-3]

■ **If intravenous access cannot be obtained, what drug(s) could be considered for this patient?**

Rectal **diazepam (0.5 mg/kg)** can be administered to the patient in status epilepticus without intravenous access. Because of the difficulty in obtaining intravenous access in an actively seizing patient, this route may be preferred in the prehospital or "at-home" settings. In addition, midazolam administered buccally, intramuscularly, or intranasally has been advocated as an alternative to rectal diazepam in the initial management of status epilepticus.[4-7] Also, an intraosseous line may be placed and drugs administered effectively via this route.

Progression

The patient receives lorazepam 0.1 mg/kg IV (second dose of benzodiazepine) for continued seizure activity. Shortly after administration of the lorazepam, the seizure activity slows.

Repeat Vital Signs

Pulse: 100

Respiratory Rate: 9

Blood Pressure: 90/70

Temperature: 37.5°C (99.5°F)

Oxygen Saturation: 89% via face mask

ASK YOURSELF

■ **What is the physiologic status now, and why?**

The child has impending respiratory failure secondary to the sedative effect of the benzodiazepines given. A second dose of benzodiazepines is appropriate in the initial management of the patient in status epilepticus. However, it is important to recognize the potential for airway compromise due to respiratory depression as a side effect of the cumulative doses of the benzodiazepines given.

■ **What interventions are needed at this time? What complications might be expected?**

Interventions:

- The patient is now unable to maintain her airway. Preparation should be made to secure the airway via RSI. *Note:* Many patients may receive BMV for a brief period until the respiratory depressive effects of administered benzodiazepines abate and adequate breathing returns. However, some patients will have significant respiratory depression and require endotracheal intubation. For these patients, with presumed full stomachs, the principals of RSI apply, and additional sedative and paralytic drugs may be indicated.
- Preoxygenate the patient with 100% O_2 via BMV. Apply cricoid pressure.
- RSI—modified; an induction drug/paralytic may not be needed.
  1. #2 Miller blade
  2. **Midazolam 0.1 mg/kg IV** or **etomidate 0.3 mg/kg IV** (only if further sedation is needed)
  3. **Rocuronium 0.6 to 1 mg/kg IV** or **succinylcholine 1 to 1.5 mg/kg IV**

- End-tidal CO_2 monitor
- Listen for equal breath sounds.
- Chest radiograph to confirm ET tube placement.
- Secure ET tube, vent G-tube or place NG tube to decompress stomach

Potential Complications:

- Vomiting, copious secretions; requires suctioning, especially if cricoid pressure not used
- Unable to visualize cords if not properly suctioned
- Failure to decompress stomach results in impaired ventilation.
- Barotrauma induced by excessive tidal volume could precipitate a pneumothorax, requiring anterior needle aspiration or chest tube placement.
- Esophageal or right mainstem intubation, necessitating BMV and reintubation.

Vital Signs After Intubation

Pulse: 105

Respiratory Rate: 20 (bagged)

Blood Pressure: 100/72

Temperature: 37.4°C (99.3°F)

Oxygen Saturation: 100% in 100% O_2

ASK YOURSELF

■ After intubation, what other medications should be administered?

At this point, a long-acting anticonvulsant drug should be considered. Fosphenytoin, the prodrug of phenytoin, is an excellent choice in this instance. Although fosphenytoin is more expensive than phenytoin, it has several advantages that favor its use as a first-line emergent anticonvulsant. Fosphenytoin is less toxic to the tissues and causes fewer cardiac side effects than phenytoin because of the lack of ethylene glycol, which is used as a diluent in phenytoin. In addition, fosphenytoin is compatible with any intravenous solution (including dextrose) and can be infused rapidly or given via the intramuscular route if intravenous access is not available. The initial drug cost is higher for fosphenytoin, but an economic outcome evaluation has shown overall institutional cost savings compared with phenytoin.[8] Fosphenytoin is dosed in phenytoin equivalents (PE) at 15 to 20 PE/kg. An additional dose of 10 PE/kg may be given if needed.[1-3,9,10]

Intravenous loading with an anticonvulsant drug is also important because the patient could continue to experience subclinical seizure activity that is masked by paralytics used during RSI.

If seizure activity persists, additional medications such as phenobarbital or a continuous infusion of benzodiazepine or barbiturate may be considered.

Objectives of This Scenario

1. Recognize the condition of status epilepticus.

Status epilepticus is rather broadly defined depending on the sources consulted. However, for practical purposes, any child who is continuously seizing for a period of 20 to 30 minutes or is experiencing repetitive or persistent episodes of seizure activity without any intervening periods of consciousness between episodes should be considered to be in status epilepticus. When transport time to the hospital is factored in, it also may be prudent to consider that any child who arrives at the emergency department still actively seizing is in status epilepticus and should be managed accordingly.

2. Discuss the initial management of the patient in status epilepticus.

As with any acutely ill or injured patient, immediate attention should focus on the ABCs of resuscitation when managing the patient in status epilepticus. A rapid glucose assay should be performed early to guide initial management of the seizure. Hypoglycemia can be a direct cause of seizure activity or result from the hypermetabolic physiologic state caused by ongoing seizure activity. Additional priorities should obviously center around terminating the seizure activity. Benzodiazepines should be considered initially in the management of the patient in status epilepticus. **Lorazepam** has an onset of action of approximately 2 to 3 minutes and a duration of action of from 12 to 24 hours. **Diazepam** has an onset of action of approximately 1 to 3 minutes with a 5- to 15-minute duration of action. In addition, diazepam can be given rectally in the event that intravenous access is not available. **Midazolam**, another benzodiazepine, also may be considered; several studies have advocated its use during management of status epilepticus.[4-7] This drug can be given intranasally, buccally, intravenously, or intramuscularly. Second-line drugs to consider include phenytoin, fosphenytoin, and phenobarbital.

3. Recognize subtherapeutic drug levels as a likely cause of seizures in the patient with a known seizure disorder.

If a child presents in status epilepticus and is currently being treated with an anticonvulsant medication, it is important to consider that the child may have subtherapeutic drug levels. Phenytoin, carbamazepine, valproic acid, and phenobarbital are all commonly used anticonvulsants whose levels can be quickly determined at most laboratories. It is important to note that actual "therapeutic" levels for these drugs can in fact be above or below the recommended dosage boundaries. However, it is important to rule out other important causes of seizures (CNS infection, trauma, metabolic abnormality) regardless of anticonvulsant levels.

References

1. Issacman DJ. Central nervous system. In Gaushe-Hill M, Fuchs S, Yamamoto L, eds: *APLS The Pediatric Emergency Medicine Resource*. 4th ed. Sudbury, Mass: American Academy of Pediatrics, American College of Emergency Physicians, Jones and Bartlett; 2004:168-175.
2. Freedman SB, Powell EC. Pediatric seizures and their management in the emergency department. *Clin Pediatr Emerg Med*. 2003;4.
3. Chiang V. Seizures. In Fleisher GR, Ludwig S, eds. *Textbook of Pediatric Emergency Medicine*. 4th ed. Philadelphia, Pa: Lippincott Williams & Wilkins; 2000:573-579.
4. Chamberlain JM, Altieri MA, Futterman C, et al. A prospective, randomized study comparing intramuscular midazolam with intravenous diazepam for the treatment of seizures in children. *Pediatr Emerg Care*. 1997;13:92-94.
5. Vilke GM. Midazolam for the treatment of out-of-hospital pediatric seizures. *Prehosp Emerg Care*. 2002;6:215-217.
6. Fisgin T, Gurer Y, Tezic T, et al. Effects of intranasal midazolam and rectal diazepam on acute convulsions in children: prospective randomized study. *J Child Neurol*. 2002;17:123-126.
7. Scott RC, Besag FM, Neville BG. Buccal midazolam and rectal diazepam for treatment of prolonged seizures in childhood and adolescence: a randomised trial. *Lancet*. 1999;353:623-626.
8. Marchetti A, Magar R, Fischer J, et al. A pharmacoeconomic evaluation of intravenous fosphenytoin (Cerebyx) versus phenytoin (Dilantin) in hospital emergency departments. *Clin Therapeut*. 1996;18:953-966.
9. Haslam RH. Nonfebrile seizures. *Pediatr Rev*. 1997;18:39-49.
10. Sabo-Graham T, Seay AR. Management of status epilepticus in children. *Pediatr Rev*. 1998;19:306-310.

SCENARIO #32

Seizure

Frances W. Craig, MD

Brief Presenting History

An 18-month-old boy is rushed into the emergency department in his mother's arms, unresponsive and with his arms and legs jerking in a rhythmic fashion.

Pediatric Assessment Triangle

Appearance: Pale, unresponsive, arms and legs jerking, eyes deviated left

Work of Breathing: Rapid, shallow respirations

Circulation to the Skin: Perioral cyanosis, delayed capillary refill time

Initial Vital Signs

Pulse: 180

Respiratory Rate: 44

Blood Pressure: 110/68

Temperature: 37.6°C (99.7°F)

ASK YOURSELF

- **How much should this 18-month-old weigh?**

  An estimated weight for an 18-month-old child is 12 kg. One can use the length-based Broselow Pediatric Emergency Tape or a pediatric table to determine weight based on age. See Appendix A.

Physical Examination

Airway: Patent, but copious oral secretions

Breathing: Rapid, shallow respirations with minimal chest wall excursion, lungs clear bilaterally without wheezes

Circulation: Skin pale and cool to the touch, capillary refill time 3 seconds centrally and 4 seconds peripherally

Disability: Eyes closed, the patient not responding to voice, extremities jerking rhythmically

ASK YOURSELF

- **What is the initial assessment? What is the patient's physiologic status?**

  Patient presents with active, generalized tonic-clonic seizure, respiratory distress, and compensated shock.

- **What interventions are needed at this time?**
  - Administer 100% O_2 by face mask for respiratory distress
  - Place the patient on a cardiorespiratory monitor with pulse oximetry.
  - Attempt intravenous access.

Progression

Intravenous access is unsuccessful, and three drops of blood are obtained.

ASK YOURSELF

- **What should you do with the three drops of blood?**

  Perform a rapid glucose determination.

- **What additional history would help you make the diagnosis?**

  Has this child had prior seizures? If so, have anticonvulsants been prescribed, and is he taking them? Have there been recent changes in medications or dosages? Is there a history of recent trauma, particularly head injury? Has the child been ill recently—in particular, has he had vomiting or diarrhea? Are there any medications in the home, either the child's or belonging to other household occupants? What was the child's behavior like leading up to this incident?[1,2]

- **What is the differential diagnosis of seizure activity in this patient?**

  Trauma should be apparent by history and physical examination, although in the case of nonaccidental trauma (ie, abuse), an accurate trauma history can be more difficult to ascertain.

  An infectious cause (meningitis, encephalitis, acute/viral febrile illness resulting in febrile seizure) is usually distinguishable by the child's recent history and fever on presentation. In the case of CNS infections, the physical examination often will reveal altered mental status (prolonged postictal phase) or meningismus.

  Inborn errors of metabolism are less likely to present at this age. They usually manifest in the first 6 months of life but should be considered in patients who have a history of vomiting or diarrhea and who have a metabolic acidosis with hypoglycemia. A metabolic etiology should be suspected in patients taking medications that might lead to electrolyte disturbances (eg, lithium, diuretics) or if various toxic ingestions are possible (especially alcohol, β-blockers, oral hypoglycemics, salicylates, and insulin). A serum bedside glucose level is quick and inexpensive to obtain, so it should be checked on all patients presenting with a nonfebrile seizure.[1-4]

Additional History and Physical Examination Findings

The patient was well previously. He lives with both parents and a 4-year-old sibling, none of whom have been ill or are taking any medications. He has had no vomiting or diarrhea. The child was in the care of his grandparents the previous night, and the grandfather takes glyburide for type II diabetes.

Past Medical History: Well, no prior seizure history

Medications: None

Allergies: None known

Physical Examination: No evidence of head trauma, breathing rapid and shallow in the face of ongoing seizure activity, capillary refill time 4 seconds, abdomen soft and nondistended; extremities mottled and exhibiting tonic-clonic activity

ASK YOURSELF

- **What interventions are needed at this time?**
  - Attempt intravenous line placement; if unsuccessful, place an intraosseous line.
    1. Begin fluid resuscitation with **normal saline 20 mL/kg.**
  - Administer a benzodiazepine to stop seizure activity.
    1. **Lorazepam 0.1 mg/kg IV/IO** (IO if IV access cannot be obtained quickly)
    2. **Diazepam 0.5 mg/kg PR** or **0.1 to 0.3 mg/kg IV/IO**

  For additional first-line anticonvulsant benzodiazepine options please see Scenario #31, pages 244-245.

Repeat Vital Signs

Pulse: 152

Respiratory Rate: 26

Blood Pressure: 90/40

Oxygen Saturation: 100% on face mask O_2

Progression

After a second dose of lorazepam, the seizure has stopped, but the child's breathing is now at a rate of 8 breaths/min, with occasional periods of apnea.

ASK YOURSELF

- **What is the child's current physiologic status?**

  Impending respiratory failure, likely due to the respiratory suppressive effects of the benzodiazepine (lorazepam).

- **What interventions are needed at this time?**
  - BMV with 100% O_2
  - Cricoid pressure
  - Preparation for intubation.

Laboratory Test Result: Rapid glucose of 25

ASK YOURSELF

- **What is the most likely diagnosis?**

  Seizure secondary to hypoglycemia, most likely due to ingestion of the grandfather's oral hypoglycemic agent.

- **What interventions are needed at this time? What complications might be expected?**

  Interventions:
  - This patient has developed respiratory insufficiency secondary to hypoventilation. Continue to support breathing using BMV with 100% O_2 and continue cricoid pressure. Preparations should be made for modified RSI if this condition persists.
  - Treat hypoglycemia with **0.5 to 1 g/kg of dextrose** using **2 to 4 mL/kg D_{25}W IV/IO.**

  Potential Complications:
  - Persistent hypoglycemia: Most oral hypoglycemic agents have half-lives in the range of 12 to 24 hours. Thus, even after a bolus of glucose, the serum levels can drop again, necessitating repeat glucose boluses, ongoing glucose drips, or even pharmacologic intervention such as **octreotide**, a long-acting analogue of somatostatin that antagonizes insulin release, depending on the severity of hypoglycemia and the half-life of the particular hypoglycemic agent ingested.[5]
  - Recurrent seizure activity: This is unlikely if the underlying cause is managed (ie, treat the hypoglycemia), but if seizure activity recurs despite normoglycemic state, consider loading with **fosphenytoin 10 to 20 mg PE/kg IV.**

Progression

Patient begins to breathe spontaneously; seizure activity has stopped.

Repeat Laboratory Test Result: Rapid glucose of 57

ASK YOURSELF

- **What disposition and additional management would be expected for this patient?**

  Repeat dextrose bolus or place on a continuous infusion of dextrose. This patient will require hospital admission or prolonged observation with frequent glucose checks until the hypoglycemic effects of glyburide have resolved.

Objectives of This Scenario

1. Recognize that management of seizures begins with the ABCs.

In an actively seizing patient, proper midline positioning with a jaw thrust and suctioning of secretions or vomitus is required. An oral or a nasopharyngeal airway can help to support the airway. Oxygen is administered to prevent hypoxic injury, but the patient may need more assistance to maintain adequate ventilation, especially in the face of respiratory depression or apnea induced by anticonvulsant medications. Often, this respiratory effect is short lived, and properly performed BMV will see the patient through this transient event. However, if the period of depression is more prolonged or if multiple doses of suppressive agents were required to stop the seizure activity, endotracheal intubation may be indicated with appropriate RSI technique.

Hypotension can occur secondarily to an underlying

process such as dehydration or vasodilation from prolonged seizure activity or as a result of the anticonvulsant medications. This is generally managed well with isotonic fluid replacement (**normal saline** or **lactated Ringer at 20 to 40 mL/kg**).

2. Formulate a differential diagnosis of seizure.

The challenge of treating seizures is to simultaneously stabilize the patient, direct therapy, and conduct a diagnostic evaluation to reveal the underlying cause of the seizure. Identifying an etiology will help guide initial management and interventions, as well as the ongoing care of the patient.

Important etiologies include CNS infection (meningitis, encephalitis); trauma and child abuse; metabolic causes such as hyponatremia, hypoglycemia, hypocalcemia, and inborn errors of metabolism; ingestions; anoxia/hypoxia; previously known seizure disorders; intracranial lesions (spontaneous bleeds, tumor mass, hydrocephalus); and ventriculoperitoneal shunt malfunction. Consideration should be given to the patient's prior history, risk for exposures, and age when approaching the evaluation. Electrolytes, CBC, and emergency neuroimaging are generally low yield in the child with first-time, unprovoked seizure, unless the seizure is focal, the child's age places him or her at risk for metabolic aberration (generally <6 months old), history reveals prolonged vomiting or diarrhea, or physical examination reveals focal neurologic findings.[1,6-8]

Hypoglycemia presents with a spectrum of symptoms, from lethargy to seizure to coma. Infants with immature livers and decreased ability to make glucose from stores of glycogen are especially susceptible to hypoglycemia when stressed or during prolonged periods of decreased intake. Potential causes of hypoglycemia include sepsis, especially in infants; decreased intake, especially in conjunction with vomiting and diarrhea; inborn errors of metabolism; and ingestions, especially of alcohol, salicylates, β-blockers, oral hypoglycemic agents, and insulin.[5,9]

3. Manage seizures secondary to hypoglycemia.

Prolonged seizures (duration >30 minutes) represent a true emergency. The initial management of any seizure relies on benzodiazepines as first-line treatment. If an underlying etiology such as hypoglycemia is identified, it must be corrected to prevent ongoing seizure activity. Seizures secondary to hypoglycemia should be treated with a rapid infusion of dextrose. Dextrose 25% as D_{25} water may be pushed through a peripheral intravenous or intraosseous line. The dose is **0.5 to 1 g/kg**, which is equivalent to **2 to 4 mL/kg of $D_{25}W$**. Greater concentrations such as 50% dextrose can cause venous sclerosis and potential infiltration if given in a peripheral vein, because of the high solute concentration. Infants may be given **$D_{10}W$ 5 to 10 mL/kg IV**. If the cause of hypoglycemia is drug related, it may be necessary to initiate a D_5- or D_{10}-containing continuous infusion at maintenance rate for a time period dictated by the half-life of the ingested agent. Patients cannot be discharged from the hospital until they are normoglycemic while off any supplemental (intravenous) dextrose.[1,2,5]

References

1. Reuter D, Brownstein D. Common emergent pediatric neurologic problems. *Emerg Med Clin North Am.* 2002;20:155-176.
2. Chang VW. Seizures. In: Fleisher GR, Ludwig S, eds. *Textbook of Pediatric Emergency Medicine.* 4th ed. Philadelphia, Pa: Lippincott Williams & Wilkins; 2000:573-579.
3. Freeman JM. Less testing is needed in the emergency room after a first afebrile seizure. *Pediatrics.* 2003;111:194-196.
4. Valencia I, Sklar E, Blanco F, et al. The role of routine laboratory tests in children presenting to the emergency department with unprovoked seizures. *Clin Pediatr.* 2003;42:511-517.
5. Schnachner H, Silfen M. Endocrine emergencies. In: Crain EF, Gershel JC, eds. *Clinical Manual of Emergency Pediatrics.* 4th ed. New York, NY: McGraw-Hill; 2003:165-168.
6. Hirtz D, Ashwal S, Berg A, et al. Practice parameter: evaluation of first nonfebrile seizures in children—report of the Quality Standards Committee of the American Academy of Neurology, The Child Neurology Society, and the American Epilepsy Society. *Neurology.* 2000;55:616-623.
7. Kenney R, Taylor J. Absence of serum chemistry abnormalities in pediatric patients presenting with seizures. *Pediatr Emerg Care.* 1992;8:65-66.
8. Sharma S, Riviello JJ, Harper MB, et al. The role of emergent neuroimaging in children with new-onset afebrile seizures. *Pediatrics.* 2003;111:1-5.
9. Osterhoudt KC, Shannon M, Henretig FM. Toxicologic emergencies. In: Fleisher GR, Ludwig S, eds. *Textbook of Pediatric Emergency Medicine.* 4th ed. Philadelphia, Pa: Lippincott Williams & Wilkins; 2000:887-889.

SCENARIO #33

Seizure

Amy L. Drendel, DO, and David C. Brousseau, MD, MS

Brief Presenting History

A 6-year-old girl is brought in by her mother. She has been lethargic and dizzy for the past 12 hours. She began to seize at home 5 minutes ago, and her mother brought her straight to the emergency department. The mother denies any history of trauma.

Pediatric Assessment Triangle

Appearance: Pale, actively seizing

Work of Breathing: Shallow respirations, stertor

Circulation to the Skin: Cool

Initial Vital Signs

Pulse: 120

Respiratory Rate: Irregular

Blood Pressure: 96/58

Temperature: 37°C (98.6°F) axillary

ASK YOURSELF

- **How much should this 6-year-old weigh?**

  An estimated weight for a 6-year-old is 20 kg. One can use the length-based Broselow Pediatric Emergency Tape or a pediatric table to determine weight based on age. See Appendix A.

Physical Examination on Arrival to the Emergency Department

Airway: Stertorous breath sounds with secretions in the mouth

Breathing: Shallow respirations with diminished effort, poor aeration with transmitted sounds

Circulation: Cool skin, capillary refill time 3 seconds; femoral pulses 2+ and equal

Disability: Unresponsive and actively seizing with symmetric generalized tonic-clonic movements of all extremities, pupils equal and reactive to light 4 to 2 mm bilaterally

ASK YOURSELF

- **What is the initial assessment? What is the patient's physiologic status?**

  This patient presents with a history of altered mental status, seizure, and respiratory insufficiency.

- **What is your approach to the seizing patient?**

  Initially, attention must focus on the ABCs because much of the morbidity and mortality associated with seizures can be attributed to hypoxia and its complications.[1] Oxygen 100% should be initiated in all patients. The child's airway should be positioned to reduce obstruction if there is no history of trauma. Secretions should be gently suctioned from the airway. An appropriately sized bag-mask device should be immediately available at the bedside. Intravenous access should be attempted and blood obtained for analysis. After initial resuscitative measures have been accomplished and a cursory history and physical examination aimed at identifying the etiology of the seizure are complete, specific therapy aimed at terminating seizure activity and preventing its recurrence should begin.

■ **What interventions are needed at this time? What complications might be expected?**

Interventions:

- Proper positioning of the head to open airway
- Suction
- Administer 100% O_2 by face mask.
- Assess ventilation and support as needed.
- Consider placement of nasal or oral airway.
- Place the patient on a cardiorespiratory monitor with pulse oximetry.
- Attempt intravenous access and obtain blood sample for analysis. Obtain rapid glucose level; consider tests for sodium, calcium, and phosphorus; renal and hepatic function; anticonvulsant drug level (if appropriate); or serum and urine toxicology based on findings from history and physical examination.
- Control hyperthermia as needed (**acetaminophen 15 mg/kg PR**).

Potential Complications:

- Oxygen not applied and child experiences oxygen desaturation
- Inappropriate positioning of patient leads to mechanical obstruction and desaturations

■ **Only three drops of blood are obtained. What should you do with the three drops of blood?**

Perform rapid bedside glucose determination.

Progression

The patient continues to seize. She has irregular respirations but improved aeration after interventions.

ASK YOURSELF

■ **What is the appropriate treatment for seizures at this time?**

- Administration of a benzodiazepine: **lorazepam 0.1 mg/kg IV**, maximum 4 mg/dose, may repeat once in 5 to 10 minutes *or* **diazepam 0.1 to 0.3 mg/kg IV**, maximum 10 mg/dose, may repeat once in 5 to 10 minutes or if no intravenous access, **diazepam 0.5 mg/kg PR**, maximum 20 mg *or* **midazolam 0.05 to 0.15 mg/kg IM**, maximum 6 mg/dose[2] *Note*: For additional first-line anticonvulsant benzodiazepine options, see Scenario #31, pages 244-245.

■ **What complications might be expected?**

- Intravenous access unsuccessful; consider intramuscular or rectal administration.
- Loss of intravenous access; consider intramuscular or rectal administration, and consider intraosseous placement.
- Apnea occurs requiring BMV and possible intubation.

Progression

Patient continues to seize 5 minutes after initial dose of benzodiazepine.

ASK YOURSELF

■ **What interventions are needed at this time?**

- Administration of a *second dose* of **lorazepam 0.1 mg/kg IV**, maximum 4 mg/dose, 5 to 10 minutes after initial dose *or* **diazepam 0.1 to 0.3 mg/kg IV**, maximum 10 mg/dose, 5 to 10 minutes after initial dose
- Administration of **fosphenytoin 20 mg PE/kg** IV or IM, 3 mg/kg/min, maximum 1,000 mg *or* **phenytoin 20 mg/kg IV**, 1 mg/kg/min, maximum 1,000 mg. *Note:* If administered more rapidly than 1 mg/kg/min, arrhythmia or hypotension can occur with phenytoin. Local irritation and phlebitis can accompany intravenous administration.
- Other toxin antidotes should be considered on a case-by-case basis.

- **In this case of benzodiazepine-induced apnea, should a reversal agent (flumazenil) be administered?**

  No, reversal of apnea induced by benzodiazepines administered for seizure activity with flumazenil is contraindicated because of the risk of seizure recurrence.

Progression

The child stops seizing after administration of the second dose of benzodiazepine.

ASK YOURSELF

- **What should be done at this time?**

  Reassess ABCs, support as needed, and obtain additional history.

Additional History and Physical Examination Findings

The patient has been ill for the past 12 hours complaining of a headache and nausea with vomiting. Her mother states that her daughter seemed worse and became confused and combative this morning. The child's two older brothers have also been "coming down" with similar symptoms, although the oldest brother took advantage of the first snow of the season and went sledding this morning and now denies symptoms. The parents report that this is the first time they have used the furnace all winter. Parents again deny a history of trauma and report no fever, recent upper respiratory tract symptoms, history of seizures, medication use, or any medications in the home.

Repeat Vital Signs

Pulse: 135

Respiratory Rate: 18 irregular

Blood Pressure: 104/60

Temperature: 37.8°C (100°F)

Oxygen Saturation: 100% with 100% O_2 via face mask

Family History: No seizure disorder

General: No evidence of trauma

HEENT: No eye deviation, no papilledema, tympanic membranes opaque, nares patent, mucous membranes moist; no gag reflex present

Lung: Irregular respiration with fair aeration

Abdomen: Nontender, nondistended, soft with bowel sounds

Neurologic: No active seizure, deep tendon reflexes 3+ throughout, opens eyes and withdraws to pain, moans incomprehensible words

Skin: No lesions, no rashes

ASK YOURSELF

- **What is the physiologic status now?**

  The patient is no longer actively seizing, however, her respiratory status has deteriorated. Often, these patients require BMV for a brief period until the respiratory depressive effects of the administered benzodiazepines abate and adequate breathing returns. However, some patients will have significant respiratory depression and require endotracheal intubation. For these patients, with presumed full stomachs, the principles of RSI apply, and additional sedative and paralytic drugs may be indicated.[3]

- **What is the differential diagnosis for seizures in pediatrics?**

  Precipitants of seizures in children[1] include CNS infection, trauma, metabolic abnormality (hypoglycemia), ingestion/exposure, intracranial lesion (tumor or congenital anomaly), hypoxia/hypercarbia, cerebrovascular (nontraumatic bleed) accident, seizure disorder/anticonvulsant medication change, and fever/infection (febrile seizure).

  This patient presents with seizures and altered mental status of unknown etiology. There is no history of fever in this patient, making serious bacterial infections or meningitis less likely.[4,5] The child has no history of seizure disorder, congenital disorders, or anoxia, removing these precipitants from consideration. Inadvertent or intentional drug ingestions or exposures are important etiologies to be considered, especially when the cause is not readily apparent, as in this child with altered mental status. Metabolic derangements, including hypoglycemia and electrolyte derangements, should be investigated.[6,7] Although there is no history of trauma, head injury and child abuse also should be considered. Progressive neurologic disorder and tumor should be considered, although the acute onset of symptoms makes these entities less likely.

Laboratory Test Results

Serum Glucose: 135

Electrolytes: Normal

Renal and Liver Functions: Normal

Toxicology Screen: No evidence of toxin

ASK YOURSELF

■ What is the likely diagnosis?

Toxin-related seizure. Given the patient's initial symptoms of headache, nausea, and vomiting, which progressed to altered mental status and seizure, in the setting of first-time seasonal furnace exposure and family members with similar symptoms and exposure, her most likely diagnosis is carbon monoxide poisoning.

■ How can you confirm the diagnosis? Do symptoms correlate with a patient's carboxyhemoglobin (COHb) level?

The most useful diagnostic test is a COHb level. Normal levels range from 0% to 5%, as carbon monoxide is a natural byproduct of the breakdown of protoporphyrin to bilirubin.[8] COHb levels of 6% to 10% are seen in one-pack-per-day smokers.[9] High levels confirm exposure, but levels do not correlate well with severity of symptoms in a substantial number of cases.[10] Most hospitals determine the carbon monoxide level by co-oximetry, which can be performed on arterial or venous blood samples.[1] Arterial samples allow for the measurement of the arterial oxygen saturation. Pulse oximetry does not detect the presence of COHb. The pulse oximeter misinterprets COHb as oxyhemoglobin, thus falsely elevating the oxygen saturation.[11] Carbon monoxide levels in the ambient air in the patient's home can also be evaluated by fire department personnel.

Progression

The patient's COHb level is 27%, and the diagnosis of carbon monoxide–induced seizure is made. Arterial blood gases measured before the administration of oxygen reveal a metabolic acidosis with decreased oxygen saturation (compared with pulse oximeter reading).

ASK YOURSELF

■ What is the appropriate initial treatment and disposition for a patient with carbon monoxide poisoning?

Treatment:

- Remove patient from exposure to carbon monoxide.
- Evaluate ABCs and provide support as needed.
- Provide 100% O_2 to maximize oxygen delivery and reduce the half-life ($t_{1/2}$) of carbon monoxide.[1,12]

$t_{1/2}$ COHb with 21% oxygen	4 hours
$t_{1/2}$ COHb with 100% oxygen	60 to 90 minutes
$t_{1/2}$ COHb with 3 atm hyperbaric therapy	15 to 30 minutes

- Administer oxygen until COHb concentration is less than 5% and the patient has regained fully normal neurologic functions.

Disposition:

Asymptomatic children with a COHb level of less than 8% should be observed for 12 hours. Symptomatic children should be administered oxygen until the COHb level is less than 5%. If symptoms persist, consideration should be given to the use of hyperbaric therapy.

■ What are the indications for hyperbaric therapy?

Recommendations by *APLS: The Pediatric Emergency Medicine Resource*[1] include the following indications for hyperbaric therapy:

- CPR at the scene
- Abnormal level of consciousness on presentation
- Unconscious at scene; report of seizure
- COHb level greater than 25%

Indications given in a review article by Ernst and Zibrak[10] include the following:

- Coma
- Any period of unconsciousness
- Any abnormal score of the CO neuropsychological screen battery
- COHb levels greater than 40%
- Pregnancy and COHb level greater than 15%
- Signs of cardiac ischemia or arrhythmia
- History of ischemic heart disease and COHb level greater than 20%
- Recurrent symptoms for up to 3 weeks
- Symptoms that do not resolve with normobaric oxygen after 4 to 6 hours

The decision to use hyperbaric therapy should be made as early as possible so arrangement can be made for a safe and rapid transfer. A detailed neurologic examination should always be performed to document abnormalities, which can be subtle.

■ Why was this child so severely affected compared with other members of her family?

Children are often more severely affected. The amount of gas absorbed is dependent on the minute ventilation, duration of exposure, and concentrations of carbon monoxide in the environment.[10] Children have a significantly higher minute ventilation than do adults due to their higher respiratory rates and thus frequently are more severely affected. This patient was most likely more severely affected than her brothers because she was younger and closer to the source of the carbon monoxide.

Objectives of This Scenario

1. Manage initial presentation of seizure.

The mortality rate in children with prolonged seizure is 1% to 3%. Seizure duration of longer than 1 hour, especially in association with hypoxia, has been associated with permanent neurologic injury.[1] This is a true medical emergency. Priority should be given to the ABCs. Once the patient is stabilized, attention should be given to administration of medication to stop seizure activity and to evaluation for the etiology of the seizure. In children, in particular, the history and physical examination should be used to rule out common etiologies, including fever and metabolic, toxin-related, or traumatic causes.

2. Consider the toxicologic etiology of seizure.

In an afebrile child with new-onset seizure, one should always consider toxic ingestion as a possible etiology. A mnemonic for the many causes of toxic seizure is **OTIS CAMPBELL**.[13]

Organophosphates

Tricyclic antidepressants

Isoniazid (INH), insulin

Sympathomimetics, salicylates

Camphor, cocaine, calcium channel blockers, cyanide, carbon monoxide

Amphetamines, arsenic, antidepressants, anticholinergics

Methylxanthines, MAO inhibitors

PCP, propoxyphene, phenol, propranolol, pesticides

Benzodiazepine withdrawal, botanicals, buproprion

Ethanol withdrawal

Lithium, lindane

Lidocaine, lead

3. Recognize carbon monoxide poisoning.

Carbon monoxide exposure is one of the most common causes of morbidity from poisoning in the United States.[10] The rate of accidental death is higher in the north and peaks during winter months.[10] Sources of exogenous carbon monoxide include motor vehicle exhaust fumes, poorly functioning heating systems, and inhaled smoke.[14] Reported scenarios that should raise suspicion for carbon monoxide poisoning include the use of a charcoal grill for heating, riding in the back of a car or truck in poor repair, and being in kerosene-heated homes.[10] Signs and symptoms mimic nonspecific viral illness. There are no pathognomonic signs or symptoms that identify carbon monoxide poisoning; a high level of suspicion is essential to make the diagnosis.[10] The classic findings of cherry-red lips, cyanosis, and retinal hemorrhages occur rarely.[1]

References

1. Dieckmann RA. Pediatric assessment. In: Gausche-Hill M, Fuchs S, Yamamoto L, eds. *APLS: The Pediatric Emergency Medicine Resource.* 4th ed. Sudbury, Mass: American Academy of Pediatrics, American College of Emergency Physicians, Jones and Bartlett Publishing Co; 2004:40.
2. Chamberlain JM. A prospective randomized study comparing IM midazolam and IV diazepam for the treatment of seizure in children. *Pediatr Emerg Care.* 1997;13:92-94.
3. Lee BS, Gausche-Hill M. Pediatric airway management. *Clin Pediatr Emerg Med.* 2001;2:91-106.
4. Green SM, Rothrock SG, Clem KJ, et al. Can seizures be the sole manifestation of meningitis in febrile children? *Pediatrics.* 1993;92:527-534.
5. Teach SJ, Geil PA. Incidence of bacteremia, urinary tract infection and unsuspected bacterial meningitis in children with febrile seizures. *Pediatr Emerg Care.* 1995;15:9-12.
6. Farrar HC, Chande VT, Fitzpatrick DF, et al. Hyponatremia as the cause of seizures in infants: a retrospective analysis of incidence, severity and clinical predictors. *Ann Emerg Med.* 1995;26:42-48.
7. Nypaver NM, Reynolds SL, Tanz RR, et al. Emergency department laboratory evaluation of children with seizures: dogma or dilemma? *Pediatr Emerg Care.* 1992;8:13-16.
8. Coburn RF. Endogenous carbon monoxide production. *N Engl J Med.* 1970;282:207-209.
9. Stewart R, Baretta ED, Platte LR, et al. Carboxyhemoglobin levels in American blood donors. *JAMA.* 1974;229:1187-1195.
10. Ernst A, Zibrak J. Carbon monoxide poisoning. *N Engl J Med.* 1998;339:1603-1608.
11. Barker SJ, Tremeper KK. The effect of carbon monoxide inhalation on pulse-oximetry and transcutaneous Po_2. *Anesthesiology.* 1987;66:677-679.
12. Tomaszewski C. Carbon monoxide. In: Goldfrank LR, Flomenbaum NE, Lewin NA, et al, eds. *Goldfrank's Toxicologic Emergencies.* 7th ed. New York, NY: McGraw-Hill; 2002:1478-1490.
13. Erickson TB, Aks SE, Williams RH. Toxicology update: a rational approach to managing poisoned patients. *Emerg Med Pract.* 2001;6.
14. Meredith T, Vale A. Carbon monoxide poisoning. *BMJ.* 1988;296:77-79.

SCENARIO #34

Seizure

Elizabeth S. Jacobs, MD

Brief Presenting History

A 2-year-old girl is brought in by her foster mother. She has been vomiting for 2 days and has become progressively less responsive.

Pediatric Assessment Triangle

Appearance: Pale, eyes closed, localizes painful stimuli

Work of Breathing: Grunting, shallow respirations

Circulation to Skin: Mottled

Initial Vital Signs

Pulse: 190

Respiratory Rate: 40

Blood Pressure: 60/30

Temperature: 38°C (100.4°F) axillary

ASK YOURSELF

- **What is the interpretation of these vital signs? What is the initial assessment?**

These vital signs and patient presentation are consistent with respiratory distress and decompensated shock. *Respiratory distress* is defined as the presence of an increased respiratory effort, rate, and work of breathing (in this case, the child is both tachypneic and grunting).[1] *Shock* is defined as a mismatch between oxygen delivery and tissue metabolic demand. Clinical signs of shock and respiratory failure result from end-organ dysfunction caused by hypoxia and acidosis. Further, decompensated shock is present when signs of shock are associated with systolic hypotension. A quick way to calculate the minimum normal (fifth percentile) systolic blood pressure (SBP) for children is as follows[1]:

- Term neonates (0 to 28 days): SBP = 60 mm Hg
- Infants aged 1 to 12 months: SBP = 70 mm Hg
- Children aged 1 to 10 years: SBP = 70 mm Hg + (2 × age [years])
- Children older than 10 years: SBP = 90 mm Hg

Systolic blood pressure must exceed the fifth percentile for age to be considered compensated. In a 2-year-old child, hypotension would be defined by an SBP less than 74 mm Hg.

Physical Examination on Arrival to the Emergency Department

Airway: Patent

Breathing: Grunting with labored, irregular respirations; no wheezing or crackles

Circulation: Skin mottled and cool to the touch, capillary refill time greater than 4 seconds both centrally and peripherally, pulses weak

Disability: Eyes closed; does not respond to voice, but moans with pain and opens eyes briefly; pupils equal and reactive to light

ASK YOURSELF

■ What is the neurologic status of this patient?

The patient has altered mental status with respiratory distress and decompensated shock. Normal, healthy children older than 2 months should be able to focus on their parent's face. A child's neurologic response can be characterized by the **AVPU** description: **A**lert; **R**esponsive to **V**oice; **R**esponsive to **P**ain; **U**nresponsive.

Responsiveness only to painful stimuli, in this case, is an ominous sign of cortical hypoperfusion due to decompensated shock.

■ What interventions are needed at this time?

- Apply 100% O_2 with nonrebreather face mask.
- Place the patient on a cardiorespiratory monitor with pulse oximetry.
- Establish intravenous access and initiate **isotonic fluid bolus of 20 mL/kg.**

Isotonic fluids can be either in the form of crystalloid solutions or colloid solutions. Initial volume resuscitation begins with isotonic crystalloid, normal saline, or lactated Ringer solution. These fluids are readily available; however, only approximately one third of crystalloid solutions remain in the intravascular space.

After 40 to 60 mL/kg of isotonic crystalloid has been given, the administration of colloid solutions should be considered; examples are 5% albumin, fresh frozen plasma, whole blood, or synthetic colloid solutions. These solutions remain in the intravascular compartment longer; however, they can cause sensitivity reactions and other complications. Blood products are indicated only for replacement of blood loss and coagulopathies.[2] Fluid response is assessed by resolution of hypotension and improvement in perfusion. Fluids should be given rapidly in 20-mL/kg bolus increments until vital signs and clinical status improve.

■ If unable to establish peripheral intravenous access, what is the next step?

Intraosseous needle placement should be attempted after 90 seconds or three unsuccessful attempts at peripheral intravenous placement. Initial attempts should be made just distal to the tibial tuberosity along the medial flat surface of the anterior, proximal tibia. Alternative sites include the distal femur, medial malleolus, and anterior superior iliac spine.[3]

Additional History and Physical Examination Findings

The foster mother is concerned because the patient had an unsupervised visit with her birth family 3 days earlier. The patient had been removed from the home because of an unexplained femur fracture. The patient has had progressively worsening vomiting over the past 2 days and an increasingly distended abdomen. There is no history of diarrhea or ill contacts.

Past Medical History: No significant chronic illnesses

Medications: None

Allergies: None known

Physical Examination: Pale with cool extremities, abdomen rigid and distended with absent bowel sounds; no evidence of bruising, but tenderness to palpation and involuntary guarding; liver and spleen cannot be palpated.

Progression

Patient is now unresponsive.

Repeat Vital Signs

Pulse: Absent

Heart Rate: 100

Respiratory Rate: 6

Blood Pressure: 50/25

ASK YOURSELF

■ What is the patient's physiologic status now?

Decompensated shock with impending respiratory failure. *Respiratory failure* is defined as the state of inadequate oxygenation, ventilation, or both.

■ What is the most likely diagnosis?

Nonaccidental trauma involving either or both closed head injury and blunt abdominal trauma. Child abuse is a common mechanism in the critically ill child. The leading cause of death in victims of child abuse is head trauma. In one series of patients, 80% of all deaths due to head trauma in children younger than 2 years were the result of abuse. The second leading cause of death is inflicted abdominal trauma, with an estimated mortality rate of 40% to 50%. These patients often have a delayed presentation because initial symptoms such as poor feeding or listlessness often are mild. A high index of suspicion should be maintained when children present with nonspecific signs and symptoms and an unclear etiology of their injuries.[4]

■ What interventions are needed at this time? What complications might be expected?

Interventions:

- Begin BMV with 100% O_2 using cricoid pressure.
- Prepare for RSI.
- Institute cervical spine precautions.
- Continue volume expansion with second **intravenous bolus of 20 mL/kg of normal saline or lactated Ringer** delivered over 2 to 3 minutes.
- RSI
  1. #2 Miller or # 2 Macintosh blade, 4.5 uncuffed ET tube
  2. Preoxygenation
  3. Cricoid pressure
  4. **Lidocaine 1 mg/kg IV** reduces the increase in intracranial pressure that occurs with laryngoscopy and should be given as an adjunct in suspected head trauma.
  5. **Atropine 0.02 mg/kg IV** reduces bradycardia from vagal stimulation that occurs with laryngoscopy or hypoxia.
  6. **Midazolam 0.1 mg/kg IV** or **etomidate 0.3 mg/kg IV** acts as a sedative agent to induce unconsciousness; a side effect of midazolam is hypotension, so a sedative without cardiovascular effects, such as etomidate, may be preferred. Thiopental should be avoided because of association with hypotension.
  7. **Succinylcholine 1 to 1.5 mg/kg IV** or **rocuronium 0.6 to 1 mg/kg IV** to induce paralysis for intubation.
- Attach and read end-tidal CO_2 monitor.
- Call for chest radiograph to confirm ET tube placement.
- Secure ET tube and place NG tube.
- Draw blood for ABGs, CBC, electrolytes, coagulation studies, and type and cross for blood products.

Potential Complications:

- The risk for aspiration is great, especially in a patient with a distended abdomen. Cricoid pressure should help avoid this complication.

Repeat Vital Signs

Heart Rate: 150 with very weak pulses

Respiratory Rate: 20 on ventilator

Blood Pressure: 70/40

Oxygen Saturation: 100% on 100% O_2 by ventilator

Initial Laboratory Values

ABG: pH 7.15, Pco_2 25, Po_2 170, HCO_3^- 30, base excess –17

Hemoglobin: 6.2 g/dL

Progression

Successful intubation with 4.5 ET tube confirmed with end-tidal CO_2 monitor. Patient develops a generalized motor seizure.

ASK YOURSELF

- **What interventions are needed at this time?**
  - Reassess ABCs and obtain a rapid glucose determination.
  - Continue seizure control with **lorazepam 0.1 mg/kg IV/IO**
  - Initiate third bolus of isotonic fluid (20 mL/kg) or begin blood products if available.
  - If no response to bolus, consider initiation of **dopamine infusion 10 mcg/kg/min** to maintain blood pressure.
  - Arrange for cervical spine series, head CT, and abdominal CT.
  - Obtain emergent surgical consultation for suspected solid-organ injury. Neurosurgical consultation may be necessary as well depending on results of the head CT and cervical spine series.
  - When stabilized, initiate nonaccidental trauma work-up: Skeletal survey (to screen for occult fractures), ophthalmologic consultation (to assess for retinal hemorrhages), and involvement of social services/law enforcement.

Progression

Glucose is 98, and seizures continue despite lorazepam 0.2 mg/kg IV.

ASK YOURSELF

- **What is the most likely cause of this seizure?**

  In this patient with suspected nonaccidental trauma, the most likely cause of seizure is increased intracranial pressure from blood or edema. Other etiologies to be considered are CNS infection, metabolic derangement (especially hypoglycemia), an ingestion, hypoxia/hypercarbia, other nontraumatic causes of increased intracranial pressure (due to a tumor, hydrocephalus/ventriculoperitoneal shunt malfunction, or nontraumatic bleeding), and seizure disorder.

- **What interventions are needed at this time?**
  - Reassess and support ABCs.
  - Load with either fosphenytoin 20 mg PE/kg IV or phenobarbital 20 mg/kg IV.

Objectives of This Scenario

1. Recognize seizure as the presentation of closed head injury and nonaccidental trauma.

The differential diagnosis of seizure in a 2-year-old was discussed. Early determination of blood glucose is essential to rule out hypoglycemia, which can be rapidly treated. Patients with suspected meningitis should be treated with empiric antibiotics immediately, without delay for diagnostic testing. Trauma is a common cause of seizure in pediatric patients; when the history does not fit the presentation, the diagnosis of nonaccidental trauma must be entertained. Febrile seizures and seizure disorder are common causes of seizures in childhood. However, these are diagnoses of exclusion and may be considered only after the more serious etiologies are ruled out. Priorities in the initial management are support of the ABCs and anticonvulsant therapy beginning with benzodiazepines. Early CT imaging and subsequent neurosurgical intervention when indicated are essential.

2. Recognize and manage decompensated shock.

The patient in this scenario presents with a blood pressure consistent with decompensated shock. The calculation for the minimum systolic blood pressure of a child is (2 × age [in years]) + 70 mm Hg. The cause for decompensated shock in this case is from hypovolemia due to blood loss in the abdomen. It should be emphasized that intracranial hemorrhage in a child with fused sutures should not result in sufficient intravascular blood loss to cause hypotension.

Although blunt abdominal trauma is an infrequent manifestation of identified cases of abuse (<1%), it is the second leading cause of death after head trauma.[5,6] It can be difficult to recognize, often with delayed presentation and vague symptoms. The treatment for decompensated shock is two or three sequential boluses of 20 mL/kg of isotonic crystalloid (either normal saline or lactated Ringer) followed by plasma or whole blood. If the patient is still hypotensive, vasoactive agents must be initiated to aid in maintaining blood pressure and systemic perfusion. Indications for operative intervention include hemodynamic instability despite maximal resuscitation, transfusion of greater than 50% of total blood volume, radiographic evidence of pneumoperitoneum, intraperitoneal bladder rupture, grade V renovascular injury, gunshot wound to the abdomen, evisceration of intraperitoneal or stomach contents, and signs of peritonitis.[7]

3. Recognize and manage impending respiratory failure.

The patient in this scenario progressed from grunting and tachypnea to impending respiratory failure. At this point the child needed assistance with BMV and endotracheal intubation. With a distended abdomen, the patient is at high risk for vomiting and aspiration. To help prevent this, cricoid pressure should be applied and maintained until ET tube placement is confirmed. For medications and RSI techniques, please see "Evaluation and Management: Airway."

References

1. Recognition of respiratory failure and shock. In: Hazinski MF, ed. *PALS Provider Manual.* Dallas, Tex: American Heart Association; 2002:23.
2. Fluid therapy and medications for shock and cardiac arrest. In: Hazinski MF, ed. *PALS Provider Manual.* Dallas, Tex: American Heart Association; 2002:128.
3. Vascular access. In: Hazinski MF, ed. *PALS Provider Manual.* Dallas, Tex: American Heart Association; 2002:155.
4. Berkowitz CD, Carroll ML. Child maltreatment. In: Gausche-Hill M, Fuchs S, Yamamoto L, eds. *APLS: The Pediatric Emergency Medicine Resource.* 4th ed. Sudbury, Mass: American Academy of Pediatrics, American College of Emergency Physicians, Jones and Bartlett Publishing Co; 2004:330.
5. Cooper A, Floyd T, Barlow B, et al. Major blunt abdominal trauma due to child abuse. *J Trauma.* 1988;28:1483-1487.
6. Jain AM. Emergency department evaluation of child abuse. *Emerg Med Clin North Am.* 1999;17:575-593.
7. Tepas JJ, Fallat ME, Moriarty TM. Trauma. In: Gausche-Hill M, Fuchs S, Yamamoto L, eds. *APLS: The Pediatric Emergency Medicine Resource.* 4th ed. Sudbury, Mass: American Academy of Pediatrics, American College of Emergency Physicians, Jones and Bartlett Publishing Co; 2004:310.

SCENARIO #35

Headache

Kathryn D. Emery, MD

Brief Presenting History

A 7-year-old boy presents with a chief complaint of headache of 4 days' duration that became worse this morning. His parents report that for the past day, he has complained of nausea, dizziness, and blurry vision. They have brought him in now because after vomiting this morning, he has just been moaning and crying.

Pediatric Assessment Triangle

Appearance: Rocking and moaning

Work of Breathing: Crying but otherwise breathing easily

Circulation to the Skin: Flushed

Initial Vital Signs

Pulse: 120

Blood Pressure: 148/100

Respiratory Rate: 22

Temperature: 37°C (98.6°F) tympanic

Physical Examination on Arrival to the Emergency Department

Airway: Patent, moving air easily

Breathing: Lungs clear, no crackles or rales

Circulation: Capillary refill less than 2 seconds with strong peripheral pulses; tachycardia, no murmurs; symmetric, strong radial and femoral pulses, no bruits

Disability: Responds to voice but unable to follow commands

ASK YOURSELF

- **What is the initial assessment? What is the patient's physiologic status?**

  The patient presents with altered mental status and hypertension.

- **What is Cushing triad? Does this patient have it?**

  Cushing triad is a late finding of increased intracranial pressure characterized by hypertension, bradycardia, and irregular respirations.[1] This patient has hypertension only.

- **What could be causing his altered mental status?**

  In general, altered mental status has a wide differential that most commonly includes infection, specifically meningitis or encephalitis; trauma, head injury; ingestion; and metabolic and uremic encephalopathy. See "Evaluation and Management: Neurologic Emergencies, Altered Mental Status" for a more complete list.

  In this patient, hypertension, either primary or secondary, must be strongly considered.

Additional History and Physical Examination Findings

The parents deny any fever in the patient other than at the time he had a sore throat 2 weeks earlier. The patient has had slightly decreased oral intake; parents are unaware of any change in urinary pattern. There is no history of trauma. There are no medications in the house, and because the patient has been in bed for the past 24 hours, the parents are fairly certain he has not had access to any drugs other than acetaminophen.

Past Medical History: This healthy child has no history of respiratory problems. Birth history is unremarkable (no history of umbilical artery catheterization). The patient has no previous history of headaches.

Medications: The patient takes no medications on a routine basis. He has no known allergies.

Physical Examination: Four extremity blood pressures are approximately equal (140s/110s). There is no evidence of upper respiratory tract infection, oropharyngeal or neck trauma, or neck stiffness, and Kernig and Brudzinski signs are negative. Ophthalmoscopic examination reveals papilledema.

ASK YOURSELF

■ What is the most likely diagnosis? What are the goals for emergent treatment?

The patient has signs of increased intracranial pressure—hypertension and papilledema—yet his vital signs, other than blood pressure, are within normal limits. Although hypertensive encephalopathy is not a common problem in pediatric patients, it is an important diagnosis to consider in this case. The results from the investigations outlined later will be helpful in establishing this diagnosis. The goal is to determine the etiology and duration of hypertension, which will dictate how aggressively the hypertension should be alleviated. Identifying an underlying condition that has caused the hypertension is essential. Because this patient displays signs of end-organ involvement (ie, altered mental status), the need for rapid intervention is indicated.

■ Differentiate between hypertension, hypertensive urgency, and hypertensive emergency.

Hypertension is characterized by systolic, diastolic, or mean arterial pressure greater than 2 standard deviations above the mean for the age and sex of the patient as measured on at least three occasions.

Hypertensive urgency is characterized by severe elevations in systolic and/or diastolic blood pressure but without signs of end-organ damage.

Hypertensive emergency is characterized by elevations in both systolic and diastolic blood pressure with evidence of end-organ damage such as encephalopathy, congestive heart failure, pulmonary edema, or acute renal failure.[2]

■ How is blood pressure most accurately measured?

It is important to use the proper pediatric blood pressure cuff size. The bladder should be two thirds of the length of upper arm and must encompass the circumference of the arm. Cuffs that are too small can lead to inaccurately elevated readings.

■ What interventions are needed at this time? What complications might be expected?

Interventions:

- Oxygenate, provide quiet and comfort, elevate head of bed.
- Place the patient on a cardiorespiratory monitor with pulse oximetry.
- Check sphygmomanometer cuff size.
- Provide intravenous access, but do not administer fluids.
- Laboratory studies: electrolytes, BUN/creatinine, urinalysis/urine cultures, CBC, chest radiograph, head CT, *Streptococcus* screen
- Administer **sodium nitroprusside, diazoxide, labetolol,** or **esmolol.** All are good antihypertensive agents in this case. Any child with findings consistent with a hypertensive emergency should have his or her blood pressure controlled with an intravenous infusion. The blood pressure should be reduced initially to a mean arterial pressure of 120 mm

Hg in patients whose initial mean pressure is higher. It has been recommended that mean arterial pressure not be lowered below 100 mm Hg during the initial 24 to 48 hours of therapy in adults with hypertensive emergencies.[3]

- Consider placing an arterial line for continuous blood pressure monitoring.

Potential Complications:

- If intravenous fluids are given, patient develops congestive heart failure or pulmonary edema.
- Stroke ensues if hypertension is not controlled.
- If hypertension is chronic and aggressively medicated, hypotension can occur, which can result in ischemia, especially of the brain and heart.

Repeat Vital Signs

Pulse: 109

Blood Pressure: 130/100

Respiratory Rate: 22

Oxygen Saturation: 97%

Progression

Patient develops generalized tonic-clonic seizure activity.

ASK YOURSELF

- **What interventions are needed at this time? What complications might be expected?**

Interventions:

- Reassess ABCs and treat seizure with **lorazepam 0.1 mg/kg IV**
- Consider increasing the antihypertensive drug dose in use or adding a second agent.

Potential Complications:

- Seizure persists; seizures may be recalcitrant without blood pressure control.
- Hypotension, secondary to antihypertensive drug administration
- Aspiration and subsequent respiratory insufficiency leading to need for intubation

Progression

Seizure persists.

Repeat Vital Signs

Pulse: 132

Blood Pressure: 135/97

Respiratory Rate: 30 and shallow

Oxygen Saturation: 89%

ASK YOURSELF

- **What interventions are needed at this time? What complications might be expected?**

Interventions:

- Increase oxygen delivery; determine if airway is maintainable.
- Continue monitoring blood pressure.
- Repeat **lorazepam**; consider **fosphenytoin 20 mg PE/kg IV.**

Potential Complication:

- Seizure persists, requiring phenobarbital, may lead to respiratory arrest necessitating intubation.

Progression

Detectable seizure activity stops.

Repeat Vital Signs

Pulse: 115

Blood Pressure: 128/89

Respiratory Rate: 18

Oxygen Saturation: 97%

ASK YOURSELF

- **What interventions are needed at this time? What complications might be expected?**

Interventions:

- Continue to monitor ABCs and blood pressure.
- Place arterial line if not already done.
- Monitor urine output; place Foley catheter.

Possible Complications:

- Hypotension, requiring adjustment of antihypertensive agent
- Stroke from prolonged hypertension

What are some of the causes of hypertension in children?

In contrast to hypertension in adults, hypertension in children is usually secondary to a disease process. Among these are renal causes such as glomerulonephritis and renovascular disease; endocrine disorders including pheochromocytoma and neuroblastoma; neurologic disease such as meningoencephalitis, tumor, and increased intracranial pressure; cardiovascular disease including aortic thrombosis and coarctation of the aorta; and drugs such as cocaine, amphetamines, and phenlyephrine.[3]

Poststreptococcal glomerulonephritis is the most common type of glomerulonephritis seen in the United States in children, usually between the ages of 3 and 7 years. It typically presents with the onset of nephritis 8 to 14 days after streptococcal pharyngitis, as in this child. In most patients, regression of the disease is good with treatment of blood pressure, which usually returns to normal within 3 to 6 weeks.[4]

Objectives of This Scenario

1. Recognize hypertension as a cause of altered mental status in a pediatric patient.

The differential diagnosis of altered mental status in pediatrics is large. See "Evaluation and Management: Neurologic Emergencies, Altered Mental Status" for a more complete list. Although uncommon, hypertension and hypertensive encephalopathy must be considered. It is important to consider not only the magnitude of elevation in blood pressure but also the percent change from baseline. The history and physical examination in this patient make more common causes of altered mental status less likely.

2. Recognize and treat a hypertensive emergency.

Commonly used drugs for acute hypertension are listed in Table 1.[5] The choice of drug to be used is determined by etiology and duration of hypertension.

Sodium nitroprusside is contraindicated in renal insufficiency predominantly because thiocyanate poisoning can occur. Both **esmolol** and **labetalol** should be avoided in patients with asthma because of their β_2 effects.

Management of hypertension begins with support of the ABCs. The blood pressure should be lowered promptly but gradually. In adults, the mean arterial pressure is lowered by approximately 25% or the

Table 1.
Commonly Used Agents to Treat Acute Hypertension

Drug	Mode of Action	Dose	Onset of Action
Diazoxide	Direct dilation of arterioles	1 to 3 mg/kg to maximum of 150 mg IV push	1 to 5 minutes
Sodium nitroprusside	Direct arterial and venous dilation, reduces preload and afterload	Continuous infusion of 0.3 to 0.5 mcg/kg/min, triate to maximum dose of 10 mcg/kg/min	Immediate
Esmolol	β-Blocker	500 mcg/kg load over 1 minute, then 50 to 250 mcg/kg/min continuous infusion	Immediate
Labetalol	α/β-Blocker	0.2 to 1 mg/kg dose; maximum dose 20 mg or 0.4 to 1 mg/kg/hr continuous infusion	5 Minutes

diastolic pressure is reduced to 100 to 110 mm Hg over minutes to hours, depending on the etiology and extent of involvement.[6] In a patient presenting with headaches and vomiting due to hypertension, the blood pressure may be lowered over hours, whereas hypertension in the actively seizing patient or one with impending herniation requires more aggressive treatment and alleviation of hypertension over a few minutes.

While treating acute hypertension, it is important to carefully monitor the patient for hypotension and neurologic deficits. A rapid reduction in blood pressure can result in permanent neurologic damage. This can result in CNS infarctions. The areas particularly susceptible are those perfused by end arteries such as the visual cortex.[3]

3. Manage hypertensive encephalopathy.

In hypertensive encephalopathy, autoregulation of cerebral blood flow is disrupted, which leads to either overregulation with exaggerated vasospasm and *ischemic injury* **or** underregulation with increased cerebral flow and *cerebral edema*.

No single symptom or sign is diagnostic. Symptoms include nausea and vomiting, headaches, altered mental status, visual disturbances, seizures, and stroke. The diagnosis is confirmed by rapid improvement after a decrease in blood pressure.

Treatment of hypertensive encephalopathy is aimed at reducing blood pressure in a rapid fashion until signs of ongoing end-organ damage resolve. For this reason, fast-acting intravenous agents with a short duration of action are considered first-line therapies.[5] Seizures may be resistant to traditional seizure therapy with benzodiazepines. Seizure control is unlikely until hypertension is controlled.

References

1. Battan FK, Anderson MS. Emergencies and injuries In: Hay WW, Hayward AR, Levin MJ, et al, eds. *Current Pediatric Diagnosis and Treatment.* 16th ed. New York, NY: Lange Medical Books/McGraw-Hill, 2003:320.
2. Fivush B, Neu A, Furth S. Acute hypertensive crises in children: emergencies and urgencies. *Curr Opin Pediatr.* 1997;9:233-236.
3. Groshong T. Hypertensive crisis in children. *Pediatr Ann.* 1996;25:368-376.
4. Eddy A. Glomerular disorders. In: Rudolph CD, Rudolph AM, Hostetter MK, et al, eds. *Rudolph's Pediatrics.* 21st ed. New York, NY: McGraw-Hill; 2002:1677-1678.
5. Sagraves R. Hypertensive emergencies in children. *Pediatr Pharmacol.* 2000;14:312-316.
6. Calhoun DA, Oparil S. Treatment of hypertensive crisis. *N Engl J Med.* 1990;323:1177-1183.

SCENARIO #36

Trauma – Altered Mental Status

Tien T. Vu, MD

Brief Presenting History

An 18-month-old boy was an unrestrained backseat passenger involved in a roll-over motor vehicle collision. The boy was found 10 feet from the car by paramedics. He was alert and crying at the scene and vomited once en route to the hospital. He arrived in the emergency department 30 minutes after the trauma.

Pediatric Assessment Triangle

Appearance: Irritable, vigorous

Work of Breathing: Strong cry, respirations unlabored

Circulation to the Skin: Flushed, well perfused

Initial Vital Signs

Pulse: 150

Respiratory Rate: 20

Blood Pressure: 105/70

Temperature: 37°C (98.6°F) tympanic

ASK YOURSELF

■ **What are the normal heart rate and blood pressure for an 18-month-old?**

The median blood pressure for an 18-month-old is approximately 96/60, with lower extremity blood pressures usually measuring 10 to 14 mm Hg higher. The normal heart rate range for a child of this age is 80 to 150 but may be increased with crying, pain, dehydration, shock, or fever.[1,2] See Appendix A.

Physical Examination on Arrival to the Emergency Department

Airway: Patent, moving air freely, with minimal secretions in mouth

Breathing: No work of breathing, but slightly irregular because of crying; clear breath sounds bilaterally with symmetric chest rise

Circulation: Skin flushed, capillary refill time 1 to 2 seconds peripherally with 1+ to 2+ palpable distal pulses

ASK YOURSELF

■ **Where would you best be able to feel the central pulse on this 18-month-old patient?**

Femoral and brachial pulses are easily palpable in infants and young children; carotid pulses can be more difficult to palpate in younger children because of their body habitus.[1]

Disability: Eyes open to stimulation. Moving all extremities equally with no obvious deformities, but large parietal/occipital scalp hematoma noted

ASK YOURSELF

- **What is the initial assessment? What is the patient's physiologic status?**

  The patient presents with altered mental status (irritability), and there is concern for closed head injury; vital signs are currently within normal limits for age.

- **What physical examination findings are important specifically in children with concern for a closed head injury?**

  In the emergency care setting, management of suspected traumatic brain injury in children focuses on prevention of secondary insults caused by hypoxia/ischemia from inadequate oxygenation, ventilation, or perfusion. Appropriate management of the ABCs in the trauma patient with head injury is crucial. Airway and breathing assessment is the first step. Respiratory abnormalities such as apnea, Cheyne-Stokes respirations (respirations with increasing and then decreasing depth, alternating with apneic periods), or hyperventilation can signal severe neurologic dysfunction and may necessitate early airway protection.[3] An abbreviated neurologic evaluation using the AVPU method (see Scenario 34, page 258) or modified Glasgow Coma Scale (GCS) score (see Appendix C) is appropriate for pediatric trauma victims.[4] Pupillary responses and signs of head injury such as skull deformity or large scalp hematoma, especially in young children, should increase suspicion for intracranial injury.[5-7]

Additional History and Physical Examination Findings

Paramedics witnessed some twitching of extremities that lasted a few seconds while en route.

Past Medical History: Born full term, but developmentally delayed by report; no history of a seizure disorder

Medications: None

Allergies: None known

Physical examination: Pulse oximetry 90% on room air. Child is irritable, with inconsolable crying. Boggy hematoma is noted on left parietal/occipital scalp; it is difficult to assess for underlying skull deformity. Pupils are 2 mm bilaterally and reactive. Gurgling oral secretions with crying are noted. Abdomen is soft and flat with minimal bowel sounds, with a small area of ecchymosis on left side. There are a few abrasions on face and arms. The child is on a backboard without a cervical collar and spontaneously moving extremities.

ASK YOURSELF

- **What interventions are needed at this time? What complications might be expected?**

  Interventions:

  - Airway management: Clear oral secretions with suctioning and provide supplemental oxygen.
  - Place cervical collar or maintain manual in-line cervical spine immobilization.
  - Place the patient on a cardiorespiratory monitor with pulse oximetry and blood pressure measurement.
  - Attempt intravenous access.
  - Notify trauma surgery and neurosurgery.
  - Trauma series radiographs: lateral cervical spine, chest, and pelvis
  - Complete primary and secondary surveys.

  Potential Complications:

  - First intravenous access attempt unsuccessful. Given patient's apparent stability, another attempt to establish peripheral intravenous access should be made. Intraosseous line placement would be appropriate if quick access is unobtainable and patient is deteriorating.

- **What laboratory studies would be helpful at this time?**

  For the head-injured and multitrauma patient, hemoglobin/hematocrit, PT/PTT, type and hold, and possibly venous blood gases would be helpful. Amylase has not proved to be particularly useful in pediatric blunt abdominal trauma in the immediate, emergency setting.[8] However, at many institutions, amylase and liver function tests are obtained in the work-up of trauma patients and may be considered.[9]

Repeat Vital Signs

Pulse: 80

Respiratory Rate: 12

Blood Pressure: 130/80

Oxygen Saturation: 100% with face mask oxygen

Progression

The patient has stopped crying and now responds with minimal movements only to painful stimulation. Respirations have become markedly irregular with prolonged apneic episodes. The left pupil is 5 mm dilated, laterally deviated, and minimally reactive; the right pupil is 3 mm and reactive.

ASK YOURSELF

■ What is the patient's physiologic status now?

Impending respiratory failure caused by severe neurologic disability

■ What are the most likely diagnoses?

Cushing triad of bradycardia, hypertension, and respiratory irregularity is a late finding caused by increased intracranial pressure. Asymmetric pupils signal uncal herniation from a large intracranial lesion such as a hematoma or severe cerebral edema causing impingement of the third cranial nerve.[10]

■ What interventions are needed at this time, while neurosurgery is en route? What complications might be expected?

Interventions:

- BMV with 100% O_2 using cricoid pressure; prepare for endotracheal intubation.
- Intraosseous placement if no other access available
- RSI[11,12]
  1. #1 or #2 Miller blade, 4.0 or 4.5 ET tube
  2. Preoxygenate
  3. Cricoid pressure
  4. Maintain cervical spine immobilization
  5. **Atropine 0.02 mg/kg IV/IO/ET** (This medication, given to blunt vagal response to laryngoscopy and intubation, is optional in this age group, however, given the patient's preintubation bradycardia, its use is recommended in this case; minimum 0.1 mg/dose; maximum 0.5 mg in a child, 1 mg in an adolescent.)
  6. **Lidocaine 1 mg/kg IV/IO/ET** (to blunt elevation of intracranial pressure during intubation)
  7. **Etomidate 0.3 mg/kg IV**
  8. **Rocuronium 0.6 to 1 mg/kg IV**
- Confirm ET tube placement by physical examination, end-tidal CO_2 detector, and chest radiograph.
- Mild hyperventilation; aim for Pco_2 between 30 and 35 mm Hg for acute herniation.[13]
- **Mannitol 0.25 to 1 g/kg IV** for increased intracranial pressure[14]
- Secure ET tube and place NG tube and Foley catheter.
- Consider central line placement if intravenous access is tenuous or inadequate.
- Isotonic fluid resuscitation as needed to maintain adequate blood pressure and cerebral perfusion[4]
- Obtain head CT scan when stabilized; consider CT of abdomen as well.

Potential Complications:

- Vomiting, especially if no cricoid pressure used
- Unable to visualize cords if not properly suctioned or jaw thrust inadequate. May have to remove cervical collar and maintain manual in-line cervical immobilization while intubating.
- Improperly positioned tube such as right mainstem or esophageal intubation
- Failure to place NG tube results in abdominal distention and impaired ventilation.
- Perfusion inadequate despite 40 mL/kg of normal saline or lactated Ringer. Colloid administration is recommended.

Repeat Vital Signs

Heart Rate: 140

Respiratory Rate: 30 (bagged)

Blood Pressure: 75/35

Progression

Pupils are equal but sluggishly reactive. Distal pulses are weak with prolonged capillary refill time of 4 seconds. Abdomen is slightly more distended despite nasogastric tube to suction.

ASK YOURSELF

- **What is your additional diagnosis now?**

Increased heart rate, lowered blood pressure, and prolonged capillary refill in the setting of trauma are most likely due to hypovolemic/hemorrhagic shock.[15] Potential sites of blood loss in this patient include the abdomen and the cranial vault. Abdominal ecchymosis and distention on examination, in addition to mechanism of injury, are consistent with blunt abdominal trauma and possible intra-abdominal hemorrhage. Neurologic findings of increased intracranial pressure can be due to massive intracranial hemorrhage. In contrast to adults, hypovolemic shock from intracranial bleeding is possible in infants and young children because of the compressibility of the brain and expandable nature of the cranial vault. At 18 months, most patients have fused sutures, making it unlikely that blood losses sufficient to cause hypotension would be caused by intracranial bleeding alone.

Another type of shock that is unlikely in this patient is neurogenic/spinal shock caused by a complete spinal cord injury. This produces loss of sympathetic tone resulting in bradycardia and hypotension.

- **What do you do now?**

Obtain a repeat hematocrit. Fluid resuscitate with isotonic fluids, up to 40 mL/kg, and then consider giving packed RBCs for further resuscitation. If volume resuscitation stabilizes perfusion and blood pressure, the patient may go to radiology for CT evaluation. Failure to stabilize hemodynamic status would necessitate immediate surgical intervention (probable exploratory laparotomy) to elucidate and treat ongoing blood loss. Consider FAST ultrasound examination prior to transfer to operating room to confirm the presence of intra-abdominal fluid.

Objectives of This Scenario

1. Identify closed head injury in children.

Children who have been ejected during motor vehicle collisions are at high risk for closed head injury. Impact trauma often produces external signs of head injury, but intracranial injury can also result from acceleration-deceleration or angular-rotational forces that may not be immediately obvious. Severe traumatic brain injury results in a GCS score of 8 or below and may produce obvious skull deformities or scalp hematomas, seizures, and focal neurologic deficits. Other common symptoms of closed head injury in young children include persistent vomiting, unusual behavior, and lethargy.[7]

2. Manage severe traumatic brain injury in children.

Once the primary brain injury has occurred, emergency management must focus on prevention of secondary insults.[16]

- **Maintain normocarbia and adequate oxygen delivery.** Because these patients cannot adequately protect their airways, early intubation of patients with severe head injury is recommended using RSI. Mild hyperventilation (P_{CO_2} 30 to 35 mm Hg) can be useful in the setting of elevated intracranial pressure or when signs of impending brain herniation are present. Lower P_{CO_2} levels can cause reactive vasoconstriction to a degree that would restrict cerebral blood flow and result in tissue ischemia.[13]
- **Avoid hypotension.** Hypotension can cause cerebral hypoperfusion resulting in secondary brain injury. *Cerebral perfusion pressure* is defined as the mean arterial pressure minus intracranial pressure. A cerebral perfusion pressure of greater than 40 mm Hg in children should be maintained.[17] In the face of increased intracranial pressure from brain injury and adequate volume resuscitation, vasopressors should be administered in the normovolemic, hypotensive patient.
- **Hyperosmolar therapy for evidence of elevated intracranial pressure.** Mannitol is effective for control of increased intracranial pressure, with therapeutic boluses ranging from 0.25 to 1 g/kg. Serum osmolarity should be maintained below 320 mOsm/L. Hypertonic saline also may be effective, although its use is not well studied in children. Saline 3% can be given as a bolus or as a continuous infusion at 0.1 to 1 mL/kg/hr, with monitoring for serum sodium and osmolarity.[14]

- **Other interventions for elevated intracranial pressure.** While awaiting definitive neurosurgical interventions for increased intracranial pressure, other possible inventions include head elevation to 30 degrees and barbiturate coma induction. The effectiveness of mild to moderate hypothermia for the treatment of traumatic brain injury has not been established in children.[14]
- **Seizure control.** For seizures in the emergency setting, anticonvulsants such as phenytoin or benzodiazepines may be used. Seizures increase intracranial pressure by increasing metabolic demand, causing the Valsalva effect, changing blood pressure, and releasing neurotoxic excitatory amino acids.[16] Currently, there are limited data on the prophylactic administration of anticonvulsant medications in the setting of pediatric head injury, and such use may be institution dependent.

References

1. Dieckmann RA. Pediatric assessment. In: Gausche-Hill M, Fuchs S, Yamamoto L, eds. *APLS: The Pediatric Emergency Medicine Resource.* 4th ed. Sudbury, Mass: American Academy of Pediatrics, American College of Emergency Physicians, Jones and Bartlett Publishing Co; 2004:40.
2. Silverman BK. Practical information. In: Fleisher GR, Ludwig S, eds. *Textbook of Pediatric Emergency Medicine.* 4th ed. Philadelphia, Pa: Lippincott Williams & Wilkins; 2000:1943.
3. Issacman DJ, Trainor JL, Rothrock SG. Central nervous system. In: Gausche-Hill M, Fuchs S, Yamamoto L, eds. *APLS: The Pediatric Emergency Medicine Resource.* 4th ed. Sudbury, Mass: American Academy of Pediatrics, American College of Emergency Physicians, Jones and Bartlett Publishing Co; 2004:148-150.
4. Tepas JJ, Fallat ME, Moriarty TM. Trauma. In: Gausche-Hill M, Fuchs S, Yamamoto L, eds. *APLS: The Pediatric Emergency Medicine Resource.* 4th ed. Sudbury, Mass: American Academy of Pediatrics, American College of Emergency Physicians, Jones and Bartlett Publishing Co; 2004:282-321.
5. Greenes DS, Schutzman SA. Clinical significance of scalp abnormalities in asymptomatic head-injured infants. *Pediatr Emerg Care.* 2001;17:88-92.
6. Gruskin KD, Schutzman SA. Head trauma in children younger than 2 years: are there predictors for complications? *Arch Pediatr Adolesc Med.* 1999;153:15-20.
7. Palchak MJ, Holmes JF, Vance CW, et al. A decision rule for identifying children at low risk for brain injuries after blunt head trauma. *Ann Emerg Med.* 2003;42:492-506.
8. Jobst MA, Canty TG, Lynch FP. Management of pancreatic injury in pediatric blunt abdominal trauma. *J Pediatr Surg.* 1999;34:818-823.
9. Holmes JF, Sokolove PE, Brant WE, et al. Identification of children with intra-abdominal injuries after blunt trauma. *Ann Emerg Med.* 2002;39(5):500-509.
10. Greenes DS, Madsen JR. Neurotrauma. In: Fleisher GR, Ludwig S, eds. *Textbook of Pediatric Emergency Medicine.* 4th ed. Philadelphia, Pa: Lippincott Williams & Wilkins; 2000:1271-1296.
11. King BR, King C, Coates WC. Critical procedures. In: Gausche-Hill M, Fuchs S, Yamamoto L, eds. *APLS: The Pediatric Emergency Medicine Resource.* 4th ed. Sudbury, Mass: American Academy of Pediatrics, American College of Emergency Physicians, Jones and Bartlett Publishing Co; 2004:702-707.
12. Adelson PD, Bratton SL, Carney NA, et al. Guidelines for the acute medical management of severe traumatic brain injury in infants, children, and adolescents. Chapter 9. Use of sedation and neuromuscular blockade in the treatment of severe pediatric traumatic brain injury. *Pediatr Crit Care Med.* 2003;4(3S):S34-S37.
13. Adelson PD, Bratton SL, Carney NA, et al. Guidelines for the acute medical management of severe traumatic brain injury in infants, children, and adolescents. Chapter 12. Use of hyperventilation in the acute management of severe pediatric traumatic brain injury. *Pediatr Crit Care Med.* 2003;4(3S):S45-S48.
14. Adelson PD, Bratton SL, Carney NA, et al. Guidelines for the acute medical management of severe traumatic brain injury in infants, children, and adolescents. Chapter 11. Use of hyperosmolar therapy in the management of severe pediatric traumatic brain injury. *Pediatr Crit Care Med.* 2003:4(3S):S40-S44.
15. Fitzmaurice L, Gerardi MJ. Cardiovascular system. In: Gausche-Hill M, Fuchs S, Yamamoto L, eds. *APLS: The Pediatric Emergency Medicine Resource.* 4th ed. Sudbury, Mass: American Academy of Pediatrics, American College of Emergency Physicians, Jones and Bartlett Publishing Co; 2004:137-138.
16. Mazzola CA, Adelson PD. Critical care management of head trauma in children. *Crit Care Med.* 2002;30(11S):S393-S401.
17. Adelson PD, Bratton SL, Carney NA, et al. Guidelines for the acute medical management of severe traumatic brain injury in infants, children, and adolescents. Chapter 8. Cerebral perfusion pressure. *Pediatr Crit Care Med.* 2003;4(3S):S31-S33.

SCENARIO #37

Trauma – Shock

Glenn Faries, MD

Brief Presenting History

A 7-year-old child is transported to the emergency department by his parents in a private vehicle. He was riding on his bicycle along some trails close to his house when he crashed.

Pediatric Assessment Triangle

Appearance: Awake and alert; conversing appropriately but anxious and pale

Breathing: Tachypneic without any evidence of respiratory distress

Circulation to the Skin: Pale and cool, somewhat mottled

Initial Vital Signs

Pulse: 178

Respiratory Rate: 45

Blood Pressure: 100/65

Temperature: 36.3°C (97.3°F) axillary

Oxygen Saturation: 91% in room air

ASK YOURSELF

- **How much should this 7-year-old weigh?**

  An estimated weight for a 7-year-old is 22 kg. Use the length-based Broselow Pediatric Emergency Tape, or a pediatric table (see Appendix A) to determine weight based on age.

Physical Examination on Arrival to the Emergency Department

Airway: Patent; blood at external nares and in mouth; one loose upper central incisor

Breathing: Tachypneic; no accessory muscle use; breath sounds full, without adventitious sounds bilaterally

Circulation: Cool and clammy; central capillary refill time 2 to 3 seconds, peripheral 4 seconds

Disability: Eyes open; pupils equal, round, and reactive from 4 mm to 2 mm

ASK YOURSELF

- **What is the initial assessment? What is the patient's physiologic status?**

  The patient presents in compensated shock, as manifest by significant tachycardia and compromised perfusion to the skin with normal blood pressure for age. See Appendix A.

- **What is the most likely cause of his compensated shock?**

  Shock, whether compensated or decompensated, in the setting of trauma most frequently implies hypovolemia resulting from blood loss. The blood loss can be external, such as with open wounds, or it can be internal, resulting from fractures of the large long bones (eg, femur). It also can result from internal injury to organs or to blood vessels. Cardiogenic shock, related to injury to the myocardium, is possible but lower on the list of differential diagnoses because of the lack of physical findings. Another possibility is neurogenic shock resulting from a lack of vascular tone caused by a head or spinal cord injury, but this is an uncommon finding in pediatric patients and unlikely in this patient without neurologic deficit. Soft tissue injuries (eg, burns) also can cause significant fluid shift resulting in hypovolemic, nonhemorrhagic shock.

- **What additional history and physical findings would help you establish the diagnosis?**

The mechanism of injury could be helpful; however, physiologic findings are usually more predicative of injury. If it is possible to assess where the child is feeling pain (eg, leg, abdomen, chest), this would be helpful. Careful examination of the chest is important. Diminished breath sounds in the face of respiratory distress indicate conditions that could require emergent intervention, such as a tension pneumothorax or hemothorax. Once his ABCs, including neurologic status, are assessed, examination of the abdomen and extremities could provide insights into the etiology of shock.

Additional History and Physical Examination Findings

The child was riding his bicycle with friends along single-track paths by his house. He reports wearing a helmet and remembers hitting a protruding root and then flipping over the handlebars, landing in some trees. He hit his abdomen on the handlebars. He was able to get up and walk at the scene and did not lose consciousness. He complains of abdominal, neck, and left knee pain.

Past Medical History: Asthma but otherwise negative

Medications: Fluticasone regularly, albuterol on an as-required basis

Immunizations: Up to date

Allergies: Peanuts

Physical Examination: The patient has a forehead contusion and facial abrasions without deformity. There is midline tenderness over C3 to C5. The abdomen has a large contusion in the epigastrium and left upper quadrant. The abdomen is slightly distended and tender to palpation throughout. The pelvis is stable, without crepitus. Genitalia are normal with no blood at the urethral meatus. There are multiple abrasions on the extremities and a laceration just below his left knee.

ASK YOURSELF

- **What interventions are needed at this time? What complications might be expected?**

Interventions:

- Immobilize cervical spine. See "Evaluation and Management: Trauma and Environmental Emergencies."
- Oxygen 100% on nonrebreather
- Place the patient on a cardiorespiratory monitor with pulse oximetry.
- Obtain vascular access; use two large-bore intravenous catheters if possible. Begin fluid resuscitation with **20 mL/kg normal saline**.
- Laboratory evaluation: CBC, type and cross, urinalysis; consider amylase/lipase, liver transaminases. Screening laboratories for blunt abdominal trauma differ across institutions and the data do not strongly support one, universally accepted approach.[1,2]
- Initial radiologic imaging: Chest radiograph and lateral neck and anteroposterior pelvis films

Potential Complications:

- Vomiting, requiring log roll (protect cervical spine) and suctioning
- Pulse oximeter not giving a reading because of poor perfusion
- Intravenous attempts unsuccessful, consider intraosseous placement

Repeat Vital Signs

Pulse: 192

Respiratory Rate: 48

Blood Pressure: Not obtainable

Oxygen Saturation: Not registering

Progression

The patient has become increasingly somnolent and intermittently agitated. He is more pale and diaphoretic. The breathing is rapid and shallow, with occasional grunting, and his abdomen is more distended.

ASK YOURSELF

■ What has happened?

The child has developed decompensated shock. He displays clinical evidence of inadequate organ perfusion, including mental status changes and diminished skin perfusion as manifested by the inability to pick up a reading on the pulse oximeter. His blood pressure has become unobtainable, indicating significant volume loss. As evidenced by his increasing respiratory difficulty, he is also experiencing impending respiratory failure. His level of consciousness has deteriorated to the point that he is unlikely to be able to maintain airway protective reflexes.

■ What interventions are needed at this time? What complications might be expected?

Interventions:

- Begin positive pressure ventilation with bag-mask and 100% O_2. Maintain in-line cervical-spine immobilization and apply cricoid pressure. Prepare for RSI.
- Obtain immediate vascular access. If attempts at intravenous access are unsuccessful, place an intraosseous line. Administer **normal saline 20 mL/kg** solution as rapidly as possible.
- Call for O-negative blood.
- RSI
  1. **Etomidate 0.3 mg/kg IV/IO** or **midazolam 0.1 mg/kg IV/IO**
  2. **Lidocaine 1 mg/kg IV/IO**
  3. **Rocuronium 0.6 to 1 mg/kg**
- Direct visualization of the larynx with a #2 blade
- Insert 5.5 ET tube.
- Auscultate chest.
- End-tidal CO_2 monitor
- Call for chest radiograph to confirm ET tube placement; secure ET tube.
- Place orogastric tube; an NG tube *must not be used* in a patient with evidence of midface trauma.
- Assess response to fluid bolus; repeat if necessary.
- Insert Foley catheter.

Potential Complications:

- Vomiting during intubation attempt, especially if no cricoid pressure: requires log roll and suctioning
- Right mainstem intubation
- Placement of NG tube instead of orogastric tube in patient with potential facial/basilar skull injury, resulting in intracranial complications
- Failure to adequately fluid resuscitate patient, resulting in inability to stabilize patient and ultimately pulseless electrical activity
- Attempts to place intraosseous line in injured leg, (if a fracture exists) leads to infiltration of fluids into soft tissues.
- Overaggressive bagging leads to pneumothorax.

Repeat Vital Signs

Pulse: 60 (sinus bradycardia)

Respiratory Rate: Bagged but oxygen saturation unobtainable

Blood Pressure: Unobtainable, femoral pulse only faintly palpable

ASK YOURSELF

■ What is the most likely cause of this patient's deterioration?

Causes include lack of adequate volume resuscitation and a postintubation complication as represented by the mnemonic DOPE[3]:

Displaced ET tube

Obstruction of tube

Pneumothorax

Equipment failure

- **What interventions are needed at this time?**
  - Reassess airway
  - Increase volume resuscitation. To crystalloid infusion add O-negative blood 10 mL/kg IV/IO rapidly.

Progression

Poor air exchange, diminished breath sounds bilaterally

ASK YOURSELF

- **What interventions are needed at this time?**
  - Suctioning ET tube yields a large amount of thick secretions.

Progression

There is return of oxygenation and improved circulation after the tube obstruction is cleared and volume resuscitation increased. After 60 mL/kg isotonic crystalloid and 20 mL/kg blood, the vital signs have stabilized.

Repeat Vital Signs

Pulse: 120

Respiratory Rate: Bagged

Blood Pressure: 105/65

Temperature: 36.2°C (97.2°F)

Oxygen Saturation: 100% in 100% O_2

Radiographic Results

Chest Radiograph: ET tube just above the carina without evidence of pneumothorax or parenchymal lung injury

Lateral Neck Film: Normal

Pelvis Film: Negative for fracture

ASK YOURSELF

- **What should be the next step in the management of this patient? How do you decide on disposition?**

  The child needs further work-up to determine the cause of his bleeding. After reassessment of the ABCs, if the patient remains hemodynamically stable, he requires further imaging to evaluate the abdomen. If he is hemodynamically unstable despite aggressive fluid resuscitation, he should be taken to the operating room for emergent exploratory laparotomy.

  The FAST examination is commonly used in adults to assess intra-abdominal injuries. However, even in adults, intra-abdominal injuries are underdiagnosed,[4] resulting in the recommendation that abdominal CT scan be used in hemodynamically stable patients. The FAST examination has been shown to be quite sensitive for identifying intra-abdominal fluid in children.[5-7] These data suggest that the best use for the FAST exam may be to identify intra-abdominal bleeding and to facilitate timely operative intervention in the hemodynamically unstable pediatric patient with blunt abdominal trauma.

Objectives of This Scenario

1. Recognize mechanisms leading to blunt trauma and that resuscitation begins with ABCs.[8-11]

Bicycle-related injuries are an important and common cause of significant trauma, including blunt abdominal trauma. Children often exhibit lack of judgment, and this, combined with improperly using or failing to use safety devices, leaves them open to significant injury. Common injuries include traumatic brain injury, blunt abdominal and chest trauma, and extremity trauma. Assessment and control of the **airway** with attention to cervical spine immobilization is the first priority. Oxygen 100% should be applied as you are assessing **breathing**. Assess **circulation** and obtain adequate vascular access as soon as possible. Ideally, this should be done with two large-bore intravenous lines, but if attempts are unsuccessful, consider early placement of an intraosseous line to initiate fluids. Address any concerns discovered during the primary survey. A rapid neurologic assessment and complete exposure of the patient to evaluate all injuries are then indicated. Reassessment of the ABCs should occur frequently, and all identified injuries should be addressed.

2. Aggressively manage hypovolemic shock with fluid resuscitation.[8-11]

Keep in mind that low blood pressure is a late finding in shock. Initial fluid resuscitation should begin with **20 mL/kg isotonic crystalloid solution**. This should be given rapidly and repeated if the patient shows persistent signs of poor perfusion. These signs include tachycardia, diminished or thready pulses, prolonged capillary refill time or cool mottled skin, or other evidence of inadequate end-organ perfusion such as mental status changes or poor urine output.

If the patient continues to show evidence of poor perfusion despite 40 to 60 mL/kg isotonic crystalloid, then colloid should be considered.[12] In the setting of trauma, where the etiology of the hypovolemia is most likely acute blood loss, type O-negative whole blood should be transfused if cross-matched, type-specific whole blood is not yet available. Other blood substitutes also may be of benefit acutely.

As this therapy is being undertaken, steps must be initiated to determine the cause of the bleeding. Abdominal injuries, chest injuries, vascular injuries, and long bone injuries (especially the femur) are common sources of significant blood loss. Intracranial hemorrhage does not generally cause significant hypotension except in infants with open skull sutures.

3. Know the management and differential diagnosis of blunt abdominal trauma.[8-11]

The differential diagnosis of bleeding and shock due to blunt abdominal trauma is wide. Lacerations to the liver and spleen are common causes of intraperitoneal bleeding,[10] as are bowel disruption and mesenteric vessel injury. Retroperitoneal bleeding is not easy to detect on physical examination. The organs involved include primarily the kidneys and renal vessels but also include the adrenals and the bladder. Bleeding into the pelvis is also important and can be caused by a fractured pelvis. Other specific injuries include duodenal hematoma, pancreatic injuries (both commonly seen when a child is struck in the abdomen with the handlebars of a bicycle),[11] and the lap belt complex (combined injuries to the pancreas, hollow viscera, and spine), which is caused by the sudden flexion of a child's torso around the fulcrum provided by an automobile lap belt when a child is restrained in a lap belt only, without the shoulder harness.[13]

As described earlier, the initial management of trauma begins with attention to the ABCs. A hematocrit may be helpful but may be misleading early on. Large volumes of blood can be lost without a significant initial decrease in hematocrit. Urinalysis showing blood in the urine can be helpful as a screen for intra-abdominal trauma as well as an indicator of renal injury. Pancreatic enzymes and liver function tests also can be of some benefit.[1,2] A CT scan of the patient's abdomen is the gold standard for evaluation of intra-abdominal injuries. The efficacy and indications of diagnostic ultrasound (FAST exam) in pediatric blunt abdominal trauma remain unclear, however it is used in some emergency departments.[5-7] Diagnostic peritoneal lavage is not usually performed in children, because most injuries can be managed nonoperatively and thus it does not afford any additional decision-making information. However, in the hemodynamically unstable patient, like the FAST exam, the technique may be use to rapidly evaluate for intra-abdominal bleeding.[14]

The cornerstone of management of a hypotensive pediatric patient with blunt abdominal trauma is aggressive volume resuscitation. If this does not achieve hemodynamic stability, operative intervention to determine the ongoing cause of blood loss and to correct it if possible may be a life-saving measure.

References:

1. Jobst MA, Canty TG, Lynch FP. Management of pancreatic injury in pediatric blunt abdominal trauma. *J Pediatr Surg.* 1999;34(5):818-823.
2. Holmes JF, Sokolove PE, Brant WE, et al. Identification of children with intra-abdominal injuries after blunt trauma. *Ann Emerg Med.* 2002;39(5):500-509.
3. Zaritsky AL, Nadkarni VM, Hickey RW, et al, eds. *PALS Provider Manual.* Dallas, Tex: American Academy of Pediatrics and American Heart Association; 2002:108-109.
4. Miller MT, Pasquale MD, Bromberg WJ, et al. Not so FAST. *J Trauma.* 2003;54:52-59.
5. Soudack M, Epelman M, Maor R, et al. Experience with focused abdominal sonography for trauma (FAST) in 313 pediatric patients. *J Clin Ultrasound.* 2004;32:53-61.
6. Suthers SE, Albrecht R, Foley D, et al. Surgeon-directed ultrasound for trauma is a predictor of intra-abdominal injury in children. *Am Surg.* 2004;70(2):164-167.
7. Holmes JF, Brant WE, Bond WF, et al. Emergency department ultrasonography in the evaluation of hypotensive and normotensive children with blunt abdominal trauma. *J Pediatr Surg.* 2001;36(7):968-973.
8. Rothrock SG, Green SM, Morgan R. Abdominal trauma in infants and children: prompt identification and early management of serious and life-threatening injuries. Part I: injury patterns and initial assessment. *Pediatr Emerg Care.* 2000;16(2):106-115.

9. Rothrock SG, Green SM, Morgan R. Abdominal trauma in infants and children: prompt identification and early management of serious and life-threatening injuries. Part II: specific injuries and ED management. *Pediatr Emerg Care*. 2000;16(3):189-195.

10. Gaines BA, Ford HR. Abdominal and pelvic trauma in children. *Crit Care Med*. 2002;30(11 suppl):S416-S423.

11. Saladino RA, Lund DP. Abdominal trauma. In: Fleisher GR, Ludwig S, eds. *Textbook of Pediatric Emergency Medicine*. 4th ed. Philadelphia, Pa: Lippincott Williams & Wilkins; 2000:1361-1367.

12. Zaritsky AL, Nadkarni VM, Hickey RW, et al, eds. *PALS Provider Manual*. Dallas, Tex: American Academy of Pediatrics and American Heart Association; 2002:259-260.

13. Newman KD, Bowman LM, Eichelberger MR, et al. The lap belt complex: intestinal and lumbar spine injury in children. *J Trauma*. 1990;30(9):1133-1138.

14. Pediatric trauma. In: *Advanced Trauma Life Support. Student manual*. 7th ed. Chicago, Ill: Committee on Trauma, American College of Surgeons; 2002:243-262.

SCENARIO #38

Trauma – Pulseless Electrical Activity

Ethan S. Wiener, MD

Brief Presenting History

A 5-year-old boy is brought in by ambulance in a cervical collar and on a rigid spine immobilization board. The patient was a helmeted passenger on the back of an all-terrain vehicle traveling at 30 to 35 miles per hour when it hit a ditch. The boy was thrown into a tree.

Pediatric Assessment Triangle

Appearance: Awake and responsive, but very agitated

Work of Breathing: Labored respirations with subcostal and suprasternal retractions

Circulation to the Skin: Extremities cool and mottled

Initial Vital Signs

Pulse: 150

Respiratory Rate: 40

Blood Pressure: 90/55

Temperature: 37.3°C (99.°F) axillary

ASK YOURSELF

- **How much should this 5-year-old weigh?**

  An estimated weight for a 5-year-old is 20 kg. Use the length-based Broselow Pediatric Emergency Tape or a pediatric table to determine weight based on age. See Appendix A.

Physical Examination on Arrival to the Emergency Department

Airway: Patent, moving air freely, small amount of blood on gums and lips, with crusted blood in the nares

Breathing: Using accessory muscles; breath sounds audible bilaterally

Circulation: Skin mottled and cool to the touch, capillary refill time 3 to 4 seconds

ASK YOURSELF

- **Where would you best feel the central pulse on this 5-year-old patient?**

  The femoral pulse is the preferred central pulse to palpate in this case. Carotid pulses can be difficult to palpate in younger children with chubby necks, especially with a cervical collar in place.

- **What is the initial assessment? What is the patient's physiologic status?**

  The child presents in moderate respiratory distress and tachycardia with a normal blood pressure for age but with delayed capillary refill consistent with compensated shock.[1]

Disability: Eyes are open and looking around, but the patient is very agitated and inconsolable. He moves all extremities equally.

ASK YOURSELF

- **What additional history and physical findings would be important in the early assessment of this child?**

  History: Although the mechanism of injury is thought to be important and is always obtained, it is not very predictive of intracranial injury. Mental status since the time of injury, vomiting, and scalp hematoma (in those <2 years old) are among elements from the history that are helpful in determining the level of concern for intracranial injury and potential need for neurosurgical intervention.[2,3] History of medications and fluids received during transport is important. Estimation of urine output can help to grossly assess renal perfusion and cardiac output.

  Physical Examination: Breath sounds to evaluate for pneumothorax and hemothorax are important but can be normal and misleading initially in pediatric patients with intrathoracic pathology.[4] Stridor can be a clue to upper airway injury and compromise. Assessment of heart rate and perfusion of the skin are important to evaluate circulation; color, temperature, and capillary refill time should be noted. Quality of pulses and heart tones should be assessed. Hypotension, defined as blood pressure below the fifth percentile for age, is diagnostic of decompensated shock and has not yet occurred in this patient.[5] Blood pressure readings within the "normal" range for age do not rule out compensated shock, which fact emphasizes the importance of evaluating perfusion; hypotension is a late finding in pediatric shock.[1] Mental status and pupil size and reactivity can be clues to intracranial injury. Pupil size and reactivity can be misleading in patients who have received narcotics, paralytic agents, or other medications.

Additional History and Physical Examination Findings

The patient had no loss of consciousness at the time of injury and has vomited once in transit. The father was transported to a different facility. The child received no medications en route. He has received 400 mL normal saline (20 mL/kg) IV so far.

Past Medical History: Not known

Medications: Not known.

Allergies: Not known.

Physical Examination: In general, the patient is anxious appearing and confused. The head is atraumatic except for crusted blood from nares. Pupils are equal, round, and reactive to light and accommodation; extra-ocular movements are intact. The neck is nontender to palpation, and a cervical collar is in place. There is bruising over his right chest. Breath sounds are audible bilaterally but slightly decreased on the right. There is no stridor, and heart tones are normal. The abdomen is not distended; there are positive bowel sounds and slight diffuse tenderness. The rectal tone is normal, and the patient is heme negative. The pelvis is stable. The patient follows commands and moves all extremities. There is obvious deformity to his right distal forearm and 1+ to 2+ pulses in all extremities.

ASK YOURSELF

- **What are the immediate concerns for this patient at this time?**

  Attention to the ABCs is the immediate concern, and initiation of appropriate interventions is paramount. This is the cornerstone of the primary survey, which also includes a rapid neurologic evaluation for disability. Early and complete exposure is important to assess for other external signs of trauma (bruising/lacerations/obvious fractures) that may give clues to internal injuries.[6,7]

- **What interventions are needed at this time? What complications might be expected?**

  Interventions:

  - Administer 100% O_2 via nonrebreather face mask for respiratory distress despite adequate initial pulse oximeter reading.
  - Place the patient on a cardiorespiratory monitor with pulse oximetry.
  - Place two large-bore intravenous lines and begin aggressive fluid resuscitation with **normal saline 20 mL/kg** (volume resuscitation is required in this patient with compromised perfusion even though the patient may have a closed head injury as well).

- Laboratory tests: ABGs, CBC, type and cross, and PT/PTT (in cases of possible intracranial bleed).
- Call blood bank for O-negative blood.
- Call for surgical consultation immediately (trauma and neurosurgery).
- Call for portable chest, pelvis, and lateral cervical spine radiographs.

Potential Complications:

- Vomiting, necessitating suction and log roll, while maintaining in-line immobilization of the cervical spine
- If intravenous access is not obtained after two attempts and the patient is hemodynamically compromised, attempt intraosseous or central venous access

Repeat Vital Signs

Pulse: 162

Respiratory Rate: 48

Blood Pressure: 82/45

Oxygen Saturation: 88% despite 100% oxygen via nonrebreather face mask

Laboratory Results

ABG: pH 7.30, Pco_2 40, Po_2 60, base excess –6, hematocrit 33

Progression

The patient is acutely more dyspneic and suddenly unresponsive. Pulses now are not palpable, but sinus tachycardia is noted on electrocardiographic monitor. The child is experiencing decreasing oxygen saturations despite being on 100% oxygen.

ASK YOURSELF

■ What is the physiologic status now?

Patient is in a pulseless arrest rhythm—pulseless electrical activity (PEA).

■ What is the most likely cause of PEA in this case?

There are several important diagnoses to consider that are rapidly treatable causes of PEA associated with blunt trauma. In the chest or abdomen, the patient could be bleeding from a major vessel or organ injury and have significant and acute hypovolemia due to exsanguination. Other causes of PEA associated with trauma that must be considered are tension pneumothorax and cardiac tamponade.[4-6] These conditions are life threatening but can frequently be diagnosed on careful physical examination and have life-saving interventions.

Progression

Electrocardiographic monitor now shows a narrow complex rhythm at a rate of 90 and falling. No breath sounds are heard over the right side of the chest. The trachea is deviated to the left (this was not initially detected because of the cervical collar).

ASK YOURSELF

■ What interventions are needed at this time? What complications might be expected?

Interventions:

- Begin CPR: BMV with 100% O_2 and chest compressions
- Perform needle thoracentesis on the right side of patient's chest to treat presumed tension pneumothorax. See "Evaluation and Management: Breathing."
- Prepare for chest tube insertion if thoracentesis is positive for rush of air.
- Prepare for RSI.
- Repeat **normal saline 20 mL/kg IV** bolus (continue aggressive fluid resuscitation).

Potential Complications:

- Hemothorax secondary to puncture of the internal mammary artery, a subcostal vessel, or mediastinal structures is possible but unlikely if proper procedures are followed.

Progression

Needle thoracostomy results in a large rush of air and the return of palpable pulses. The patient is still unresponsive and has agonal respirations, persistent hypoxia, and hypotension.

Repeat Vital Signs

Pulse: 70

Respiratory Rate: 8

Blood Pressure: 75 and palpable

ASK YOURSELF

■ What interventions are needed at this time? What complications might be expected?

Interventions:

- Institute RSI while maintaining in-line cervical spine immobilization.
  1. Miller #2 laryngoscopy blade and 5.0 uncuffed ET tube
  2. Preoxygenate and continue cricoid pressure.
  3. **Etomidate 0.3 mg/kg IV** or **midazolam 0.1 mg/kg IV**
  4. **Rocuronium 0.6 to 1 mg/kg IV** or **succinylcholine 1 to 1.5 mg/kg IV**
  5. **Atropine 0.02 mg/kg IV** (minimum, 0.1 mg) should be administered before succinylcholine in children younger than 5 years to prevent bradycardia and excessive secretions.
- Evaluate tube placement with auscultation of the chest in the axillae, observation of chest wall rise, and end-tidal CO_2 monitor.
- Secure ET tube and place NG tube.
- Place thoracostomy tube (20 to 32 French) if not already done. See "Evaluation and Management: Breathing."
- Call for chest radiograph to confirm ET tube and thoracostomy tube placement.
- Repeat ABGs and hematocrit.

Potential Complications:

- Vomiting if BMV is performed without applying cricoid pressure
- Right mainstem intubation results in ineffective ventilation.
- Tube falls out if not properly cared for and secured in place.
- Chest tube placed inferior to rib results in chest wall bleeding. This procedure can also result in diaphragmatic injury if not performed correctly using appropriate landmarks.

■ What additional complications might be expected for this patient with blunt thoracic trauma?

Hemothorax can occur; the chest tube may drain a large amount of blood indicating intrathoracic blood and air. A large amount of blood in the chest can indicate a need for surgical intervention. *Pulmonary contusions* could lead to difficulties with oxygenation and ventilation. *Cardiac tamponade* caused by pericardial bleeding can be responsible for PEA and necessitates an emergent pericardiocentesis. This is a more common complication in penetrating injury than in blunt trauma. Injuries to the *great vessels* and *bronchial tree* can be challenging to diagnose but represent true surgical emergencies.

Progression

Pulse becomes regular at 130 with assisted ventilations at 20 to 30 breaths per minute. If hemodynamically stable, the patient may go to radiology department for CT scans of the head, chest, and abdomen to evaluate for occult bleeding and injury. If the patient is unstable or if there is persistent bloody chest tube output, he may go directly to the operating room for thoracotomy and/or exploratory laparotomy.

Objectives of This Scenario

1. Recognize mechanisms and results of multiple blunt trauma.

Common mechanisms for major blunt traumatic injuries are motor vehicle collisions, automobile-versus-pedestrian injuries, falls, or, as in this case, an accident involving an open vehicle (bicycle, motorcycle, ATV). The injury and death rate associated with ATV usage is high and disproportionately affects young riders, especially adolescents, who experience more severe injuries and more head injuries than other age groups.[8]

Resuscitation begins with the primary survey and the ABCs. Assessment and control of the **airway** with attention to cervical spine immobilization is the first priority. Oxygen 100% is administered as **breathing** is evaluated. **Circulation** is assessed; two large-bore intravenous lines are placed, and fluid resuscitation is begun. After a rapid neurologic examination, the patient is exposed so that all injuries can be evaluated. All problems identified in the primary survey are addressed in the resuscitation phase. The patient is completely examined in the secondary survey and other problems are identified.[6,7]

Aggressive fluid resuscitation is a critical part of the initial management of the injured child with signs of hemodynamic instability.[1,4,6,7] Initial fluid resuscitation consists of **isotonic crystalloid 20 mL/kg** administered rapidly and repeated if reassessment reveals persistent tachycardia or poor perfusion, as evidenced by diminished pulses, prolonged capillary refill time, cool, mottled skin, or, in severe cases, altered mental status resulting from decreased cerebral perfusion. Hypotension is a late finding of shock (ie, decompensated shock) in the pediatric patient and is a sign of impending cardiovascular collapse.[1,4,6,7] If hypotension persists despite 40 mL/kg of isotonic crystalloid, the addition of colloid must be considered. Type O-negative whole blood should be used if cross-matched, type-specific whole blood is not available.

Associated findings on secondary survey must be considered. Early notification of the surgery trauma team is essential. The trauma, orthopedic, and neurosurgeons are responsible for the definitive care phase of trauma.

2. Formulate the differential diagnosis of respiratory distress in blunt thoracic trauma and initiate treatment.

Respiratory distress in blunt chest trauma can be secondary to one or more of the following: pneumothorax, tension pneumothorax, hemothorax, pulmonary contusion, cardiac tamponade, flail chest, and aortic or bronchial disruption.[9,10] Significant abdominal distention from gastric air or intra-abdominal blood also can lead to respiratory distress by restricting downward diaphragmatic movement.

Tension pneumothorax should be suspected in patients presenting with respiratory distress and unilateral chest findings. Decreased breath sounds, deviation of the trachea or heart sounds, and hyperresonance to percussion all suggest the presence of air in the pleural cavity. Dullness to percussion may be elicited in patients with hemothorax. Either of these can impede venous return to the heart, resulting in loss of cardiac output and circulatory collapse. Thoracentesis is a life-saving procedure in these cases, and there is no rationale to wait for radiologic confirmation. Tube thoracostomy is indicated after a needle thoracentesis.[4,9]

Injuries to the thoracic aorta and great vessels must be suspected when great force is involved such as occurs in motor vehicle crashes and falls from great heights. Fractures of the first or second ribs or scapula suggest significant force was involved and should raise suspicion for possible injury to the great vessels. Chest radiographic findings that are important to recognize include widening of the mediastinum, blurring of the aortic knob, and depression of the left mainstem bronchus.[11,12] Often one sees pulmonary contusion, hemothorax or pneumothorax, and injury to the heart and great vessels or trachea and bronchial tree in the absence of bony abnormalities, even where massive forces are applied to the thorax, as occurs in a motor vehicle collision.[9,10] This is due to the elastic quality and compressibility of the bony structures of the pediatric chest wall.

Paradoxical chest wall movement leading to ineffective ventilation is the result of flail chest injuries. Fractures to adjacent ribs or multiple ribs cause a portion of the chest to be no longer affixed to the thorax. During inspiration, the flail segment moves independently of the chest, resulting in severe respiratory distress that requires positive pressure ventilation and immediate tube thoracostomy. Flail chest is relatively uncommon in children because of the elasticity of the chest wall.[9,10]

3. Identify and manage pulseless arrest in the victim of blunt thoracic trauma.

Pulseless arrest in the victim of blunt trauma has a finite number of etiologies. The first to consider, and the one that must be addressed before it becomes a life-threatening condition, is inadequate circulatory volume due to hypovolemia. Aggressive fluid resuscitation, as discussed earlier, will prevent many cases of arrest in preparation for definitive care.

When a patient goes into a pulseless arrest, the first objective is to determine if this is a wide- or narrow-complex rhythm or if asystole has occurred. The algorithms for these dysrhythmias differ significantly. See "Evaluation and Management: Circulation." After CPR is initiated, wide-complex pulseless rhythms are treated with defibrillation, asystole is treated with epinephrine, and narrow-complex pulseless arrest, or PEA, is treated by addressing the underlying cause.

It is important here to remember the four Hs (**h**ypoxemia, **h**ypovolemia, **h**ypothermia, and **h**ypokalemia or hyperkalemia) and four Ts (**t**ension pneumothorax, cardiac **t**amponade, **t**oxins/drugs/poisons, and pulmonary **t**hromboembolism) of reversible pulseless arrest.[13]

Lifesaving procedures in these circumstances include thoracentesis/tube thoracostomy and pericardiocentesis.

References

1. Bell L. Shock. In: Fleisher GR, Ludwig S, eds. *Textbook of Pediatric Emergency Medicine.* 4th ed. Philadelphia, Pa: Lippincott Williams & Wilkins; 2000:47-57.
2. Palchak M, Holmes J, Vance CW, et al. A decision rule for indentifying children at low risk for brain injuries after blunt head trauma. *Ann Emerg Med.* 2003;42:492-506.
3. Greenes DS, Schutzman SA. Clinical significance of scalp abnormalities in asymptomatic head-injured infants. *Pediatr Emerg Care.* 2001;17(2):88-92.
4. Tepas J, Fallat M, Moriarty T. Trauma. In: Gausche-Hill M, Fuchs S, Yamamoto L, eds. *APLS: The Pediatric Emergency Medicine Resource.* 4th ed. Sudbury, Mass: American Academy of Pediatrics, American College of Emergency Physicians, Jones and Bartlett Publishing Co; 2004:268-323.
5. Recognition of respiratory failure and shock. In: Zaritsky AL, Nadkarni VM, Hickey RW, et al, eds. *PALS Provider Manual.* Dallas, Tex: American Academy of Pediatrics and American Heart Association; 2002:23-42.
6. Pediatric trauma. In: *Advanced Trauma Life Support. Student Manual.* 7th ed. Chicago, Ill: Committee on Trauma, American College of Surgeons; 2002:243-262.
7. Trauma resuscitation and spinal immobolization. In: Zaritsky AL, Nadkarni VM, Hickey RW, et al, eds. *PALS Provider Manual.* Dallas, Tex: American Academy of Pediatrics and American Heart Association; 2002:253-286.
8. Smith LM, Pittman MA, Marr AB, et al. Unsafe at any age: a retrospective review of all-terrain vehicle injuries in two level I trauma centers from 1995 to 2003. *J Trauma.* 2005;58:783-788.
9. Bliss D, Silen M. Pediatric thoracic trauma. *Crit Care Med.* 2002;30:S409-S415.
10. Kadish H. Thoracic trauma. In: Fleisher GR, Ludwig S, eds. *Textbook of Pediatric Emergency Medicine.* 4th ed. Philadelphia, Pa: Lippincott Williams & Wilkins; 2000:1341-1360.
11. Sivit CJ. Pediatric thoracic trauma: imaging considerations. *Emerg Radiol.* 2002;9:21-25.
12. Gittelman MA, Gonzalez-del-Rey J, Brody AS, et al. Clinical predictors for the selective use of chest radiographs in pediatric blunt thoracic trauma evaluations. *J Trauma.* 2003;55:670-676.
13. Rhythm disturbances. In: Zaritsky AL, Nadkarni VM, Hickey RW, et al, eds. *PALS Provider Manual.* Dallas, Tex: American Academy of Pediatrics and American Heart Association; 2002:185-228.

SCENARIO #39

Trauma – Altered Mental Status and Shock

Carlos A. Delgado, MD

Brief Presenting History

An 8-year-old boy fell about 20 feet out of his tree house. Witnesses report that he was unconscious for approximately 10 minutes at the scene. He was brought to the emergency department by paramedics who had placed him on a full spine board, with the cervical spine immobilized.

Pediatric Assessment Triangle

Appearance: Moaning, intermittently poorly responsive; has a large contusion and laceration to the right parietal region with moderate amount of blood to dressing

Work of Breathing: Symmetric chest excursion, unlabored

Circulation to the Skin: Capillary refill 3 seconds centrally

Initial Vital Signs

Pulse: 150

Respiratory Rate: 24

Blood Pressure: 110/70

Temperature: 37.6°C (99.7°F) axillary

Physical Examination

Airway: Patent, moving air freely, no secretions in the mouth

Breathing: Equal breath sounds throughout lung fields

Circulation: Skin mottled and cool to the touch, capillary refill time 3 seconds centrally and 4 seconds peripherally

Disability: Eyes closed, patient responding to pain, pupils equal and reactive to light 4 mm to 2 mm bilaterally, moving all extremities when reacting to pain

ASK YOURSELF

- **How much should this 8-year-old weigh?**

  An estimated weight for a 8-year-old is 25 kg. Use the length-based Broselow Pediatric Emergency Tape or a pediatric table to determine weight based on age. See Appendix A.

- **What is the initial assessment? What is the patient's physiologic status?**

  This patient sustained injury with a mechanism that increases the potential for multiple blunt trauma and displays altered mental status and compensated shock.

- **What causes of altered mental status should be considered in this patient?**

  First and foremost, a closed head injury must be considered in any patient who has fallen. As in this case, in which multiple trauma is suspected, the shock state and hypoperfusion to the brain due to hypovolemia secondary to active significant intrathoracic or intra-abdominal blood loss may also explain the altered mental status. An ingestion, intentional or inadvertent, may have precipitated the fall and also should be considered. Seizures can result in altered mental status and in this case also could have led to the fall, emphasizing the importance of obtaining a complete history.

Additional History and Physical Examination Findings

The fall was witnessed by a 9-year-old friend who was present at the treehouse. The patient cried briefly but became still and unresponsive soon after the fall. The friend denies ingestions or seizure activity.

Past Medical History: Seasonal allergies, otherwise noncontributory

Medications: None

Allergies: None known

Physical Examination: The abdomen is tender and distended. There is a left forearm deformity.

ASK YOUSELF

■ **What interventions are needed at this time?**

- ABCs
  1. **Airway:** Check for patency; suction as needed; maintain in-line cervical spine immobilization.
  2. **Breathing:** Administer oxygen, and assess work of breathing and quality of breath sounds.
  3. **Circulation:** Recognize compensated shock; place two large-bore peripheral intravenous lines and begin fluid resuscitation with **normal saline 20 mL/kg IV.**
- Place the patient on a cardiorespiratory monitor with pulse oximetry.
- Laboratory studies: glucose, CBC, ABGs, urinalysis, and type and cross-match blood. Consider PT/PTT, electrolytes, liver function tests, amylase.

Progression

Respirations are now are irregular and shallow, with oxygen saturation of 90% on face mask oxygen. Femoral pulse is thready, blood pressure is 80/40, and the patient is now unresponsive.

ASK YOURSELF

■ **What is the physiologic status now?**

Impending respiratory failure, decompensated shock, and altered mental status.

■ **What interventions are needed at this time? What complications might be expected?**

Interventions:

- Assist breathing with BMV and 100% O_2. Prepare for RSI. Apply cricoid pressure when providing positive-pressure ventilation in the unresponsive patient.
- If intravenous access attempt is unsuccessful, place an intraosseous line. Administer **normal saline 20 mL/kg IV/IO.**
- RSI with manual in-line cervical spine immobilization
  1. #2 Miller blade, 6.0 ET tube
  2. Preoxygenate
  3. Cricoid pressure
  4. **Lidocaine 1 mg/kg IV** (assume closed head injury with increased ICP)
  5. **Etomidate 0.3 mg/kg IV/IO** or **midazolam 0.1 mg/kg IV** (Avoid thiopental in a hypotensive patient.)
  6. **Rocuronium 0.6 to 1 mg/kg IV** or **succinylcholine 1 to 1.5 mg/kg IV**
  7. End-tidal CO_2 monitor
  8. Call for chest radiograph to confirm ET tube placement
  9. Secure ET tube and place NG tube (or orogastric tube if there is evidence of facial trauma)
- Stabilize the cervical spine. Maintain head and neck in midline position.
- Obtain lateral neck and pelvis films.

Potential Complications:

- Vomiting requires suctioning, especially if cricoid pressure is not used.
- Unable to visualize cords if not properly suctioned
- Failure to place NG or orogastric tube results in abdominal distention and impaired ventilation.

■ What injuries would explain the hypovolemic shock state of this patient?

Given the lack of thoracic findings such as an asymmetric examination (decreased breath sounds), difficulty with oxygenation or ventilation, or an abnormal chest radiograph, an intra-abdominal injury would be most likely. *Note:* Because of a highly elastic chest wall, pediatric patients can have significant intrathoracic or intra-abdominal injuries without overt physical signs. In the presence of impaired perfusion, these sites must be vigorously investigated.

- Liver and spleen are most commonly injured from blunt trauma in children.
- Pancreatic and/or duodenal injuries commonly result from a direct blow to these organs. Intramural duodenal injury, however, usually presents as an acute upper intestinal obstruction and does not typically lead to significant blood loss.
- Intestinal injuries: Perforation can occur after a deceleration injury and is commonly associated with lap belt injury.
- Mesenteric vessels: Abdominal trauma can result in significant bleeding when mesenteric blood vessels are involved.
- Genitourinary injuries: Most renal injuries are minor, self-limited contusions. Lower urinary tract and bladder injuries usually occur in association with severe pelvic trauma.

Radiographs

Chest and pelvis films are normal. Lateral cervical spine radiograph reveals loss of normal lordosis with widening (7 mm) of the prevertebral space at C3. There also is a slightly angulated distal fracture of the left radius and ulna.

ASK YOURSELF

■ What is your interpretation of the cervical spine film findings?

Placement of a cervical spine collar and positioning on a backboard can affect cervical spine lordosis; however, prevertebral soft tissue swelling is suggestive of a cervical spine injury. Careful attention to in-line cervical immobilization remains paramount regardless of whether the initial lateral neck film findings are significant.

■ What other complications might be expected for this patient?

- If decompensated shock is not recognized and aggressively treated with volume, the patient will develop cardiovascular collapse.
- Possible cervical spine injury, if not properly immobilized and secured, progresses.
- Cerebral edema and increased intracranial pressure from a closed head injury

■ What disposition and additional management would be expected for this patient?

Once hemodynamic stability is achieved, the patient can be sent to radiology for CT of the head and abdomen, with completion cervical spine films and possibly CT of the cervical spine. If operative intervention is not required, the patient should be transferred to the ICU for continued management, monitoring, and serial examinations. If volume resuscitation is not adequate to stabilize circulation, the patient may require emergent operative intervention with exploratory laparotomy.

Progression

With the administration of **40 mL/kg normal saline**, perfusion improves and blood pressure is now 98/62.

Radiology Results

CT of Brain: Small epidural hematoma with parietal skull fracture

CT of Abdomen: Liver and spleen lacerations

Cervical Spine Films: Fracture of the posterior element of C2

All injuries were stabilized, and the patient was managed with close observation in the ICU. No surgical intervention was required.

Objectives of This Scenario

1. Recognize multiple blunt trauma and that resuscitation begins with the ABCs.

The patient in this scenario presented with progressed signs and symptoms of decompensated hypovolemic shock and a closed head injury. Second to motor vehicle crashes, falls are the most common mechanism associated with major blunt traumatic injuries. Resuscitation begins with the primary survey of the ABCs. The first priority is assessment and control of the **airway** with attention to cervical spine immobilization. Oxygen 100% is applied as **breathing** is evaluated. **Circulation** is assessed, two large-bore intravenous lines are placed, and fluid resuscitation begun. After a rapid neurologic examination, the patient is exposed so that all injuries can be evaluated. All problems identified in the primary survey are addressed in the resuscitation phase. The patient is completely examined in the secondary survey and other problems are identified.

During the definitive care phase, all injuries are addressed. The trauma, orthopedic, and neurosurgeons are responsible for the definitive care phase of trauma.[1-3] See "Evaluation and Management: Trauma and Environmental Emergencies."

2. Manage hypovolemic shock associated with aggressive fluid resuscitation.

Initial fluid resuscitation consists of **isotonic crystalloid 20 mL/kg** given rapidly and repeated if reassessment reveals ongoing losses or hypotension, as evidenced by tachycardia and poor skin perfusion. Low blood pressure is a late finding of shock in the pediatric patient due to compensatory mechanisms. If the patient displays ongoing signs of hypovolemia such as tachycardia, diminished pulses, prolonged capillary refill time, or cool mottled skin, aggressive fluid resuscitation must continue.[2,3]

If shock persists despite the administration of 40 mL/kg of isotonic crystalloid, strong consideration must be given to the addition of colloid. Type O-negative whole blood is used if cross-matched, type-specific whole blood is not available.

Sites of ongoing blood loss must be investigated. The abdomen, retroperitoneum, and pelvis are areas of "silent" bleeding that require evaluation by physical examination and CT scanning. Long bone fractures, especially those involving the femurs, can lead to significant bleeding.

Intracranial bleeding typically does not lead to overt hypotension, because the cranial vault is a fixed space that allows a finite amount of blood loss. However, the open sutures of an infant's skull allow the intracranial space to expand, and large amounts of blood can accumulate.

There is no role for vasopressors, steroids, or sodium bicarbonate in the initial management of hypovolemic shock in trauma. Keep in mind the 3:1 rule—patients require 300 mL of crystalloid to replace each 100 mL of blood loss.[1]

3. Recognize and manage multiple blunt trauma.

Patients presenting with significant physiologic findings associated with trauma must be considered to have injuries to multiple organ systems. As resuscitation begins and the ABCs are addressed, consideration must be given to specific problems such as closed head injury, blunt abdominal trauma, and thoracic injures. The approach to these specific injuries is addressed in the "Evaluation and Management" section devoted to trauma as well as in Scenarios #36 through #38.

4. Identify and manage a cervical spine injury.

The incidence of pediatric spinal cord injuries is relatively low, occurring in 1% to 2% of multiply injured patients.[4] Despite the low incidence, a spine injury should be suspected in all children who sustain multiple trauma or head and neck trauma and in children in whom abuse or shaken baby syndrome is suspected. The presenting signs and symptoms that should increase suspicion for a cervical spine injury include altered level of consciousness including intoxication, neck or back pain, midline cervical tenderness, limitation of range of motion, abnormal sensory motor or neurologic examination, and unexplained hypotension.[5-8] Neurogenic shock secondary to spinal trauma, although uncommon, should be suspected in patients who present with hypotension and bradycardia or in those who fail to become tachycardic in response to hypovolemia.

Diagnostic studies should include a timely cervical spine series and other spine plain radiographs as deemed necessary by the history and physical examination findings. It must be emphasized that radiographs alone are not sufficient to rule out spinal cord injuries. The syndrome of spinal cord injury without radiograph abnormalities (SCIWORA) occurs mainly in children younger than 8 years when flexibility of the spinal column predisposes patients to cord injury, despite lack of bone abnormalities.[8,9]

Spinal cord injuries are divided into two categories. *Primary* spinal cord injuries are irreversible injuries sustained at the time of injury. *Secondary* injuries are those injuries that develop over hours to days and may be distinct from the primarily injured neurons.[9] The goal in treating patients with a suspected cervical spine injury is to achieve effective immobilization and stabilization of the primary spinal injury to prevent further or more serious injury to the spinal cord. Ideal immobilization includes a semirigid cervical collar along with a full spine board and soft spacing devices between the head and securing straps.

As with all significant trauma, management of spinal cord injuries begins with aggressive support of the ABCs of resuscitation. The role of blood pressure (hypertension) in the progression of injury is unresolved. Adequate volume replacement and normotension are currently recommended.[10]

The true efficacy of the treatment of pediatric spinal cord injuries with corticosteroids is not known. However, since 1990, when a large-scale clinical trial showed significantly better recovery in patients who began treatment with methylprednisolone within 8 hours of their injury, it has become common treatment for acute spinal cord injury. Methylprednisolone is thought to reduce the damage to cellular membranes that contributes to neuronal death after injury, to reduce inflammation near the injury, and to suppress the activation of immune cells that appear to contribute to neuronal damage.[11]

Current care of acute spinal cord injury involves three primary considerations. First, cord compression, gross misalignments of the spine, and other structural problems must be diagnosed and relieved. Second, the spine must be stabilized to prevent further injury. Finally, cellular-level damage must be minimized if possible.

References

1. Pediatric trauma. In: *Advanced Trauma Life Support Student Manual.* 7th ed. Chicago, Ill: Committee on Trauma, American College of Surgeons; 2002:243-262.
2. Ruddy R, Fleisher G. An approach to the injured child. In: Fleisher GR, Ludwig S, eds. *Textbook of Pediatric Emergency Medicine.* 4th ed. Philadelphia, Pa: Lippincott Williams & Wilkins; 2000:1249-1258.
3. Ziegler M. Major trauma. In: Fleisher GR, Ludwig S, eds. *Textbook of Pediatric Emergency Medicine.* 4th ed. Philadelphia, Pa: Lippincott Williams & Wilkins; 2000:1259-1269.
4. Koboska ER, Keller MS, Rallo MC, et al. Characteristics of pediatric cervical spine injuries. *J Pediatr Surg.* 2001;36:100-105.
5. Hoffman JR, Mower WR, Wolfson AB, et al, for the National Emergency X-Radiography Utilization Study Group. Validity of a set of clinical criteria to rule out injury to the cervical spine in patients with blunt trauma. *N Engl J Med.* 2000;343:94-99.
6. Vicellio P, Simon H, Pressman BD, et al, for the Nexus Group. A prospective multicenter study of cervical spine injury in children. *Pediatrics.* 2001;108:E20.
7. Panacek EA, Mower WR, Holmes JF, et al, for the Nexus Group. Test performance of the individual NEXUS low-risk clinical screening criteria for cervical spine injury. *Ann Emerg Med.* 2001;38:22-25.
8. Tepas JJ, Fallat ME, Moriarty TM. Trauma. In: Gausche-Hill M, Fuchs S, Yamamoto L, eds. *APLS: The Pediatric Emergency Medicine Resource.* 4th ed. Sudbury, Mass: American Academy of Pediatrics, American College of Emergency Physicians, Jones and Bartlett Publishing Co; 2004:296-307.
9. Greenes DS, Madsen JR. Neurotrauma. In: Fleisher GR, Ludwig S, eds. *Textbook of Pediatric Emergency Medicine.* 4th ed. Philadelphia, Pa: Lippincott Williams & Wilkins; 2000:1291-1284.
10. Guidelines for the acute medical management of severe traumatic brain injury in infants, children, and adolescents. Chapter 4. Resuscitation of blood pressure and oxygenation and prehospital brain-specific therapies for the severe pediatric traumatic brain injury patient. *Pediatr Crit Care Med.* 2003;4(3 suppl):S12-S18.
11. Bracken MB. Steroids for acute spinal cord injury. *Cochrane Database Syst Rev.* 2002;3:CD001046.

SCENARIO #40

Trauma – Shock

Jeffrey S. Blake, MD

Brief Presenting History

A 5-year-old boy is rushed into the emergency department in his father's arms. The father states that his son was hit by a bullet from a "gang shooting" while playing in their front yard.

Pediatric Assessment Triangle

Appearance: Alert, anxious, screaming in pain, bloodstained tee-shirt

Work of Breathing: Tachypneic with moderate retractions (intercostal and suprasternal)

Circulation to the Skin: Diaphoretic, pale

Initial Vital Signs

Pulse: 160

Respiratory Rate: 52

Blood pressure: 98/62

Temperature: 37°C (98.6°F) axillary

Oxygen Saturation: 91% in room air

Physical Examination on Arrival to the Emergency Department

Airway: Patent, trachea slightly deviated to the right, no neck vein distention appreciated, no oral secretions, stridor, or subcutaneous emphysema in the neck

Breathing: Moderate use of accessory muscles, equal chest rise, bullet entry wound (nonsucking) at the left lateral chest below the nipple line with a small amount of active bleeding, absent breath sounds on the left with hyperresonance on percussion

Circulation: Pink, cool, clammy skin; capillary refill time 3 seconds; strong femoral pulses; weak peripheral pulses; normal heart sounds

Disability: Extremely agitated but following commands and responding verbally

ASK YOURSELF

- **What is the initial assessment? What is the patient's physiologic status?**

  This patient has respiratory distress with mild hypoxia and compensated shock likely secondary to a tension pneumothorax. Tachycardia in this patient could be multifactorial secondary to pain, anxiety, hypoxia, and/or shock from poor central venous blood return due to a tension pneumothorax or blood volume loss from a concurrent hemothorax. However, it should be presumed that this patient is in compensated shock until proved otherwise. Remember that children can lose up to 25% of their circulating blood volume without demonstrating severe signs of shock such as altered mental status and hypotension.[1,2]

- **What is the differential diagnosis of shock in penetrating trauma to the chest?**

  Tension pneumothorax classically presents as respiratory distress, unilaterally decreased or absent breath sounds and hyperresonance to percussion, tracheal deviation away from the affected side, and signs of poor perfusion. Jugular venous distention (JVD) also can be present but, like tracheal deviation, can be difficult to assess in children because of their relatively short and chubby necks.[3]

Cardiac tamponade can present with the Beck clinical triad of hypotension with a narrowed pulse pressure, muffled heart sounds, and JVD.[3] Tamponade initially can be confused with tension pneumothorax because they both can present with respiratory distress, signs of shock, and JVD. However, they can be differentiated by careful examination, because cardiac tamponade would not cause tracheal deviation or diminished breath sounds and likely will demonstrate muffled heart sounds.

Hemothorax would be expected to cause diminished or absent breath sounds and dullness to percussion on the affected side but should not cause tracheal deviation. Most commonly, it is due to bleeding from injured lung parenchyma, but it also can result from injury to small vessels such as the intercostals or internal mammary arteries, and, less commonly, from a hilar or great vessel injury.[1]

Great vessel injury presents as shock, often with sudden death in the field, from bleeding into the mediastinum or pleural space (hemothorax).

Abdominal organ injury is possible because of the proximity of the abdomen to the thorax. Thoracic trauma commonly involves hepatic, splenic, renal, or abdominal vascular injuries (aorta, vena cava, etc).

■ For what other injuries is this patient with a penetrating injury to the chest at risk?

Tracheobronchial rupture, pulmonary laceration/contusion, open pneumothorax ("open, sucking chest wound") or flail chest, esophageal rupture, and cervical/thoracic spinal injury should be considered.

With penetrating trauma occurring below the nipple line, abdominal injuries such as diaphragmatic injury, solid organ injury (hepatic, splenic, or renal), perforated viscus, and thoracic/lumbar spinal injury also should be considered.

■ How much should this 5-year-old weigh?

As estimated weight for a 5-year-old child is 20 kg. One can use the length-based Broselow Pediatric Emergency Tape or a pediatric table to determine weight based on age. See Appendix A.

■ What interventions are needed at this time? What complications might be expected?

Interventions:

- Call for immediate surgical consultation.
- Cervical and thoracolumbar spine immobilization
- Supplemental oxygen via face mask
- **Immediate needle thoracostomy** (using a 14- to 18-gauge needle at the second intercostal space, in the midclavicular line) followed by **tube thoracostomy** (insertion of chest tube at intercostal space 4-5, in the lateral chest wall just anterior to the midaxillary line)[3]
- Apply direct pressure to bleeding chest wound to achieve hemostasis.
- Establish intravenous access with two large-bore intravenous lines (≥20 gauge).
- Volume resuscitation with **normal saline** or **lactated Ringer solution at 20 mL/kg**, via rapid push, and reassessment of circulation.
- Send blood for type and cross for **2 units of packed RBCs**.
- Place a Foley catheter to monitor urinary output.

Potential Complications:

- Failure to recognize tension pneumothorax or delay in intervention (eg, waiting for radiographic confirmation before performing needle thoracostomy)
- Intravenous access unobtainable; placement of intraosseous line indicated in that case[2,4]
- Fluid-resistant hypotension: Total pediatric blood volume is 80 mL/kg, and this patient could have lost at least 25% of this volume (20 mL/kg).[3] Because of the redistribution of crystalloid solutions into the extravascular space, the "3 to 1 rule" reminds us that three times as much crystalloid volume is necessary to restore intravascular volume for a given estimated blood loss. If the administration of

40 to 60 mL/kg of crystalloid fails to improve signs of shock, ongoing blood loss should be suspected. In that circumstance, blood transfusion and an urgent open thoracotomy are indicated.

- Persistent pneumothorax after placement of chest tube: Consider tracheobronchial injury, air leak at the skin around the chest tube, improper tube position, or a leaking underwater-seal apparatus.

Progression

Needle thoracostomy produced a "rush of air" followed by rapid resolution of the patient's hypoxia and a dramatic improvement in his labored breathing and tachycardia. A chest tube is placed (200 mL of blood drained initially and then tapered off), intravenous access is established, and fluid administration is initiated.

ASK YOURSELF

- **What further physical findings would help to determine the extent of this patient's injuries?**

  Secondary Survey: A head-to-toe search for other injuries should be conducted, including a search for the bullet exit wound to establish the bullet trajectory. A *mediastinal traversing wound* is one with an entrance wound in one hemithorax and an exit wound or a missile lodged in the contralateral hemithorax. Such an injury pattern puts the patient at an increased risk of having injuries to mediastinal structures including the heart, great vessels, tracheobronchial tree, and esophagus.[2]

Additional History and Physical Examination Findings

Past Medical History: Negative, time of last meal unknown

Medications: None

Allergies: None known

Physical Examination: No exit wound or other injury found; abdomen soft, nontender, nondistended with normal bowel sounds; normal mental status, and intact motor/sensory function throughout

Progression

Thirty minutes later, the patient is much more comfortable, is still not hypoxic, and has only minimally labored breathing, but he remains tachycardic despite receiving a total of 40 mL/kg of normal saline. Urine output has been marginal. Chest radiograph shows proper chest tube placement, no visible pneumothorax, small left-sided pulmonary contusion and pleural fluid collection, normal mediastinum, and a bullet lodged in the left posterior thoracic wall. Several minutes later, the patient becomes unresponsive and even more tachycardic and hypotensive, and the nurse tells you that the chest tube drainage has significantly increased totaling 160 mL (8 mL/kg) over the past 30 minutes. The breath sounds are decreased on the left with no hyperresonance to percussion. There is no tracheal deviation or JVD.

ASK YOURSELF

- **What is the most likely cause of this patient's acute deterioration?**

  This patient has progressed to decompensated shock, most likely resulting from a massive hemothorax given the large amount of chest tube blood output (2 to 4 mL/kg/hr or more is considered excessive).[3] However, due to the possibility of multiple thoracic injuries, any cause of hypovolemic or obstructive shock (massive hemothorax, cardiac tamponade, tension pneumothorax) should be considered.

- **What interventions are needed at this time? What complications might be expected?**

  Interventions:

  - Repeat ABCs.
  - Endotracheal intubation with RSI (**etomidate** and **succinylcholine** or **rocuronium** would be appropriate choices in this hypotensive patient)
  - Search for other causes of hypotension; physical examination suggests massive hemothorax.

- Blood transfusion: **Packed RBCs 20 mL/kg** (use type O negative if type-specific blood not yet available)
- Preparation for open thoracotomy in the operating room.

Potential Complications:

- Esophageal intubation: Ensure that vocal cords are visualized before advancing ET tube and always confirm ET tube placement with auscultation and an end-tidal CO_2 detector.

■ When is an emergent open thoracotomy indicated in the emergency department?

Patients who sustain penetrating trauma to the chest and develop cardiac arrest in transit to or in the emergency department are eligible for thoracotomy in the emergency department. It is also indicated in patients with penetrating chest injuries who fail to respond to aggressive fluid resuscitation (although the thoracotomy may be better performed in the operating room) and in victims of blunt trauma who arrest in the emergency department. Although this dramatic procedure could be a life-saving intervention in this subset of patients, the mortality rate is still extremely high.[5] It is not indicated for patients with blunt trauma who arrest in the field.

Objectives of This Scenario

1. Recognize and manage tension pneumothorax.

Thoracic injuries are the second most common cause of traumatic death in children, following CNS injuries. Penetrating thoracic wounds carry a 14% mortality rate.[4,6] The immediate goal of the primary survey is to quickly identify and treat any immediate threats to life, namely a loss or pending loss of airway, hypoventilation, apnea, tension pneumothorax, massive hemopneumothorax, and cardiac tamponade.[4] The diagnosis of tension pneumothorax is made clinically, and immediate intervention is indicated; avoid waiting for radiographic confirmation.

2. Recognize, evaluate, and treat compensated shock in a penetrating trauma victim.

Having a high suspicion for the development of shock in penetrating trauma and recognizing and treating shock in its early, or compensated, phase are paramount. Knowing that shock in trauma is almost always hypovolemic, resulting from blood loss, helps to narrow the differential diagnosis. However, "obstructive" shock can occur as well, such as with tension pneumothorax (where shifting of the mediastinum compresses the vena cava, limiting central venous blood return to the heart) or with cardiac tamponade (where stroke volume is limited by underfilling of the left ventricle).[1] Needle thoracostomy followed by tube thoracostomy was the treatment of choice in this patient who presented with shock secondary to a tension pneumothorax.

3. Recognize fluid-resistant shock and the need to provide a definitive airway.

Unresponsive patients in the setting of trauma require endotracheal intubation to definitively control their airway. Furthermore, trauma patients who present in shock may not respond to fluid resuscitation because of ongoing blood loss or the development of other injuries that result in shock. Therefore, a rapid reassessment of their circulatory status after fluid resuscitation and consideration of other causes of shock is warranted. In this patient, a massive hemothorax complicated his course. For a hemothorax, thoracotomy is indicated for initial chest tube drainage of more than 20 mL/kg or for continued drainage of more than 2 mL/kg/hr for more than 2 hours.[3,4]

References

1. Kadish H. Thoracic trauma. In: Fleisher GR, Ludwig S, eds. *Textbook of Pediatric Emergency Medicine*. 4th ed. Philadelphia, Pa: Lippincott Williams & Wilkins; 2000:1341-1360.
2. Pediatric trauma. In: *Advanced Trauma Life Support (ATLS) for Doctors*. 6th ed. Chicago, Ill: American College of Surgeons Committee on Trauma; 1997:289-310.
3. Tepas JJ III, Fallat ME, Moriarty TM. Trauma. In: Gausche-Hill M, Fuchs S, Yamamoto L, eds. *APLS: The Pediatric Emergency Medicine Resource*. 4th ed. Sudbury, Mass: American Academy of Pediatrics, American College of Emergency Physicians, Jones and Bartlett Publishing Co; 2004:268-319.
4. Stafford PW, Blinman TA, Nance ML. Practical points in evaluation and resuscitation of the injured child. *Surg Clin North Am*. 2002;82:273-301.
5. Practice management guidelines for emergency department thoracotomy. Working Group, Ad Hoc Subcommittee on Outcomes, American College of Surgeons, Committee on Trauma. *J Am Coll Surg*. 2001;193:303-309.
6. Cooper A, Barlow B, DiScala C. Mortality and truncal injury: the pediatric perspective. *J Pediatr Surg*. 1994;29:33-38.

SCENARIO #41

Environmental Emergency

Arleta B. Rewers, MD, PhD, MSPH

Brief Presenting History

A 3-year-old boy is found on the ground beneath a second-story window of a burning house.

Pediatric Assessment Triangle

Appearance: Awake, agitated, crying

Work of Breathing: Unlabored, mild wheezing; intermittent inspiratory stridor with agitation

Circulation to the Skin: Skin red and warm with blisters

Initial Vital Signs

Pulse: 145

Respiratory Rate: 40

Blood Pressure: not obtainable due to agitation

Temperature: 37°C (98.6°F) axillary

Physical Examination on Arrival to the Emergency Department

Airway: Patent, moving air freely, carbonaceous material in mouth and nose

Breathing: Fast, breath sounds equal with mild expiratory wheeze and crackles, intermittent inspiratory stridor

Circulation: Capillary refill time 3 seconds peripherally, femoral pulses 1+ and 2+

Disability: Eyes open, making eye contact, crying, highly agitated, moves all extremities

ASK YOURSELF

- **What is the initial assessment? What is the patient's physiologic status?**

  Patient presents with respiratory distress and compensated shock with burns, probable smoke inhalation, and exposure to noxious substances.[1]

- **What could be causing this patient's respiratory distress and shock?**

  Carbonaceous material in the mouth and nose with respiratory distress indicates injury to the upper airways. Shock is common in burns secondary to capillary leak and distributive shock. Traumatic etiologies must always be considered and seem likely in this case in which the patient is found on the ground beneath a second-story window.

- **What additional history would help you establish a diagnosis?**

  More information on the time and circumstances of the house fire would be helpful in establishing the diagnosis. Patients exposed to smoke inhalation can present with unlabored respirations initially and develop laryngeal edema slowly over the next few hours. Upper airway edema reaches its peak 2 to 8 hours after injury.[2] Also, it is important to ascertain the patient's status during the fire and rescue, particularly whether there was loss of consciousness, which could be associated with hypoxia, carbon dioxide poisoning, or a closed head injury, or other signs of altered mental status.

Additional History and Physical Examination Findings

The child was home alone with a teenaged babysitter while his parents were visiting friends. The fire started about 2 hours ago on the second floor in the patient's bedroom where he was playing. The babysitter was watching TV in the family room on the first floor. She called 911 after seeing flames on the staircase. The patient was very agitated and confused when he was found.

Past Medical History: Healthy child with no history of respiratory problems

Medications: None

Allergies: None known

Physical Examination: He has erythema with blisters over the face, neck, and arms; the skin over the chest extending to the back is pale and leathery. His hair is burned, the scalp has a boggy area over the right occipital region. The eyebrows are singed, carbonaceous material is present in the mouth and nose. There are no obvious extremity abnormalities, but the hands and feet are becoming edematous.

ASK YOURSELF

■ What is the status of this patient's airway?

This patient presents with upper airway edema due to smoke inhalation and impending respiratory failure. At this point, the determination must be made as to whether this airway is maintainable. Due to the potential progression of the airway edema, this patient requires advanced airway support. Recommendations have been made to electively intubate all patients with potential for progressive airway edema associated with inhalation injury (ie, erythema/burns or carbonaceous materials in the mouth or nose).[3]

■ What interventions are needed at this time? What complications might be expected?

Interventions:

- Prepare for RSI
- 100% O_2 by face mask with bag-mask.
- Cervical spine immobilization, full spine board
- Place the patient on a cardiorespiratory monitor with pulse oximetry
- Obtain IV access, 2 large-bore catheters through burned skin if necessary, begin **normal saline 20 mL/kg IV**.
- RSI
  1. Preoxygenate
  2. Cricoid pressure
  3. **Etomidate 0.3 mg/kg IV** or **midazolam 0.1 mg/kg IV**
  4. **Rocuronium 0.6 to 1 mg/kg IV** or **succinylcholine 1 to 1.5 mg/kg IV**
  5. **Fentanyl 2 to 5 mcg/kg IV** (only if patient is deemed hemodynamically stable; probably would be withheld in this patient with compromised perfusion)
  6. **Lidocaine 1 mg/kg IV** (if head injury is suspected)
  7. Laryngoscope Miller/Mac #2 or #3 and 4.5 to 5.0 ET tube
- End-tidal CO_2 monitor
- Secure ET tube and place NG tube.
- Call for chest radiograph to confirm ET tube placement and to obtain baseline study

Potential Complications:

- Vomiting; requires log roll and suction, especially if cricoid pressure is not used
- Supraglottic edema present, requiring a smaller ET tube
- Inability to visualize cords if not properly suctioned
- Failure to place NG tube results in abdominal distention and impaired ventilation.
- Intubation attempts fail because of airway edema, requiring attempts at BMV and, if unsuccessful, cricothyrotomy.

Repeat Vital Signs

Pulse: 180

Respiratory Rate: 20

Blood Pressure: 80/45

Oxygen Saturation: 100% intubated

Capillary refill time 5 seconds centrally

Pulses 1+ and 2+ radial and femoral

Progression

Patient has developed significant generalized edema of the skin.

ASK YOURSELF

■ What is the physiologic status now?

Shock has become decompensated. Shock associated with burns is caused by diffuse capillary leakage and typically occurs in patients with burns extending over 20% body surface area (BSA).[4] It is also important to consider blood loss due to trauma as a cause of shock in this patient who was in a house fire.

■ What is the proper fluid resuscitation for patients with burns?

Initially, **10 to 20 mL/kg lactated Ringer** or **normal saline** is administered as a bolus when the severity and extent of burns are being assessed. The Parkland formula is typically used during first 24 hours.[4] **Isotonic crystalloid 2 to 4 mL/% BSA** partial- and full-thickness burn multiplied by the child's weight in kilograms is recommended over the first 24 hours: half during the first 8 hours and half during the next 16 hours. The Parkland formula does not include maintenance fluid requirements, which must be added to these calculations.[5]

■ What interventions are needed at this time? What complications might be expected?

Interventions:

- Seek additional intravenous access, central venous line in patients with severe burns.
- **Lactated Ringer** or **normal saline 20-mL/kg** bolus should be given over 30 minutes.
- Provide aggressive fluid resuscitation using the Parkland formula.
- Consider **5% albumin** and **dopamine 2 to 10 mcg/kg/min** if the patient remains hypotensive after **40 mL/kg isotonic crystalloid**.
- Place urinary catheter and monitor urine output.
- Obtain CBC, electrolytes, BUN, creatinine, liver function tests, ABGs, carboxyhemoglobin and cyanide levels, and urinalysis.

Potential Complications:

- Inability to place intravenous line through burned skin
- Failure to adequately provide fluid resuscitation can lead to cardiovascular collapse.

Laboratory Results

ABG: pH 7.22, P_{CO_2} 60, P_{O_2} 56, Na^+ 139, K^+ 4.2, HCO_3^- 17, glucose 159, hematocrit 37, carboxyhemoglobin 10%

Repeat Vital Signs

Pulse: 120

Blood Pressure: 95/50

Capillary refill time 3 seconds centrally, pulses 1+ and 2+ radial and femoral

Oxygen Saturation: 85% intubated on 100% O_2

Progression

Patient is becoming progressively more difficult to ventilate. Chest excursion is poor, and breath sounds are bilaterally decreased.

ASK YOURSELF

■ What is the most likely diagnosis?

The patient has developed impaired ventilation due to restriction in expansion of the chest caused by full-thickness burns of the trunk and eschar formation.

■ What interventions are needed at this time? What complications might be expected?

Interventions:

- Emergent escharotomy; longitudinal incisions are made through the devitalized, burned skin to allow reexpansion of the thoracic cavity.[6]

Possible complications:

- Pneumothorax due to overaggressive bagging

- Failure to recognize need for escharotomy leading to respiratory arrest

Progression

With escharotomy, the patient's ventilatory status improves. Secondary survey reveals a 6-cm depressed, boggy area on the right side of the occiput. Abdomen is full. Capillary refill time remains 4 seconds.

Repeat Vital Signs

Pulse: 185

Blood pressure: 75/50

ASK YOURSELF

What is the most likely diagnosis?

Poor response to volume and abdominal distention strongly suggest intra-abdominal bleeding. Presence of a 6-cm depressed, boggy area on the right side of the occiput suggests head injury with skull fracture and possibility of intracranial injury.

What interventions are needed at this time? What complications might be expected?

Interventions:

- Continue aggressive volume replacement: consider **20 mL/kg of crystalloid** or **O-negative blood.**
- Manage closed head injury with possible increased intracranial pressure.
- When hemodynamically stable, go to radiology for CT scan of abdomen and head.
- If patient is unstable, move directly to the operating suite.

Potential Complications:

- Generalized tonic-clonic seizure
- Failure to adequately fluid resuscitate leading to cardiovascular collapse

Objectives of This Scenario

1. Recognize and manage the airway altered by heat and smoke inhalation.

Smoke inhalation is a leading cause of morbidity and mortality in burn victims.[7] Inhalation of hot gas containing noxious substances results in burns of the pharynx and upper airway and also can produce systemic intoxication. Dry air has little effect on the lower airway, but the steam heat can also lead to lower airway injury. Thermal injury may lead to edema and upper airway obstruction within the several hours after initial exposure. To prevent respiratory arrest due to loss of airway patency, the airway must be controlled early in the course. The presence of facial burns, intraoral erythema, singed nasal or facial hairs, and carbonaceous debris provides evidence of airway burns and indications for aggressive control of the airway via endotracheal intubation.[3] Failure to secure the airway may lead to respiratory arrest or need for emergent, surgical airway.

2. Recognize and manage the complications of severe burns and smoke inhalation.

Hypoxia from smoke inhalation is the most common cause of death in the first hours after a burn.[7] Maintenance of adequate oxygenation and ventilation is essential. Careful attention must be paid to the patient's level of consciousness. Continuous pulse oximetry and ABG determinations are also helpful in monitoring the level of hypoxia or hypercarbia.

Carboxyhemoglobinemia. In patients exposed to smoke, CO toxicity should be suspected. Patients should be placed on 100% oxygen immediately. For children with carboxyhemoglobin greater than 25%, consider transfer to a facility with hyperbaric capabilities.

Hypovolemia and **electrolyte imbalance** occur early in children with severe burns. Children with burns exceeding 15% to 20% of BSA require aggressive intravenous fluid resuscitation. The initial fluid resuscitation consists of isotonic crystalloid solution such as **lactated Ringer** or **normal saline 10- to 20-mL/kg bolus** followed by ongoing fluids calculated using the Parkland formula. Urine output should be maintained at a minimum of 1 mL/kg/hr. Electrolyte levels and urinalysis should be followed frequently as ongoing losses are potentially great. Failure to recognize myoglobinuria or hemoglobinuria and need for alkalinization of urine can lead to renal injury.[4]

Capillary leakage in the severely burned patient leads to anasarca and pulmonary edema. It is important to secure at least two sites of intravenous access early in the course before developing edema makes this task more difficult. Vasopressors can be required to improve shock from this mechanism. Volume resuscitation is vital, especially if occult traumatic bleeding is suspected. The use of positive end-expiratory pressure will improve oxygenation in patients with pulmonary edema; however, barotrauma is a complication to be considered.

Burn patients can require significant amounts of narcotics to **control pain**. The doses should be given in small increments with careful monitoring of vital signs.[4]

3. Recognize and manage underlying trauma-related injuries.

Traumatic injuries resulting from falls and from falling debris must always be suspected in fires. Management begins with immobilization of the cervical spine. Careful examination of the head, chest, abdomen, pelvis, back, and extremities for evidence of trauma is essential. Aggressive fluid resuscitation is often required, followed by diagnostic CT scanning and surgical intervention as indicated.[8]

References

1. Dieckmann RA. Pediatric assessment. In: Gausche-Hill M, Fuchs S, Yamamoto L, eds. *APLS: The Pediatric Emergency Medicine Resource.* 4th ed. Sudbury, Mass: American Academy of Pediatrics, American College of Emergency Physicians, Jones and Bartlett Publishing Co; 2004:20-48.

2. Erickson TB. Toxicology: ingestions and smoke inhalation. In: Gausche-Hill M, Fuchs S, Yamamoto L, eds. *APLS: The Pediatric Emergency Medicine Resource.* 4th ed. Sudbury, Mass: American Academy of Pediatrics, American College of Emergency Physicians, Jones and Bartlett Publishing Co; 2004:234-262.

3. Finkelstein JL, Schwartz SB, Madden MR, et al. Pediatric burns. An overview. *Pediatr Clin North Am.* 1992;39:1145-1163.

4. Joffe MD. Burns. In: Fleisher GR, Ludwig S, eds. *Textbook of Pediatric Emergency Medicine.* 4th ed. Philadelphia, Pa: Lippincott Williams & Wilkins; 2000:1427-1434.

5. Coren C. Burn injuries in children. *Pediatr Ann.* 1987;16:328-339.

6. Schiller WR. Burn management in children. *Pediatr Ann.* 1996;25:431-438.

7. Parish RA. Smoke inhalation and carbon monoxide poisoning in children. *Pediatr Emerg Care.* 1986;2:36-41.

8. Tepas JJ III, Fallat ME, Moriarty TM. Trauma. In: Gausche-Hill M, Fuchs S, Yamamoto L, eds. *APLS: The Pediatric Emergency Medicine Resource.* 4th ed. Sudbury, Mass: American Academy of Pediatrics, American College of Emergency Physicians, Jones and Bartlett Publishing Co; 2004:268-319.

SCENARIO #42

Environmental Emergency

Noel S. Zuckerbraun, MD, and Richard A. Saladino, MD

Brief Presenting History

A 6-year-old boy falls through ice while walking home from school with his older siblings. He is rescued by bystanders after being in the water for 10 minutes. Emergency medical technicians arrive on the scene at 15 minutes. The patient is in full arrest.

Pediatric Assessment Triangle

Appearance: Pale, lips white, unresponsive, appears dead

Work of Breathing: No spontaneous breaths

Circulation to the Skin: Skin pale and very cold

Initial Vital Signs

Pulse: 0

Respiratory Rate: 0 (bag-mask ventilation)

Blood Pressure: unobtainable

Oxygen Saturation: unobtainable

ASK YOURSELF

- **How much should this 6-year-old weigh?**

  An estimated weight for a 6-year-old is 22 kg. One can use the length-based Broselow Pediatric Emergency Tape or a pediatric table to determine weight based on age. See Appendix A.

- **What other vital sign should be measured?**

  Temperature, which is 29.5°C (85.1°F) rectal

Physical Examination on Arrival to the Emergency Department

Airway: Airway patent, trachea midline

Breathing: Breath sounds full and equal with BMV

Circulation: Pulseless, pale skin with capillary refill time of greater than 5 seconds

Disability: Pupils dilated and fixed

ASK YOURSELF

- **What is the initial assessment? What is the patient's physiologic status?**

  The patient is in cardiopulmonary arrest after a submersion in icy water. He is hypothermic with a rectal temperature of 29.5°C. Standard thermometers read to only 34°C; if the proper type of thermometer is not used, the temperature will be incorrectly recorded as 34°C.

- **What other associated problems should be considered at this time?**

  For all submersion victims, the possibility of underlying trauma should be considered, and the cervical spine should be immobilized.

Additional History and Physical Examination Findings

Past Medical History: Healthy child

Medications: None

Allergies: None known

ASK YOURSELF

- **What interventions are needed at this time? What complications might be expected?**

Interventions:

- BMV with 100% O_2 should be continued using cricoid pressure and maintaining cervical spine precautions. Preparations should be made for intubation.
- Begin chest compressions.
- Place the patient on a cardiorespiratory monitor with pulse oximetry.
- Perform endotracheal intubation with cervical spine precautions: #2 straight blade, 5.0 cuffed ET tube
- Check end-tidal CO_2. If quantitative end-tidal CO_2 is available, a goal of 28 to 30 is desired.
- Call for chest radiograph to confirm ET tube placement.
- Secure ET tube and place NG or orogastric tube (use orogastric tube for patients with facial trauma).
- Obtain intravenous access and begin fluid resuscitation with **normal saline 20 mL/kg.**
- Place rectal or esophageal continuous temperature probe[1] and begin *active rewarming.*
  - Remove wet clothing, and apply warm blankets.
  - Increase the humidified temperature of inspired oxygen to 44°C.
  - Heat intravenous fluids to 40° to 42°C. Deliver fluids through a fluid warmer using tubing that is as short as possible.
  - Perform gastric or rectal lavage with warmed normal saline heated to 40° to 44°C.

Potential Complications:

- Right mainstem intubation or ET tube dislodged if not properly handled
- Intravenous access not achieved after three attempts or 90 seconds, necessitating intraosseous placement
- If no warming or only passive rewarming (warm blankets) occurs and not active external core rewarming (warmed humidified air via ET tube, warmed intravenous fluids, and various lavage techniques), patient progresses from pulseless electrical activity to ventricular fibrillation. *Note:* At temperatures of less than 30°C, the myocardium is resistant to defibrillation and pharmacologic agents. At these temperatures, defibrillation should be attempted only once. If unsuccessful, CPR should be continued until the patient's temperature is above 30°C.[2]

Progression

The temperature has risen to 31°C. The cardiorespiratory monitor shows sinus bradycardia but no pulses are palpable.

ASK YOURSELF

- **What is the physiologic status now?**

Improving hypothermia with respiratory failure and pulseless electrical activity (PEA).

- **What are the causes of PEA?**

The 4 Hs and the 4 Ts: hypoxia, hypothermia, hypovolemia, and hyper- or hypokalemia and tamponade, tension pneumothorax, toxins, and thromboembolism.

- **What interventions are needed at this time? What complications might be expected?**

Interventions:

- Continue CPR with chest compressions and positive pressure ventilation using a peak end-expiratory pressure (PEEP) of 5 cm H_2O. Continue warming.
- Recheck pulses. Central pulses are now present. Patient is bradycardic with pulse of 50.
- Continue CPR.
- **Epinephrine 0.1 mL/kg, 1:10,000 IV/IO,** or **1:1,000 ET**

- An intraosseous line should have been placed if intravenous access was not already obtained.
- Continue rapid resuscitation with intravenous fluids, with an additional **normal saline 20 mL/kg IV.**
- Place Foley catheter to monitor urine output.
- Continue active rewarming.

Potential Complications:

- Persistent hypoxia and difficult bag ventilation if PEEP not used
- Persistent hypotension if intravenous fluid resuscitation is inadequate
- Pulseless ventricular tachycardia necessitating defibrillation with 2 J/kg if rewarming not continued

■ Why might you expect to have difficulty ventilating and oxygenating this patient?

Aspiration of water occurs in 90% of drowning victims, causing surfactant washout and subsequent atelectasis. In response to the hypoxia, reflex-mediated pulmonary hypertension with intrapulmonary shunting ensues. This results in an increased ventilation-perfusion mismatch and oxygen requirement. The patient may have decreased lung compliance and hence bag ventilation can be difficult. For these reasons, PEEP of 5 to 10 cm H_2O should be used.[3]

Repeat Vital Signs

Pulse: 140

Respiratory Rate: 20

Blood Pressure: 70/40

Oxygen Saturation: 95% (positive pressure ventilation with 100% oxygen)

Temperature: 32°C (89.6°F)

Progression

Pulses are present. The monitor shows sinus tachycardia. The patient remains unresponsive.

ASK YOURSELF

■ What is the physiologic status now?

This patient is now in a perfusing sinus tachycardia rhythm. He remains in decompensated shock. His hypothermia continues to slowly improve with active warming measures.

■ What interventions are needed at this time? What complications might be expected?

Interventions:

- Give third bolus of **normal saline 20 mL/kg**; consider giving **blood (10 mL/kg)** in patients with suspected multiple trauma[4] and/or beginning **dopamine 10 mcg/kg/min.**
- Check rapid glucose, blood gases, and blood metabolic panel.
- Continue active rewarming.

Potential Complications:

- Persistent hypotension if fluid resuscitation inadequate or blood and/or dopamine not instituted
- Seizure from hypoglycemia if rapid glucose not measured
- Pulseless ventricular tachycardia, necessitating defibrillation with 2 J/kg

■ What laboratory studies would be helpful at this time?

The patient has moderate to severe hypothermia associated with asphyxia from submersion. The first blood test should be a rapid blood glucose. Blood should then be sent for the following measurements: serum electrolytes, blood gas, hemoglobin, WBC count, hepatic and renal function tests, creatine kinase levels, and coagulation profile. Toxicology screening should be considered if an ingestion cannot be ruled out by history.[1]

■ What other complications might be expected for this patient?

- Persistent hypotension
- Seizure from head trauma
- Dysrhythmias can develop during rewarming. Peripheral vasodilation occurs with rewarming, allowing blood to circulate to the cold peripheral extremities. This in turn can

decrease the temperature of the circulating blood and subsequently decrease the body's core temperature. This phenomenon is known as core temperature afterdrop. *Afterdrop* can lead to complications with altered mental status and breathing and cardiac dysrhythmias. For this reason, in patients with moderate to severe hypothermia, active external rewarming techniques should be applied only to the trunk, not to the extremities.[1] The goal should be to rewarm the patient 1° to 2°C/hr to a range of 33° to 35°C.[2] If the patient is hemodynamically stable, aggressive rewarming above this range should be avoided because hyperthermia has been shown to worsen underlying cerebral injury in post–cardiac arrest patients.[5]

Objectives of This Resuscitation

1. Recognize priorities of the management of drowning.

The ABCs of resuscitation, including immobilization of the cervical spine, are always addressed first. All submersion patients have hypoxemia. With the underlying pulmonary insult and subsequent fluid resuscitation, expect the submersion victim to develop pulmonary edema and hypoxia. The goal of resuscitation is to reverse the hypoxia. Endotracheal intubation with PEEP for the treatment of pulmonary edema is the single most effective method for reversing hypoxemia. Routine use of antibiotics is not recommended with the possible exception of submersion in grossly contaminated water (e.g., sewage), for which prophylaxis can be considered.[3] Routine use of corticosteroids is not indicated.[3]

Despite results from experimental animal models, there are no important clinical or therapeutic differences between fresh water and saltwater drowning in humans.[3] Both fresh water and saltwater drowning victims need aggressive fluid resuscitation. In addition, hypothermia should be anticipated and treated in all submersion patients, including victims of warm-water drowning.

2. Recognize and treat hypothermia and complications of hypothermia.

Hypothermia is defined as a core temperature of less than 35°C. Many factors can predispose children to nonintentional hypothermia, including endocrine or metabolic derangements (hypoglycemia, hypothyroidism), infection, intoxication, intracranial pathology (trauma, congenital), submersion injury, environmental exposure, burns, and iatrogenic exposure (cold intravenous fluids, environmental exposure during treatment). Of these, submersion injury is the most common and results in the highest rate of mortality.[2] In cold water, the clinical effects are more rapid and more profound. In the emergency department, the main goals are to provide physiologic support to maintain cardiovascular stability while stopping the fall in core temperature and establishing a safe, steady rewarming rate.

The degree of hypothermia can be classified as mild, moderate, or severe. This classification helps to predict clinical findings and aid in choosing the appropriate method of rewarming.[6]

- **Mild hypothermia** (32° to 35°C): The patient may have slowed mental status and shivering as the only manifestations of hypothermia at this stage. *Passive rewarming* is usually sufficient.
- **Moderate hypothermia** (28° to 32°C): Coma occurs at temperatures less than 30°C. Cyanosis, tissue edema, and rigidity ensue. Respirations and pulses can be difficult to detect. A "J" (or Osborn) wave can now be detectable on an electrocardiogram. *Active rewarming* should be instituted.
- **Severe hypothermia** (<28°C): The patient can appear dead with dilated and unresponsive pupils and no detectable vital signs. *Active rewarming* should be instituted.

Rewarming can be performed via *passive* or *active* methods. The method used should be based on the severity of hypothermia.[6] Temperature should be continuously monitored with a rectal or an esophageal probe.

- **Passive rewarming** involves the use of warm blankets and can be used for patients with mild hypothermia.
- **Active rewarming** is required for patients with moderate to severe hypothermia and can be done with active external or active core techniques. *Active external rewarming* includes hot packs, heat lamps, and forced air external warmers.[7]

These techniques should be applied primarily to the trunk and not the extremities as application to the extremities can result in afterdrop complications (discussed earlier). *Active core rewarming* methods typically include warmed oxygen, warmed intravenous fluid (the shortest possible length of intravenous tubing must be used to ensure efficacy of this method), and lavage techniques (gastric/peritoneal/rectal lavage with warm normal saline and, in more severe cases, open thoracotomy for mediastinal lavage with warm sterile saline). Cardiopulmonary bypass is the most aggressive and most rapid method of active core rewarming.[8] Early notification of the trauma team and ICU staff is essential, especially if hypothermia is refractory to aggressive rewarming and requires peritoneal/ thoracotomy lavage or cardiopulmonary bypass.

It is important to recognize and treat ventricular tachycardia and ventricular fibrillation. Cardioactive medications and cardioversion or defibrillation attempts are typically ineffective when the core temperature is 30°C or less. At these temperatures, defibrillation should be attempted only once, and CPR should be continued until the temperature is above 30°C. At temperatures above 30°C, electricity should be used if ventricular fibrillation/ventricular tachycardia persists.[2]

In some cases of rapid severe hypothermia in icy cold water (<5°C), cerebral protection can occur. For this reason, resuscitative efforts should never be terminated until the patient's core body temperature is greater than 32°C for at least 30 minutes if possible.[2] Traditionally stated, "You are not dead until you are warm and dead."

3. Consider associated problems with submersion injuries: intoxication, head injury, and cervical spine injury.

Consider and treat intoxications secondary to alcohol and other drugs. Consider and treat traumatic injuries, which may not be readily recognizable secondary to hypothermia and altered mental status. Early consultation with the trauma team is indicated. Consider underlying medical conditions that may play a role in submersion injuries such as seizure or cardiac disorders (including long QT syndromes).

References

1. Biem J, Koehncke N, Classen D, et al. Out of the cold: management of hypothermia and frostbite. *CMAJ*. 2003;168:305-311.
2. Hodge D. Environmental emergencies. In: Gausche-Hill M, Fuchs S, Yamamoto L, eds. *APLS: The Pediatric Emergency Medicine Resource*. 4th ed. Sudbury, Mass: American Academy of Pediatrics, American College of Emergency Physicians, Jones and Bartlett; 2004:220-223.
3. Orlowski JP, Szpilman D. Drowning: rescue, resuscitation and reanimation. *Pediatr Clin North Am*. 2001;48:627-646.
4. Wetzel RC, Burns RC. Multiple trauma in children: critical care overview. *Crit Care Med*. 2002;30(suppl):S468-S477.
5. Hickey RW, Kochanek PM, Ferimer H, et al. Hypothermia and hyperthermia in children after resuscitation from cardiac arrest. *Pediatrics*. 2000;106:118-122.
6. Danzl DF, Pozos RS. Accidental hypothermia. *N Engl J Med*. 1994;331:1756-1760.
7. Steele MT, Nelson MJ, Sessler DI, et al. Forced air speeds rewarming in accidental hypothermia. *Ann Emerg Med*. 1996;27:479-484.
8. Walpoth BH, Walpoth-Aslan BN, Mattle HP, et al. Outcome of survivors of accidental deep hypothermia and circulatory arrest treated with extracorporeal blood warming. *N Engl J Med*. 1997;337:1500-1505.

SCENARIO #43

Environmental Emergency

Holly E. Perry, MD

Brief Presenting History

A 16-month-old boy is brought in to the emergency department by his 18-year-old babysitter because he is "acting funny."

Pediatric Assessment Triangle

Appearance: Flushed child with eyes closed, lying motionless on stretcher

Work of Breathing: Unlabored but rapid and shallow; breath sounds clear

Circulation to the Skin: Strong peripheral pulses; skin diffusely flushed

Initial Vital Signs

Pulse: 200

Respiratory Rate: 60

Blood Pressure: 80/60

Temperature: 41.7°C (107.1°F) rectal

Physical Examination on Arrival to the Emergency Department

Airway: Patent, without evidence of obstruction

Breathing: No retractions; good air exchange; respiratory rate rapid, but breath sounds clear

Circulation: Capillary refill time 4 to 5 seconds, strong peripheral pulses

Disability: Eyes closed with no spontaneous opening; responsive only to pain; no verbalizations

ASK YOURSELF

- **What is the initial assessment? What is the patient's physiologic status?**

  The patient presents with altered mental status, significant fever, and possible uncompensated shock.

- **What could be causing these symptoms?**

  The differential diagnosis of lethargy in a child is extensive. Two useful mnemonics are **I SPOUT A VEIN** and **AEIOU TIPS.**

  Insulin [too little or too much]

  Shock

  Psychogenic

  Opiates and other drugs

  Uremia and other metabolic abnormalities

  Trauma

  Alcohol

  Vascular

  Infection/intussusception

  Neoplasm)

  Alcohol

  Encephalopathy/endocrinopathy/electrolytes

  Insulin/intussusception

  Opiates and other drugs

  Uremia

Trauma

Infection

Psychogenic

Seizure

The presence of fever helps to narrow the diagnosis to infection, ingestion (anticholinergics such as diphenhydramine, amphetamines, salicylates, dinitrophenol, and illicit drugs, including MDMA, cocaine, and PCP), and heat stroke.

■ **What additional history would help you establish the diagnosis?**

Defining the rapidity of onset of symptoms is essential. Both sepsis and meningitis generally have a prodromal phase before the onset of lethargy. Assessing the probability that the child could have ingested a toxic substance and obtaining a list of the medications available at home or in the babysitter's possession would be useful. Last, knowing the ambient temperature and humidity to which the child was exposed would be helpful in assessing the risk for heat stroke.

Additional History and Physical Examination Findings

Child has had vomiting and diarrhea for the past 2 days with poor oral intake and fewer wet diapers than normal. He did not have a fever, but he had been "clingy" all morning, and the babysitter had been holding him almost constantly. She drove to the grocery store and left him in his car seat with the car locked and the windows slightly open while she ran into the store "for just a minute" to get some ginger ale. The child had just fallen asleep when she got to the store; he had been cranky but alert when she put him in his car seat at home. The current weather outside is cloudless and 95°F, with 80% humidity.

Past Medical History: Healthy child with no chronic medical problems

Medications: None

Allergies: None known

Physical Examination: Head is normocephalic and atraumatic. Mucous membranes parched. Pupils equal 3 mm and reactive to 2 mm bilaterally. Skin is flushed and dry; no discrete rash. Responsive to pain, nonfocal.

ASK YOURSELF

■ **What is the most likely diagnosis?**

Heat stroke is most likely given the evidence of dehydration and acute change in mental status temporally associated with environmental heat stress. Sepsis or meningitis also must be considered in the differential diagnosis. Not only is the incidence of sepsis much greater than that of heat stroke, but also the prompt administration of antibiotics could be lifesaving. Ingestion is less likely because the child did not have an opportunity to ingest any medications because he was constantly held that morning, nor does the physical examination support common causes of hyperthermia from an ingestion such as dilated pupils, which would be seen after ingestion of either an anticholinergic or a sympathomimetic agent.[1]

■ **What interventions are needed at this time? What complications might be expected?**

Interventions:

- 100% O_2 by face mask.
- Place the patient on a cardiorespiratory monitor with pulse oximetry and continuous rectal temperature probe.
- Establish intravenous access with two large-bore intravenous lines. Administer **normal saline 20 mL/kg** bolus over 10 to 20 minutes.
- Remove the patient's clothes.
- Institute active cooling measures. Place ice packs over the groin and axillae. Mist patient's entire body with cool water or wrap in a cool, wet sheet. Provide for air circulation over the patient using an electric fan. **Goal is to cool patient to 38.3°C within 1 hour.** *Note:* Antipyretics are ineffective, and cooling blankets alone are not sufficient.
- After obtaining a blood culture and considering a lumbar puncture, administer **ceftriaxone 100 mg/kg IV.**

Potential Complications:

- Unable to obtain intravenous access; in this case, start an intraosseous line.
- Patient starts shivering. Shivering must be controlled as muscular activity will produce significant heat. Benzodiazepines are the preferred agent to control shivering. Chlorpromazine has been recommended in the past, but there are a number of objections to its use. It may interfere with thermoregulation, lower the seizure threshold, further depress mental status, and exacerbate hypotension.[1]

Progression

The child becomes ashen. He develops weak pulses and an increased capillary refill time.

Repeat Vital Signs

Pulse: 240

Respiratory Rate: 50

Blood Pressure: 50/30

Temperature: 41.1°C (106°F)

Oxygen Saturation: Not recording

ASK YOURSELF

- **What has happened?**

  The patient is developing clearly uncompensated cardiogenic shock due to heat-related injury to the myocardium.

- **What is the next appropriate intervention?**

  Dobutamine 5 to 20 mcg/kg/min IV as a continuous infusion should be started. **Dobutamine** provides inotropic support but is not a vasoconstrictor, allowing for continued heat dissipation. Agents that are strong vasoconstrictors such as **epinephrine** and **norepinephrine** should not be used because they interfere with dissipation of heat. The patient may require 1 to 2 additional fluid boluses with normal saline (20 mL/kg) followed by colloid (eg, 5% albumin).

Repeat Vital Signs

Pulse: 190

Respiratory Rate: 40

Blood Pressure: 75/55

Temperature: 40.1°C (104.2°F)

Oxygen Saturation: 96%

Progression

The patient has a generalized tonic-clonic seizure.

ASK YOURSELF

- **What has happened?**

  The child has experienced a complication of heat stroke. Seizures can occur, particularly during the cooling phase.

- **What are other potential complications of heat stroke? How should they be managed?**

  The rapid rise of body temperature leads to pathologic change in every organ system. In addition to cardiogenic shock and seizures, other complications include rhabdomyolysis, acute renal failure, and disseminated intravascular coagulation (DIC). Laboratory evaluation should include electrolytes, BUN, creatinine, calcium, phosphorous, CBC, PT/PTT, creatine phosphokinase (CPK) with MB fraction, and urinalysis. If myoglobinuria occurs, adequate fluid should be given to maintain urine output at greater than 1 mL/kg/hr, and the urine should be alkalinized by administering sufficient **sodium bicarbonate.** A dose of **mannitol (0.25 to 1 g/kg)** should be considered, although this may exacerbate hypotension. In the event of DIC, **fresh frozen plasma** should be administered.[2]

- **What interventions are needed at this time?**

  - Attempt to stop the seizure with **lorazepam 0.05 to 0.1 mg/kg IV/IO.**
  - Repeat lorazepam once if seizure continues.
  - **Phenobarbital 20 mg/kg IV/IO** if seizure remains refractory to lorazepam; airway and ventilatory effort should be closely monitored under these circumstances.
  - Continue aggressive cooling measures.

■ **What is the prognosis?**

The overall prognosis depends primarily on how long the temperature has been elevated before cooling, the maximum temperature reached, and the affected individual's overall health. The mortality rate for heat stroke has been reported to range between 30% and 80%.[2]

Objectives of This Scenario

1. Describe the spectrum of heat illness.

Heat illness is divided into minor and major manifestations based on the temperature and severity of symptoms. Minor heat illness includes heat edema, heat cramps, and heat syncope. Heat exhaustion and heat stroke are the two forms of major heat illness. Heat exhaustion is a precursor to heat stroke. Symptoms include a temperature up to 39°C, malaise, headache, nausea, irritability, and dehydration. Temperature regulatory mechanisms remain intact. In contrast, normal thermoregulatory mechanisms are no longer intact with heat stroke. The patient with heat stroke usually presents with temperature higher than 41°C and altered mental status.

Heat stroke is categorized as nonexertional (classic) and exertional. Classic heat stroke is most commonly seen during periods of high environmental temperature and humidity, especially in those individuals least able to tolerate heat stress: infants, the elderly, and patients who are chronically ill or psychiatrically impaired. In contrast, exertional heat stroke occurs as a result of increased motor activity. It can occur in young healthy individuals such as athletes or military recruits. Predisposing factors include dehydration, failure to acclimatize, and poor physical conditioning.[3]

2. Understand what factors predispose to heat illness and why.

Hyperthermia occurs when the heat load exceeds the ability of the body to dissipate heat. Heat load is generated by basal metabolism, muscle activity including shivering, and environmental causes. Body heat can be dissipated by radiation, conduction, convection, and evaporation. Radiation accounts for up to 55% of heat loss and is dependent on the difference between body surface temperature and the environment. Radiation, conduction, and convection are ineffective ways to lose heat when the ambient temperature is greater than 37°C. Evaporation accounts for up to 30% of heat loss but is inefficient when the humidity exceeds 90% to 95%.[4]

Classic heat stroke is most frequently noted in the elderly and in infants.[5] The susceptibility of young children is multifactorial. In comparison to adults, sweating starts at a higher temperature. In addition, they have a larger body-surface-area-to-volume ratio than an adult so that they absorb comparatively more heat.[4] For the same reason, infants are much more susceptible to loss of body heat during periods of low environmental temperatures.

References:

1. Vassallo SU, Delaney KA. Thermoregulatory principles. In Goldfrank LR, Flomenbaum NE, et al, eds. *Toxicologic Emergencies.* 6th ed. Stamford, Conn: Appleton & Lange; 1998:285-308.
2. Bouchama A, Knochel JP. Heat stroke. *N Engl J Med.* 2002;346:1978-1988.
3. Tek D, Olshaker JS. Heat illness. *Emerg Med Clin North Am.* 1992;10:299-310.
4. Hodge D. Environmental emergencies. In: Gausche-Hill M, Fuchs S, Yamamoto L, eds. *APLS: The Pediatric Emergency Medicine Resource.* 4th ed. Sudbury, Mass: American Academy of Pediatrics, American College of Emergency Physicians, Jones and Bartlett Publishing Co; 2004:216-230.
5. Centers for Disease Control and Prevention. Heat-related illnesses and death: Missouri 1998 and United States 1979-1996. *MMWR Morb Mortal Wkly Rep.* 1999;48:469-472.

SCENARIO #44

Environmental Emergency

Guy L. Upshaw, MD

Brief Presenting History

A 10-year-old girl is brought in by her mother, who found the patient unconscious and "hardly breathing" and states, "I think she might have been shocked."

Pediatric Assessment Triangle

Appearance: Poorly responsive and limp

Work of Breathing: Shallow infrequent respirations, no retractions

Circulation to the Skin: Mottled, gray-cyanotic diffusely

Initial Vital Signs

Pulse: 150

Respiratory Rate: 8

Blood Pressure: 70/40

Temperature: 36.4°C (97.5°F) tympanic

ASK YOURSELF

- **How much should this 10-year-old weigh?**

  An estimated weight for a 10-year-old child is 32 kg. One can use the length-based Broselow Pediatric Emergency Tape or a pediatric table to determine weight based on age. See Appendix A.

Physical Examination on Arrival to the Emergency Department

Airway: Patent, poor gag reflex

Breathing: Shallow, infrequent, symmetric respirations; clear breath sounds

Circulation: Tachycardic; no murmur, rub, or gallop; skin mottled; distal extremities cool; capillary refill time 5 seconds; distal pulses thready

Disability: Responsive only to pain; withdraws extremities, briefly opens eyes; poor tone; pupils 5 mm and sluggishly reactive

ASK YOURSELF

- **What is the initial assessment? What is the patient's physiologic status?**

  She is critically ill or injured with respiratory insufficiency, decompensated shock, and altered mental status.

- **What is causing this critical instability?**

  Electric shock is most likely on the basis of the currently available history. A severe shock could profoundly injure the central nervous system, heart, and/or musculature, causing such a presentation. The differential diagnosis is otherwise quite broad. See "Evaluation and Management section on Altered Mental Status."

■ **What additional history and physical examination findings would help establish the diagnosis?**

History: Knowledge of the last known activity of the patient may be helpful as well as the presence or absence of symptoms or signs of illness before the presentation.

Physical Examination: Determining whether trauma such as shock entrance/exit burns or head injury exists is important.

Additional History and Physical Examination Findings

The mother left the kitchen while the patient was washing the dishes. Minutes later, the lights and television went out. The mother called the child and became concerned when there was no answer. She found the child on the floor beside the kitchen sink, also noting a burning smell in the air. The mother called 911 but did not wait for the ambulance. A police officer arrived to find an empty house, noting the electricity was off, as well as noting a charred electrical outlet and radio plug by the kitchen sink. Mother states the patient was acting well earlier in the day.

Past Medical History: Healthy, no chronic illness; tetanus booster at age 5

Medications: None

Allergies: None known

Physical Examination: Oxygen saturation is 68% on room air. Skin is notable for mild yellow-white lesions with surrounding erythema of the right thumb and index finger and the left palm, which are beginning to swell. The scalp and neck are without obvious trauma. The abdomen is soft and nondistended. The extremities have skin findings as above but no obvious deformities.

ASK YOURSELF

■ **What is the most likely diagnosis?**

The history and examination findings point to severe electrical injury.

■ **What interventions are needed at this time? What complications might be expected?**

Interventions:

- BMV with 100% O_2
  1. Cricoid pressure if gag reflex absent
  2. Prepare for rapid sequence intubation.
- In-line cervical spine immobilization
- Place the patient on a cardiorespiratory monitor with pulse oximetry.
- Attempt intravenous access.
  1. Place intraosseous needle if intravenous attempts are unsuccessful in first 90 seconds.
  2. Rapid volume expansion with isotonic crystalloid: **normal saline** or **lactated Ringer 20 mL/kg IV/IO.**
  3. Laboratory studies: Bedside glucose, ABGs, electrolytes, BUN and creatinine, urinalysis, urine myoglobin

Potential Complications:

- Oxygen saturation remains low because of poor BMV technique
- Soft tissues swell and tense around the intraosseous line during rapid fluid administration, dislodging the intraosseous line and thereby necessitating central venous line placement or intraosseous line placement in the other tibia or distal femur.

Repeat Vital Signs

Pulse: 180

Respiratory Rate: 0

Blood Pressure: 50 and palpable

Oxygen Saturation: 92% with BMV

Progression

Patient is now apneic and unresponsive.

ASK YOURSELF

■ **What interventions are needed at this time? What complications might be expected?**

Interventions:

- Modified RSI
  1. Preoxygenate with 100% O_2

2. #2 or #3 Mac or Miller laryngoscope blade
3. 6.5 uncuffed or 6.0 cuffed ET tube
4. Continue cricoid pressure until intubated.
5. Lung examination, check monitors to confirm placement
6. End-tidal CO_2 determination
7. Call for chest radiograph to assess ET tube position.
8. Secure ET tube and place nasogastric tube.
9. ABGs. Venous blood gases are acceptable if O_2 saturation is within the normal range.

- Repeat **normal saline/lactated Ringer 20 mL/kg IV/IO** rapidly.
- Consider **dopamine continuous infusion 5 to 20 mcg/kg/min IV/IO** if perfusion does not improve.

Potential Complications:

- Patient becomes partially responsive before intubation and now requires RSI with pharmacologic sedation and neuromuscular blockade.
- Absent left lung breath sounds if ET tube placed in right mainstem bronchus
- Oxygen saturation drops if ET tube placed in esophagus or if oxygen tubing becomes disconnected.

Progression

ECG Monitor:

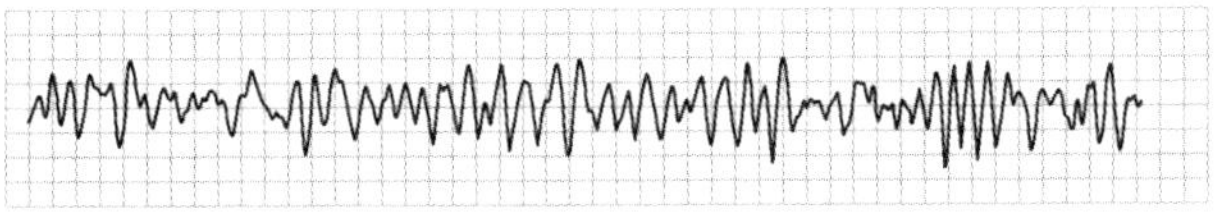

ASK YOURSELF

■ **What interventions are needed at this time? What complications might be expected?**

Interventions:

- Continue bagging 100% O_2 through the ET tube.
- Palpate femoral pulse to confirm pulselessness, and begin chest compressions.
- **Defibrillate** with **2 J/kg**, then **2 to 4 J/kg** up to 3 times as needed.
- **Epinephrine 0.01 mg/kg IV/IO** if the rhythm does not convert. (See "Evaluation and Management section on Circulation," Figure 1, for pulseless arrest algorithm.)

Potential Complications:

- Persistent ventricular fibrillation
- Seizure due to neurologic injury from electric shock or hypoxia/acidosis
- Hypotension secondary to blood loss from blunt thoracic or abdominal trauma (if the original mechanism of electrical injury had been a lightning strike or was associated with a fall from height after receiving a shock, eg, retrieving a kite from high voltage wires).

Progression

Patient converts to sinus rhythm. The pulses are palpable but perfusion remains compromised.

ASK YOURSELF

■ **What additional management and disposition would be expected?**

Continue to evaluate and treat hypotension. CT scans of the head and abdomen may be indicted to evaluate for traumatic injury and occult bleeding.

When stabilized, transfer the patient to ICU for continued critical care and cardiac monitoring.

Objectives of This Scenario

1. Recognize the presentation of electrical injury.

Electrical injury presents with a wide range of complaints from mild skin irritation and a "shock" sensation to full cardiopulmonary arrest. The extent of electrical injuries depends on the resistance and direction of electrical current through the patient's body; the type, frequency, and intensity of the current; and the duration of contact.[1,2]

In severe electrical injury, the patient's skin often has current entrance and exit wounds, which may vary from mild, superficial to full-thickness burns. Often severe shocks cause more internal injury than surface burns imply; thus, a high degree of suspicion for internal injury is warranted.[1,3-5] However, some high-voltage injuries such as lightning strikes can produce relatively small skin lesions and rarely lead to deep thermal injury as the exposure is instantaneous.[2,5]

Respiratory arrest can be secondary to electric current injury to the medullary respiratory center, tetanic contraction, or paralysis of the diaphragm and chest wall muscles, or it may accompany primary cardiac arrest.[1,2,5,6] Cardiac arrhythmias can be induced by primary respiratory arrest.[1,5,6]

Cardiac presentations include asystole (typically from high-voltage direct or alternating current), ventricular tachycardia, ventricular fibrillation (typically from low or high alternating current), sinus tachycardia, supraventricular tachycardia, various degrees of heart block, and atrial and ventricular ectopy.[1-3,5] Patients may describe "crushing" chest pain secondary to myocardial injury.[5]

Symptoms of CNS injury and/or hypoxia include loss of consciousness, confusion, poor recall, coma, seizures, and paralysis.[1,2,5,6] These effects may be transient.[2,5]

2. Recognize and treat associated traumatic injuries.

Electrical injuries can be associated with significant force. High DC voltage can throw a person. DC or AC voltage can cause falls. Lightning, which can generate 1 million V and a 30,000 K temperature within its stroke channel, can create a shock wave causing mechanical trauma.[2] These forces can result in multiple traumatic injuries including head and cervical spine injury. Tetanic muscle contractions can result in fractures, tendon rupture, and dislocations.[2,5,6] Patients who "lock on" to AC voltage can incur deep thermal injury.

Patients with significant electrical exposure should have the cervical spine immobilized and be evaluated as any other multiple trauma patient. In addition to blunt trauma, those patients in whom a deep tissue injury is suspected or those with significant skin burns require surgical consultation. Escharotomy or even fasciotomy may be necessary to restore normal tissue perfusion depending on the depth of the injury.[1,7] Fluid replacement using traditional skin burn formulas can underestimate actual needs due to third-spacing of intravascular volume into surrounding tissues.[3,7]

3. Manage the complications of electrical injuries.

Because of the multiple factors that determine the extent of electrical injuries and direction of electrical flow through the body, all patients should be aggressively evaluated for potential life-threatening complications.

Cardiopulmonary arrest is the most common cause of immediate death in severe electrical injury.[1,5,6] Rapid assessment and support of the airway, breathing, and circulation are imperative. Aggressive, prolonged resuscitation efforts are indicated as most patients with electrical injury are young and otherwise without preexisting cardiac disease. They may have neurologic injury to the brainstem, impairing respiratory drive. Thoracic muscle tetany or paralysis can cause primary respiratory arrest leading to secondary cardiac arrest.[1,2,5,6] Autonomic system injury can cause transiently fixed, dilated pupils or anisocoria, which is not indicative of overwhelming brain injury and in this instance should not dissuade further resuscitation.[2,5] Basic and advanced life support of respiratory failure and cardiac arrhythmias must be tenaciously provided.

Rhabdomyolysis can result from severe electrical injury. Resultant renal myoglobin deposition can lead to acute tubular necrosis and renal failure.[1,2,5,6] Emergency management requires aggressive hydration with Ringer lactate or normal saline to maintain urine output at no less than 1 mL/kg/hr. Alkalinization is recommended to keep blood pH at 7.35 to 7.40, and use of the osmotic diuretic mannitol can further aid in the excretion of myoglobin.[2,7] Hyperkalemia can result from the same severe muscle injury and must be managed appropriately.[3,5] See also Scenario #28.

References

1. Koumbourlis A. Electrical injuries. *Crit Care Med.* 2002;30(11 suppl):S424-S430.
2. Jain S, Bandi V. Electrical and lightning injuries. *Crit Care Clin.* 1999;15:319-331.
3. Smith ML. Pediatric burns: management of thermal, electrical, and chemical burns and burn-like dermatologic conditions. *Pediatr Ann.* 2000;29:367-378.
4. Andrews CJ, Cooper MA, ten Duis HJ, et al. The pathology of electrical and lightning injuries. In: Wecht CJ, ed. *Forensic Sciences.* New York: Matthew Bender and Co; 1995.
5. Baum CR. Electrical injuries. In: Fleischer GR, Ludwig S, eds. *Textbook of Pediatric Emergency Medicine.* 4th ed. Baltimore, Md: Williams & Wilkins; 2000:959-963.
6. American Heart Association in collaboration with International Committee on Resuscitation and Emergency Cardiovascular Care: International Consensus on Science. Electric shock and lightning strikes. *Circulation.* 2000;102(suppl I):I-250-I-252.
7. Tepas JJ III, Fallat M, Moriarty TM. Electrical trauma. In: Gausche-Hill M, Fuchs S, Yamamoto L, eds. *APLS: The Pediatric Emergency Medicine Resource.* 4th ed. Sudbury, Mass: American Academy of Pediatrics, American College of Emergency Physicians, Jones and Bartlett Publishing Co; 2004:316-321.

SCENARIO #45

Environmental Emergency

William M. McDonnell, MD, JD

Brief Presenting History

An 18-year-old man is brought to the emergency department in Leadville, Colorado, complaining of a severe headache, nausea, vomiting, cough, and dyspnea.

Pediatric Assessment Triangle

Appearance: Awake, anxious, agitated

Work of Breathing: Tachypnea with persistent cough

Circulation to the Skin: Pallor with central cyanosis

Initial Vital Signs

Pulse: 100

Respiratory Rate: 34

Blood Pressure: 140/70

Temperature: 38.5°C (101.3°F)

Oxygen Saturation: 78% on room air

Physical Examination on Arrival to the Emergency Department

Airway: Mild dyspnea

Breathing: Tachypnea, with mild retractions; diminished breath sounds with diffuse crackles more prominent in right lung fields

Circulation: Normal heart tones without murmur; strong peripheral pulses, brisk capillary refill

Disability: Awake and responsive but somewhat confused, ataxic gait

ASK YOURSELF

- **What is the initial assessment? What is the patient's physiologic status?**

  This febrile patient is hypoxic and is experiencing respiratory distress. His altered mental status and ataxia demonstrate neurologic impairment.

- **What could be causing his distress?**

  The hypoxia, tachypnea, and crackles suggest compromised pulmonary gas exchange. The differential diagnosis includes infection, acute asthma exacerbation, and pulmonary edema. The patient's headache, agitation, confusion, and ataxia also suggest a neurologic component, the differential diagnosis of which includes hypoxia, dehydration with shock, infection, intracranial hemorrhage or infarction, and cerebral edema.

- **What additional history would help you establish the diagnosis?**

  The duration and degree of fever and respiratory symptoms might help distinguish an infectious cause. Previous episodes of wheezing and respiratory distress might suggest acute asthma exacerbation. A history of trauma would help establish diagnoses of pulmonary contusion, intracranial hemorrhage, and/or cerebral edema. Determining the patient's altitude of residence, his time at the current altitude, the temporal relation between the onset of his current symptoms and arrival at current altitude, and any previous history of altitude sickness might help establish a diagnosis of acute mountain sickness (AMS).

Additional History and Physical Examination Findings

This previously healthy 18-year-old athlete flew from San Diego, California, into Denver and drove immediately to Leadville, Colorado (elevation 10,150 ft/3,000 m), 2 days ago for a mountain bike race. After substantial alcohol consumption on the night of arrival, he has been complaining of insomnia, nausea, headache, and loss of appetite. He denies sore throat, nasal congestion, or rhinorrhea. He has had no subjective fever. Although his performance in a bicycle race yesterday was poor, he denies any falls, collisions, or other trauma.

Past Medical History: No significant previous illnesses or chronic medical problems, including no asthma, wheezing episodes, or other significant respiratory problems

Medications: No chronic medications. The patient has taken several appropriate doses of ibuprofen over the past 2 days, with some transient improvement of symptoms.

Physical Examination: Head shows no evidence of trauma. Pupils are round and appropriately reactive. Nares are patent without discharge. Oral mucosa is tacky. Oropharynx is without erythema, exudates, or lesions. Neck is supple without lymphadenopathy. Tachypnea is noted at rest, with intercostal and subcostal retractions. Also noted are diffuse crackles with increased prominence in the right middle lobe, intermittent cough productive of pink-tinged frothy sputum, and tachycardia, with normal peripheral pulses. Patient is awake and alert, with appropriate verbal responses. Ataxic gait is observed. Cranial nerves, sensation, strength, and deep tendon reflexes are grossly normal.

ASK YOURSELF

■ What is the most likely diagnosis?

The history of rapid onset of symptoms shortly after travel to high altitude strongly suggests AMS and potentially the more severe acute altitude illnesses, high-altitude pulmonary edema (HAPE) and high-altitude cerebral edema (HACE). These high-altitude syndromes affect nonacclimatized travelers shortly after ascent to high altitude.[1-3] High-altitude illness also can occur in high-altitude residents after a visit to low altitude and subsequent return home.[4] AMS is characterized by nonspecific symptoms such as headache, anorexia, nausea, vomiting, fatigue, dizziness, low-grade fever, and sleep disturbance that appear shortly after rapid ascent to high altitude.[1,2,5] It is important to recognize AMS because it can progress to the life-threatening conditions of HAPE and HACE.[1,2,5]

■ What interventions are needed at this time? What complications might be expected?

Interventions:

- Supplemental oxygen
- Place the patient on a cardiorespiratory monitor with pulse oximetry.
- Obtain intravenous access and administer **isotonic crystalloid solution 20 mL/kg**
- Laboratory studies including ABG, CBC, and serum glucose
- Chest radiograph
- Electrocardiogram
- **Nifedipine 10 mg PO** may help to reduce pulmonary vascular resistance and pulmonary artery pressure.[1,2,5]
- **Dexamethasone 10 mg IV:** Treatment for HACE seems to be beneficial if instituted early, although definitive evidence of efficacy is lacking.[1-3,5]
- Prepare for medical transport to lower elevation.

Potential Complications:

- **Nifedipine** can produce hypotension.

Repeat Vital Signs

Pulse: 110

Respiratory Rate: 40

Blood Pressure: 150/70

Oxygen Saturation: 80% on 7 L O_2 by nasal cannula

Laboratory Test Results: ABGs: pH 7.48, P_{CO_2} 28, P_{aO_2} 50. CBC: WBC count 14,000, hemoglobin 13.5, hematocrit 40, platelets 380,000, glucose 125

Radiology Studies: Chest radiograph shows normal cardiac silhouette, full pulmonary arteries, diffuse patchy alveolar and interstitial infiltrates more prominent in right middle and bilateral lower lobes.

Electrocardiogram: Right ventricular strain (asymmetric ST-segment depression and T-wave inversion) in leads II, III, aVF, V_1, and V_2

Progression

Increasingly labored breathing with decreasing respiratory rate. Decreasing oxygen saturations despite supplemental oxygen. Decreasing level of consciousness, with the patient becoming drowsy and no longer verbally responsive or following commands.

ASK YOURSELF

■ What has happened?

The patient is exhibiting signs of both HAPE and HACE. He is showing respiratory insufficiency and impending respiratory failure. Cerebral edema is also evident, and without prompt intervention, he may progress to complete unresponsiveness.

Repeat Vital Signs

Pulse: 130

Respiratory Rate: 8

Blood Pressure: 100/60

Oxygen Saturation: 65% on 7 L O_2 by face mask

ASK YOURSELF

■ What interventions are needed at this time? What complications might be expected?

Interventions:

- BMV with 100% O_2 using cricoid pressure Preparations should be made for RSI.
- RSI[6]
  1. #3 Miller or #3 Macintosh laryngoscope blade, 8.0 cuffed ET tube
  2. Preoxygenate with 100% O_2 while continuing cricoid pressure.
  3. **Lidocaine 100 mg IV** to blunt increased intracranial pressure response to intubation
  4. **Etomidate 20 mg IV**, sedative with minimal cardiovascular and intracranial pressure effects
  5. **Rocuronium 60 mg IV** or succinylcholine 80 mg IV for muscle relaxation
- End-tidal CO_2 monitor, auscultate breath sounds over chest and abdomen
- Chest radiograph to confirm ET tube placement
- Secure ET tube and place NG tube.
- Measure ABGs.
- Medical evacuation to lower elevation

Potential Complications:

- Emesis during BMV requiring suctioning, especially if cricoid pressure is not applied
- Abdominal distention leading to impaired ventilation and/or emesis if an NG tube is not placed
- Right mainstem intubation if ET tube is inserted too far (beyond 24 cm)
- Desaturation and progression to cardiopulmonary arrest if esophageal intubation is unrecognized due to failure to verify ET tube placement with end-tidal CO_2 monitor, auscultation, and chest radiograph

■ What additional complications might be expected for this patient?

If this patient with severe HACE is not rapidly transported to a lower elevation, increasing cerebral edema can be expected. Progression to deep coma or death from brain herniation can occur within hours to days from the onset of symptoms.[1,5,7]

Objectives of This Scenario

1. Recognize acute mountain sickness.

This patient presented with the classic history and hallmark symptoms of AMS. The most common of the acute mountain illnesses, AMS includes the nonspecific symptoms of headache, anorexia, nausea, dyspnea, sleep disturbance, low grade fever, and malaise.[1-3,5] AMS is common, with an incidence of approximately 25% in travelers to altitudes above 6,500 ft (2,000 m).[1,5] Physical fitness is not protective, and risk factors include rapid rate of ascent, physical exertion, alcohol consumption, and cold temperatures.[1,7] There is some evidence that an antecedent viral illness also could be a risk factor.[1] The incidence of AMS in children is similar to that in adults.[8] Symptoms commonly begin in the first 12 to 24 hours after arrival at high altitude and usually peak on the second or third day.[5,7]

2. Prevent and treat acute mountain sickness.

The best preventive strategy for AMS is gradual ascent, allowing time for acclimatization.[1] Prophylactic treatment with **acetazolamide** has been shown to reduce the incidence and severity of AMS.[1-3] Some studies have suggested that *Ginkgo biloba* helps prevent or lessen the severity of AMS.[1,9]

For all patients with AMS, further ascent is contraindicated, and patients should descend to a lower altitude if symptoms worsen.[1-3,7] Rest and hydration are frequently sufficient treatment for mild AMS, and symptomatic relief may be provided by antiemetics and analgesics such as acetaminophen and ibuprofen.[1,2]

3. Recognize evolving high-altitude pulmonary edema.

HAPE is a life-threatening progression of AMS and the most common cause of fatality at high altitude.[5] HAPE is a form of hydrostatic pulmonary edema associated with marked pulmonary artery hypertension that occurs rapidly in otherwise healthy people, usually above 8,200 ft (2,500 m), impairing alveolar gas exchange.[10,11] The usual presentation includes the typical nonspecific symptoms of AMS, in conjunction with cough that may be productive of blood-tinged mucus, dyspnea at rest, crackles, and hypoxia.[3,5,11] Patients may describe a “gurgling” in their lungs.[5] Chest radiography may show patchy, peripheral infiltrates that often are asymmetric, with focal infiltrates often most prominent in the right midlung field.[4] Electrocardiography may show evidence of right ventricular strain.[1] Untreated, HAPE can rapidly progress to respiratory failure and death.[3,5,10]

4. Manage high-altitude pulmonary edema.

As with AMS, the most effective way to prevent HAPE is with gradual ascent.[1] Oral nifedipine may prevent the development of HAPE in patients who are particularly susceptible.[12] Inhaled β-adrenergic agonists also may help prevent HAPE.[13]

Although the usual treatment for HAPE includes immediate descent to lower elevation and supplemental oxygen,[1,2,5] some evidence suggests that patients with HAPE at moderate altitudes (below 10,000 ft/3,000 m) may be treated with bed rest and supplemental oxygen.[11] However, all patients who are unstable despite supplemental oxygen must be immediately transported to lower altitude. A portable fabric hyperbaric chamber (eg. Gamow bag [available at Chinook Medical Care, Durango, CO]) can be used as a temporary measure to increase pressurization and duplicate lower altitude.[1-3,5,7] **Nifedipine** may be helpful for reduction of pulmonary vascular resistance and pulmonary artery pressure.[1,2,5]

5. Recognize evolving high-altitude cerebral edema.

HACE, generally considered the end-stage progression of AMS, is characterized by ataxia and altered mental status, which may rapidly progress over hours to coma and death from brain herniation.[1,3] HACE is generally preceded by AMS symptoms and is often associated with HAPE.[5] Physical examination may reveal papilledema and retinal hemorrhages.[1] Although HACE usually occurs at altitudes above 12,000 ft (3,600 m), it has been reported at altitudes below 9,000 ft (2,700 m).[7]

6. Manage high-altitude cerebral edema.

Although potentially fatal, HACE is completely reversible with expeditious treatment.[5] The primary treatment of HACE is immediate descent or medical evacuation to lower altitude.[1,3,5] Additional therapy includes supplemental oxygen and oral or parenteral **dexamethasone**.[1-3,5] Treatment with dexamethasone seems to be beneficial in alleviating the symptoms of HACE if instituted early, although definitive evidence of efficacy is lacking.[1-3,5] As with HAPE, a portable hyperbaric chamber may be used until medical evacuation is initiated.[1]

References

1. Basnayat B, Murdoch DR. High-altitude Illness. *Lancet.* 2003;361:1967-1974.
2. Klocke DL, Decker WW, Stepanek J. Altitude-related illnesses. *Mayo Clin Proc.* 1998;73:988-993.
3. Peacock AJ. ABC of oxygen: oxygen at high altitude. *BMJ.* 1998;317:1063-1066.
4. Rabold M. High-altitude pulmonary edema: a collective review. *Am J Emerg Med.* 1989;7:426-433.
5. Yarnell PR, Heit J, Hackett PH. High-altitude cerebral edema (HACE): the Denver/Front Range experience. *Semin Neurol.* 2000;20:209-217.
6. King BR, King C, Coates WC. Critical procedures. In: Gausche-Hill M, Fuchs S, Yamamoto L, eds. *APLS: The Pediatric Emergency Medicine Resource.* 4th ed. Sudbury, MA: American Academy of Pediatrics, American College of Emergency Physicians, Jones and Bartlett Co; 2004:702-707.
7. Kuo DC, Jerrard DA. Environmental insults: smoke inhalation, submersion, diving, and high altitude. *Emerg Med Clin North Am.* 2003;21:475-497.
8. Yaron M, Waldman N, Neirmeyer S, et al. The diagnosis of acute mountain sickness in preverbal children. *Arch Pediatr Adolesc Med.* 1998;152:683-687.
9. Roncin JP, Schwartz F, D'Arbigny P. EGb 761 in control of acute mountain sickness and vascular reactivity in cold exposure. *Aviat Space Environ Med.* 1998;67:445-452.
10. Swenson ER, Maggiorini M, Mangovin S, et al. Pathogenesis of high-altitude pulmonary edema: inflammation is not an etiologic factor. *JAMA.* 2002;287:2228-2235.
11. Zafren K, Reeves JT, Schoene R. Treatment of high-altitude pulmonary edema by bed rest and supplemental oxygen. *Wilderness Environ Med.* 1996;2:127-132.
12. Bartsch P, Maggiorini M, Ritter M, et al. Prevention of high-altitude pulmonary edema by nifedipine. *N Engl J Med.* 1991;325:1284-1289.
13. Sartori C, Allemann Y, Duplain H, et al. Salmeterol for the prevention of high-altitude pulmonary edema. *N Engl J Med.* 2002;346:1631-1636.

SCENARIO #46

Environmental Emergency

Debra L. Weiner, MD, PhD, Shannon F. Manzi, PharmD, and Mark L. Waltzman, MD

Brief Presenting History

A 5-year-old boy with a history of asthma presents to the emergency department with the acute onset of cough and shortness of breath.

Pediatric Assessment Triangle

Appearance: Anxious and crying with runny nose

Work of Breathing: Rapid, labored

Circulation to the Skin: Well perfused

Initial Vital Signs

Pulse: 100

Respiratory Rate: 32

Blood Pressure: 100/70

Temperature: 37°C (98.6°F) oral

Oxygen Saturation: 94% in room air

Physical Examination on Arrival to the Emergency Department

Airway: Patent, increased nasal and oral secretions, noisy upper airway sounds

Breathing: Rapid, labored respirations with frequent coughing; breath sounds symmetric and coarse, with scattered end expiratory wheezes; no rales or rhonchi present; aeration decreased

Circulation: Capillary refill time less than 2 seconds in the extremities

Disability: Alert, responsive, anxious, but fatigued

ASK YOURSELF

- **How much should this 5-year-old weigh?**

  An estimated weight for a 5-year-old is 20 kg. One can use the length-based Broselow Pediatric Emergency Tape or a pediatric table to determine weight based on age. See Appendix A.

- **What is the initial assessment? What is this patient's physiologic status?**

  He is alert and anxious, in moderate respiratory distress without evidence of shock.

- **What would be the most common possible diagnoses for this patient?**

  The abrupt onset of severe respiratory distress with increased secretions suggests one of the following common causes of acute respiratory distress:

  - Asthma exacerbation
  - Allergic reaction to environmental allergen(s)
  - Other acute respiratory infectious illness (upper respiratory infection, croup, bronchiolitis)

Additional History and Physical Examination Findings

The boy went to a baseball game at the local outdoor stadium with his father this sunny afternoon. After the game he acutely developed symptoms on the subway platform while they waited for a train. He and his father left the subway tunnel immediately and took a cab to the emergency department. The father thinks that the child is having an asthma attack. The child ate a hotdog and peanuts just before leaving the game.

Past Medical History: Asthma

Medications: Albuterol inhaler on an as-needed basis, fluticasone inhaler daily

Allergies: Possibly to nuts

Physical Examination: Clear rhinorrhea, no intraoral swelling, no drooling, no stridor, neck supple and nontender and without adenopathy, abdomen soft and nontender, skin sunburned; pupils equal, round, 1 mm, unresponsive to light

ASK YOURSELF

■ What other diagnoses would you add to the differential?

Foreign body (ie, peanut) aspiration, heat illness, and toxic exposure.

■ What interventions are needed at this time? What complications might be expected?

Interventions

- Place the patient on a cardiorespiratory monitor with pulse oximetry.
- Apply 100% humidified oxygen.
- Suction oral secretions.
- Administer a nebulized **albuterol** treatment.
- Establish vascular access.
- Obtain a portable chest radiograph.

Potential Complications:

- Hypoxia could develop.
- Respiratory arrest could rapidly ensue.

■ What laboratory studies, if any, would you obtain?

An ABG analysis would help evaluate the patient's oxygenation, ventilation, and acid-base status.

Progression

Nebulized albuterol treatment provides some transient improvement in aeration. In addition to initial findings, patient now is intermittently agitated and stuporous, complaining of nausea, crampy abdominal pain, and muscle weakness. He is increasingly hypotonic.

Repeat Vital Signs

Pulse: 140

Respiratory Rate: 36

Blood Pressure: 100/70

Oxygen Saturation: 99% on 5 L 100% O_2 delivered via face mask

ASK YOURSELF

■ What is the physiologic status now?

The child appears to be in cholinergic crisis.[1] Features of cholinergic crisis are salivation, lacrimation, urination, defecation, gastrointestinal cramping, and emesis (SLUDGE).[2] A more comprehensive list of symptoms is captured by the acronym BAG (the) PUDDLES:

Bronchoconstriction

Apnea

Glandular secretions

Pupillary constriction

Urination

Defecation

Diaphoresis

Lacrimation

Emesis

Seizures

Clinical diagnosis is based on recognition of cholinergic toxidrome and a high index of suspicion. A history of exposure and a response to therapy further support the diagnosis.

Manifestations of a cholinergic crisis may be mild, moderate, or severe:

Mild: Miosis, eye pain, dimming of vision, blurry vision, conjunctival injection, rhinorrhea, throat and/or chest tightness, dyspnea, cough

Moderate: Increased severity of mild symptoms and blurry vision, severe nasal congestion, drooling, nausea, vomiting, diarrhea, abdominal cramping, muscle weakness, twitching of large muscle groups, headache, ataxia, confusion, drowsiness

Severe: Increased severity of moderate symptoms and involuntary urination, defecation, seizures, coma, flaccid paralysis, respiratory arrest, death

Which agents can cause cholinergic crisis?

Acetylcholinesterase inhibitors are numerous and include the following classes:

- Organophosphate pesticides[3,4] (malathion, parathion, methyl parathion, trichlorfon, tetrachlorvinphos)
- Carbamate insecticides—no CNS effects
- Nerve gas agents[5-7] (sarin, tabun, soman, cyclosarin, VX)
- Pharmacologic acetylcholinesterase inhibitors (physostigmine, neostigmine)
- Mushrooms—no nicotinic effects (*Clitocybe, Inocybe, Amanita muscaria*)

Organophosphate pesticide exposure is among the most common human toxic exposures. Organophosphates are not detected on most routine comprehensive drug screens.

What is the mechanism of action of acetylcholinesterase inhibitors?

They work via toxic accumulation of acetylcholine at nicotinic and muscarinic receptors and in the central nervous system via inhibition of acetylcholinesterase.[3] These agents also bind directly to nicotinic and cardiac muscarinic receptors, inhibit γ-aminobutyric acid (GABA) neurotransmission, and stimulate *N*-methyl-D-aspartate (NDMA) receptors.

What interventions are needed at this time? What complications might be expected?

Interventions:

- Prepare for possible intubation, avoiding ketamine (increases secretions) and succinylcholine (risk for prolonged paralysis).
- Place a second large-bore intravenous line.
- Give **atropine 0.02 mg/kg IV (maximum, 2 mg)** repeated every 5 to 10 minutes. This is a muscarinic receptor competitive antagonist that decreases secretions and alleviates wheezing and bradycardia.
- Give **pralidoxime chloride** (**2-PAM, Protopam**) **25 to 50 mg/kg IV (maximum, 1,000 mg)** over 30 minutes, repeated once in 1 to 2 hours. An oxime, it cleaves the organophosphate from the acetylcholinesterase and results in improved muscle and diaphragm strength. The oximes will enhance the activity of atropine at the muscarinic sites and are indicated for nicotinic and/or CSN manifestations.
- Give **lorazepam 0.1 mg/kg IV** to prevent/control seizures.

Potential Complications:

- Apnea
- Pneumonitis (due to inhalation of acetylcholinesterase inhibitors with hydrocarbon base or due to emesis and aspiration)
- Noncardiogenic pulmonary edema
- Respiratory failure/arrest
- Seizures
- Flaccid paralysis
- Coma
- Treatment-related complications
    1. Atropine: Hyperthermia, inspiratory stridor, delirium, arrhythmias.
    2. Pralidoxime: Tachycardia, hypertension, hyperventilation, laryngospasm, muscle weakness, muscle rigidity

What other laboratory tests should be obtained? What abnormalities may be expected?

- CBC: Leukocytosis
- Electrolytes: Hyperkalemia, hyperglycemia
- Urinalysis: Proteinuria, glycosuria
- Amylase: Elevation correlates with increased risk of respiratory failure, death
- Electrocardiography: Sinus tachycardia and later bradycardia, ST- and T-wave changes, prolonged QT, complete heart block, torsade de pointes, asystole. Arrhythmias correlate with increased risk of death.

Progression

EMS personnel announce over the radio that there has been what is thought to be a nerve gas exposure, possibly sarin, in the subway.

ASK YOURSELF

■ What interventions are needed at this time? What complications might be expected?

Interventions:

- Prepare for a mass casualty disaster including activation of hospital disaster response plan, contacting local authorities to activate community disaster response plan, and setting up triage, decontamination units, and antidote administration station.

Potential Complications:

- Health provider and health care facility contamination can occur due to exposure to contaminated patients.
- Resources may be overwhelmed if the exposure is widespread.
- Challenge of providing supportive care, decontamination, and antidote administration may overwhelm inexperienced staff.
- Hypothermia due to the nerve agent exposure and decontamination procedures may affect patients.
- There is a limited availability of medical history for young patients who are not accompanied by a parent or guardian.
- Patients and staff experience psychosocial trauma.

■ What was the most likely route of exposure? Why are you able to discern this?

The route of exposure and the dose determine the initial symptoms and time of onset after exposure to a nerve gas agent.[5-7] There are three different routes:

- *Vapor inhalation.* Onset is seconds to minutes, and initial symptoms for mild exposure include miosis, rhinorrhea, dyspnea, and tightness in the throat or chest. With moderate exposure, symptoms progress to include abdominal cramping, vomiting, diarrhea, muscle fasciculations, confusion, and agitation. Severe exposure may result in immediate loss of consciousness, apnea, seizures, and flaccid paralysis.
- *Cutaneous exposure* to liquid. Abdominal pain, nausea, and vomiting are common manifestations of exposure via any route, but they may be the first systemic effects from liquid exposure on the skin. Onset of symptoms ranges from minutes up to about 18 hours.
- *Ingestion* of nerve agents through contaminated food or water is relatively rare. Initial symptoms are nausea, vomiting, diarrhea, abdominal cramping, and weakness.

■ What would you have done differently if you had known about the chemical exposure before the child arrived in the emergency department?

Father and child should have been decontaminated.[8,9] Health care providers should first put on rubber gloves, gowns, aprons, and a self-contained breathing apparatus (SCBA) before decontamination of patients.

- For exposure to vapor, patients should remove all clothing, wash skin, and rinse hair. Clothing and other personal items should be placed in double bags that are then sealed and labeled appropriately.
- For exposure to liquid, patients should be scrubbed and rinsed twice using large amounts of soap and water with a sponge or washcloth.
- For ocular exposure to liquid, eyes should be irrigated with room temperature water for at least 15 minutes.
- For gastric contamination, consider gastric lavage if a large ingestion occurred less than 30 to 60 minutes earlier, give activated charcoal orally or via nasogastric tube, with appropriate airway protection and after seizure prophylaxis as clinically indicated. Do not induce vomiting.

Objectives of This Scenario

Management of patients with exposure to chemical agents requires an understanding of the characteristics of these agents, their clinical manifestations based on exposure route and dose, differences in risks and mechanisms of exposure and in clinical findings between adults and children, and appropriate decontamination and treatment.

1. Recognize the possibility of exposure to one or more chemical agents including their toxidromes, and know decontamination principles and agent-specific antidotes.

Recognition of exposure to a chemical agent is challenging, particularly for first cases. Clinical manifestations often are similar to those of common illnesses and vary based on dose and route of exposure (Table 1). Exposure to more than one agent may obscure classic toxidromes. Information on clinical syndromes produced by chemical agents and biologic toxins is available on the CDC website: http://www.bt.cdc.gov/agent/agentlistchem.asp and http://www.cdc.gov/mmmwr/preview/mmwrhtml/mm5239a.htm.

The chemical structure of sarin (GB or isopropyl methylphosphonofluoridate) and other nerve agents, tabun, soman, cyclosarin and VX, are similar to that of organophosphate pesticides. Nerve agents were initially developed as pesticides and are not naturally occurring substances. Nerve agents are more toxic than organophosphate pesticides, particularly with respect to CNS effects, and in fact, are the most toxic and most rapidly acting chemical warfare agents known. The effects of nerve agents are due to inactivation of acetylcholinesterase, direct binding to receptors, and interference with neurotransmitters. Sarin is a volatile, clear, colorless, odorless, and tasteless liquid that evaporates at the same rate as water.[6,7] It is the most quickly acting nerve agent. Exposure may be in the form of vapor, liquid, or ingestion. As a vapor, sarin is rapidly absorbed via the eyes and respiratory tract. The vapor is not readily absorbed through the skin. As a liquid, sarin penetrates clothing, skin, and eyes rapidly. Sarin gas was used in the terrorist attack in the Tokyo subway in 1995, resulting in 12 deaths and toxic effects in thousands. Most patients were ambulatory at the scene of the attack and were able to transport themselves to a hospital with minimal assistance. Many initially went to work and sought medical care only after symptoms progressed.

Acute onset of multisystem organ findings suggests a toxic exposure. Nerve agents affect ocular, respiratory, cardiovascular, gastrointestinal, muscle, and neurological systems due to muscarinic (neuroeffector junctions), nicotinic (skeletal myoneural junctions and autonomic ganglia), and direct CNS toxicity.[5] Onset of symptoms for vapor exposure varies from within seconds up to 30 minutes. Liquid exposure onset time is generally 30 minutes to 18 hours, and ingestion symptoms usually occur within 30 minutes.

Death usually occurs secondary to respiratory failure and can occur within minutes to hours after exposure. Even small amounts of nerve agents, particularly as liquid, can cause death. In surviving victims, some symptoms (particularly miosis, gastrointestinal effects, myalgias, headache, irritability, lethargy) may persist for weeks to months. Neurologic deficits may have

Table 1.
Clinical Findings of Nerve Agents[1,5-7,11]

Muscarinic (DUMBELS)	Nicotinic (MATCH)	CNS
Defecation, diarrhea, diaphoresis	**M**uscle weakness, fasiculations	Restlessness
Urination	**A**drenal medulla activity increase	Anxiety
Miosis	**T**achycardia	Headache
Bronchospasm, Bradycardia	**C**ramping skeletal muscles	Seizures
Emesis	**H**ypertension	Confusion
Lacrimation		Lethargy
Salivation, secretions bronchial		Coma
		Depression of respiratory and cardiovascular function

delayed onset and can persist long term, even lifelong.

Treatment for nerve agent exposure consists of immediate decontamination, supportive care, antidote administration, and ongoing care.[10] Some patients will require minimal or no care. Patients with presumed inhalational exposure and no possibility of liquid exposure who are without symptoms on arrival to a health care facility have likely not had a significant exposure since onset of symptoms is usually within seconds to minutes. Similarly, since patients with ingestion usually become symptomatic within 30 minutes, those who are asymptomatic after 30 minutes to 1 hour are at low risk. Patients with liquid exposure should be observed for 18 hours since onset of symptoms may be delayed for 18 hours.

For symptomatic patients, supportive management of airway, breathing, and circulation is based on APLS/PALS guidelines. Respiratory support is usually the most critical issue because toxicities include apnea, bronchospasm, increased airway secretions, diaphragm weakness, central respiratory depression, and possible aspiration due to vomiting. Early intubation and ventilation can be critical if coma or respiratory compromise develop. Ketamine is contraindicated in RSI because of the potential for increased secretions. Likewise, succinylcholine is contraindicated because it is metabolized to acetylcholine, increasing the potential for prolonged paralytic effect. Bronchodilators and ipratropium may have therapeutic efficacy.

Acetylcholinesterase inhibitors are among the few chemical agents for which there are antidotes. A combination of atropine, an oxime, and a benzodiazepine can be very effective even in ameliorating cardiopulmonary arrest if administered expeditiously. *It is particularly important to treat children because of their greater sensitivity to neurotoxic effects.*[10,12] Ideally, antidotes should be administered prior to arrival to the health care facility. **Atropine**, a muscarinic receptor antagonist should be administered every 5 to 10 minutes as required until bronchial secretions decrease, airway resistance improves, and cardiovascular status normalizes. **Pralidoxime chloride** restores cholinesterase activity by displacing the organophosphate from the enzyme. Pralidoxime is indicated for severe poisoning, nicotinic effects (ie, muscle weakness, cramps, fasiculations), and/or central effects (ie, coma, seizures). It is most effective if given within the first 3 hours of exposure. Recognize that antidotes usually must be administered repeatedly.

Although not antidotes, **benzodiazepines** should be used for both treatment and prophylaxis of seizures.[11] Recognize that manifestations of seizure activity can be subtle and that an EEG may ultimately be required for detection. These seizures are usually refractory to other classes of anticonvulsants; however if benzodiazepines are not effective, phenobarbital should be administered. Phenytoin has shown no effect in several animal studies and is therefore not recommended.

2. Understand that children are more vulnerable to the effects of nerve gas agents.[10]

Nerve gas vapor is approximately 5 times heavier than air. Therefore its concentration is greatest closer to the ground, potentially exposing children to increased concentrations of gas in the air they inspire. In addition, children have increased minute ventilation and will therefore have greater exposure when compared to adults. Children also are more vulnerable to absorption of liquid nerve gas because of their greater surface-area-to-volume ratio and thinner dermis.

Studies on the clinical manifestations of organophosphate toxicity demonstrate that children are less likely than adults to manifest peripheral effects such as miosis, lacrimation, increased secretions, bradycardia, gastrointestinal manifestations, and muscle fasiculations. Children are *more* vulnerable, however, to CNS effects including weakness, hypotonia, flaccidity, seizures, stupor, and coma. Children also are more likely than adults to have prolonged, even lifelong, neurologic sequelae.

3. Recognize the risk for secondary contamination of health care workers and others.

Inadvertent contamination of health care workers and a health care facility can paralyze a response to an episode of widespread toxic exposure. Chemical protective clothing is essential: rubber gloves, gown, and apron. A self-contained breathing apparatus (SCBA) is required for health care providers working in areas with potentially high concentrations of vapor. Ideally, once mass exposure has been recognized, individuals will be decontaminated offsite. Patients requiring decontamination on arrival to a health care facility should be decontaminated outside.

References

1. Erickson TB. Toxicology: ingestions and smoke inhalation. In: Gausche-Hill M, Fuchs S, Yamamoto L, eds. *APLS: The Pediatric Emergency Medicine Resource.* 4th ed. Sudbury, Mass: American Academy of Pediatrics, American College of Emergency Physicians, Jones and Bartlett Publishing Co; 2004:252-253.
2. Osterhoudt KC, Shannon M, Henretig FM. In: Fleisher GR, Ludwig S, eds. *Textbook of Pediatric Emergency Medicine.* 4th ed. Philadelphia, Pa: Lippincott Williams & Wilkins; 2000:920-921.
3. Rusyniak DE, Nanagas KA. Organophosphate poisoning. *Semin Neurol.* 2004;24:197-204.
4. Organophosphates. In: Klasco RK, ed. POISINDEX System. Greenwood Village, Colo: Thomson MICROMEDEX (edition expires 6/2004). Available at: http://www.micromedex.com/products/poisindex/. Accessed: June 2004.
5. Lee EC. Clinical manifestations of sarin gas exposure. *JAMA.* 2003;290:659-662.
6. Nerve agents. In: Klasco RK, ed. POISINDEX System. Greenwood Village, Colo: Thomson MICROMEDEX (edition expires 6/2004). Available at: http://www.micromedex.com/products/poisindex/. Accessed: June 2004.
7. Facts about sarin. CDC Web site. Available at: http://www.bt.cdc.gov/agent/sarin/basics/pdf/sarin-facts.pdf. Accessed: May 2004.
8. Rotenberg JS, Burklow TR, Selanikio JS. The decontamination of children. *Pediatr Ann.* 2003;32:261-267.
9. Henretig FM, Cieslak TJ, Kortepeter MG, et al. Medical management of the suspected victim of bioterrorism: an algorithmic approach to the undifferentiated patient. *Emerg Med Clin North Am.* 2002;20:351-364.
10. Rotenberg JS. Diagnosis and management of nerve agent exposure. Pediatr Ann. 2003;32:247-250.
11. Kales SN, Christiani DC. Acute chemical emergencies. *N Engl J Med.* 2002;350:800-808.
12. Lifshitz M, Shahak E, Sofer S. Carbamate and organophosphate poisoning in young children. *Pediatr Emerg Care.* 1999;15:102-103.

Appendix A

Normal Vital Sign Ranges by Age

Age	Weight (kg)	Respiratory Rate (bpm)	Heart Rate (bpm)	Systolic BP (mm Hg)
Premie	<3	30-60	120-160	52 ± 10
Newborn/ Neonate	3-4	30-60	90-160	60 ± 10
1-6 mo	4-6	24-30	110-180	80 ± 10
6-12 mo	6-10	24-30	110-180	89 ± 25
1-2 yr	10-13	20-24	90-150	96 ± 30
2-4 yr	13-17	20-24	75-135	99 ± 25
4-6 yr	17-20	20-24	60-130	100 ± 20
6-8 yr	20-25	12-20	60-120	105 ±13
8-10 yr	25-30	12-20	60-120	110 ± 15
10-12 yr	30-40	12-20	60-120	112 ± 15
12-14 yr	40-50	12-20	60-120	115 ± 20
14-adult	>50	10-16	60-120	120 ± 20

Standard Equipment Sizes by Age

Age	Suction Catheter (Fr)	Laryngoscope	ET Tube (mm)	Tracheostomy Tube size	NG Tube (Fr)	Foley (Fr)	Chest Tube (Fr)
Premie	6	0 Miller	2.5-3.0	00	5	5	10
Newborn/ Neonate	8	0 Miller	3.0-3.5	0	8	5	10-12
1-6 mo	10	1 Miller	3.5-4.0	0-1	8	8	10-12
6-12 mo	10	1 Miller	4.0	1-2	8	8	12-20
1-2 yr	10	1 Miller	4.5	1-2	8	8-10	16-20
2-4 yr	10-14	1-2 Miller	5.0	2-3	8-10	10	20-24
4-6 yr	14	2 Miller	5.5 ± cuffed	3	10	10	24-28
6-8 yr	14-16	2 Miller	6.0 cuffed	3-4	10	10	28
8-10 yr	16	2 Miller	6.0-7.0 cuffed	4	10-12	10-12	28-32
10-12 yr	16	2 Miller, 2 Mac	7.0 cuffed	4-5	12	12	32
12-14 yr	16	2-3 Miller, 2-3 Mac	7.0-7.5 cuffed	5-6	12	12	32-36
14-adult	16	3 Miller, 3 Mac	7.5-8.0 cuffed	6	14	12	36-42

Appendix B: Frequently Used Abbreviations

ABCs	Airway, breathing, and circulation
ABG	Arterial blood gas
ACTH	Adrenocorticotropic hormone
ALT	Alanine aminotransferase
AMS	Acute mountain sickness
AP	Anteroposterior
ARDS	Acute respiratory distress syndrome
ASAP	As soon as possible
AST	Aspartate aminotransferase
ATV	All-terrain vehicle
AV	Atrioventricular
AVM	Arterial-venous malformation
BP	Blood pressure
BPM	Beats per minute
BUN	Blood urea nitrogen
BMV	Bag-mask ventilation
CAH	Congenital adrenal hyperplasia
CBC	Complete blood count (usually includes differential and platelet count)
CHF	Congestive heart failure
CNS	Central nervous system
CO	Carbon monoxide
CPAP	Continuous positive airway pressure
CPP	Cerebral perfusion pressure
CPR	Cardiopulmonary resuscitation
CSF	Cerebrospinal fluid
CT	Computed tomography
CVP	Central venous pressure
DIC	Disseminated intravascular coagulation
DKA	Diabetic ketoacidosis
DOCA	Deoxycortisone acetate
DPL	Diagnostic peritoneal lavage
ECG	Electrocardiogram
EEG	Electroencephalogram
EMS	Emergency medical services, pre-hospital
EMT	Emergency medical technician
ENT	Ear, nose, and throat
ET	Endotracheal
FAST	Focused assessment with sonography for trauma
FFP	Fresh frozen plasma
Fr	French
GCS	Glasgow Coma Scale
HACE	High-altitude cerebral edema
HAPE	High-altitude pulmonary edema
Hct	Hematocrit
HEENT	Head, eyes, ears, nose, and throat
Hgb	Hemoglobin
HR	Heart rate
HUS	Hemolytic-uremic syndrome
ICP	Intracranial pressure
ICU	Intensive care unit
IM	Intramuscular
IO	Intraosseous
ITP	Idiopathic (or immune) thrombocytopenia
IV	Intravenous
JVD	Jugular venous distention
LOC	Loss of consciousness
mL	Milliliters
Mac	Macintosh blade
MAP	Mean arterial pressure
MCD	Mock code director
MRI	Magnetic resonance imaging
NG	Nasogastic
NICU	Newborn intensive care unit
OR	Operating room
PE	Phenytoin equivalent
PEA	Pulseless electrical activity
PEEP	Positive end-expiratory pressure
PICU	Pediatric intensive care unit
PIP	Peak inspiratory pressure
PO	Per os (mouth)
PR	Per rectum
PRBCs	Packed red blood cells
PRN	As needed
PT	Prothrombin time

PTT	Partial thromboplastin time
QTc	Calculated QT interval
RAD	Reactive airways disease
rpm	Respirations per minute
RSI	Rapid sequence intubation
RVH	Right ventricular hypertrophy
SIADH	Syndrome of inappropriate secretion of antidiuretic hormone
SIDS	Sudden infant death syndrome
SL	Sublingual
SLE	Systemic lupus erythematosus
SQ	Subcutaneous
SVR	Systemic vascular resistance
SVT	Supraventricular tachycardia
TCA	Tricyclic antidepressant
TIBC	Total iron-binding capacity
type and cross	Type and crossmatch blood
URI	Upper respiratory infection
VBG	Venous blood gas
VF	Ventricular fibrillation
VPS	Ventriculoperitoneal shunt
VSD	Ventricular septal defect
VT	Ventricular tachycardia
WBC	White blood cell

Appendix C: Glasgow Coma Scale

The Glasgow Coma Scale, or GCS, is an ordinal scale from 3 to 15. It was originally designed as a tool for the assessment of patients who have incurred traumatic brain injury.[1,2] A score of 15 represents an awake, oriented, and responsive person. A score of 3 represents a severely obtunded person. It is composed of three parameters:

- Best eye-opening response
- Best verbal response
- Best motor response

It has been modified for use in preverbal infants.

Glasgow Coma Scale[2]

Eye Opening Response (1-4)

1. No eye opening
2. Eye opening to painful stimuli
3. Eye opening to verbal command
4. Eyes open spontaneously

Verbal Response (1-5)

1. No verbal response
2. Incomprehensible or nonspecific sounds
3. Inappropriate words
4. Confused
5. Oriented

Motor Response (1-6)

1. No motor response
2. Extension to painful stimuli
3. Flexion to painful stimuli
4. Withdrawal from painful stimuli (usually a pinch to medial aspect of arm/leg)
5. Localizes painful stimuli (usually a sternal rub)
6. Follows commands

Glasgow Coma Scale Modified for Infants[3]

Eye Opening Response (1-4)

1. No eye opening
2. Eye opening to painful stimuli
3. Eye opening to verbal stimuli
4. Eyes open spontaneously

Verbal Response (1-5)

1. No verbal response
2. Moaning to painful stimuli
3. Crying to painful stimuli
4. Irritable and continuous crying
5. Cooing and/or babbling (normal activity)

Motor Response (1-6)

1. No motor response
2. Extension to painful stimuli
3. Flexion to painful stimuli
4. Withdrawal from painful stimuli
5. Withdrawal from touch
6. Spontaneous or purposeful movement

References

1. Teasdale G, Jennett B. Assessment of coma and impaired consciousness: a practical scale. *Lancet.* 1974;2:81-84.
2. Jennett B, Teasdale G. Aspects of coma after severe head injury. *Lancet.* 1977;1:878-881.
3. James HE. Neurologic evaluation and support in the child with acute brain insult. *Pediatr Ann.* 1986;15:16-22.

Appendix D: Mock Code Review Guide and Checklist

CODE CALLED — **TIME**

_____ Code leader identified, roles designated _____
_____ Gloves, masks, eye protection _____
_____ Estimated weight _____

Primary Survey – ABCs

Airway
_____ Assessment: patency established _____
_____ Neutral neck position, jaw thrust/chin lift, suction _____
_____ Cervical spine evaluated/immobilized _____

Breathing
_____ Assessment: chest rise, air exchange _____
_____ Oxygen administered _____
_____ Pulse oximeter placed _____
_____ Bag-mask ventilation initiated _____
_____ Intubation performed _____
_____ Postintubation assessment: Chest radiograph, end-tidal CO_2 _____
_____ Nasogastric/orogastric tube placed _____

Circulation
_____ Assessment: skin perfusion, capillary refill time, pulses _____
_____ Cardiorespiratory monitor placed _____
_____ Compressions: proper technique, backboard _____
_____ IV/IO access, appropriate fluid resuscitation _____
_____ Resuscitation medications _____
_____ Cardioversion/defibrillation _____

Disability
_____ Brief neurologic assessment (AVPU, pupils) _____

Exposure
_____ Remove obstructive clothing _____

_____ **REASSESS** _____

Secondary Survey
_____ History
_____ Physical examination
_____ Temperature
_____ Rapid glucose
_____ Hematocrit
_____ ABG/additional labs

Additional
_____ Assessment of fluids given
_____ Radiology
_____ Interaction with parents/guardians
_____ Additional medications (eg, pressors)
_____ Tubes: Foley, chest tube
_____ Consulting services notified when appropriate

Appendix E: Scenario Lists

In Order of Appearance (with Diagnosis)

By Diagnosis (with Scenario Title)

Index

Page references followed by "f" indicate figure, and by "t" indicate table.

T